Psychotherapy for Ischemic Heart Disease

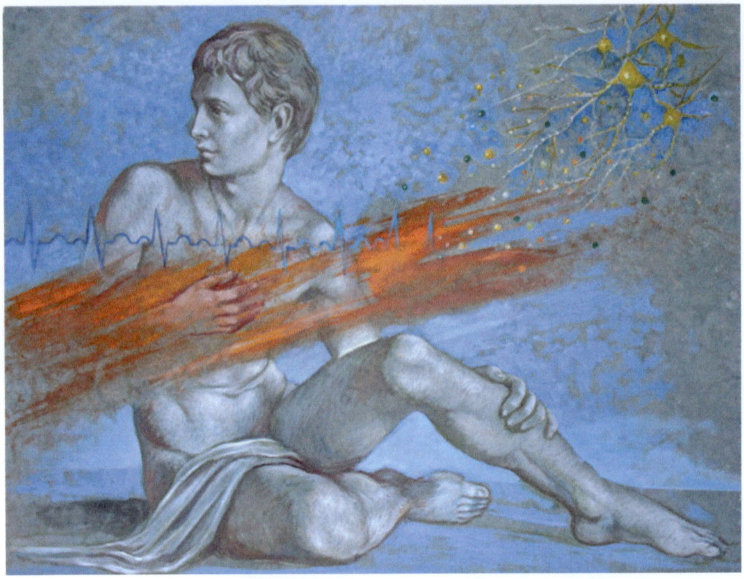

This picture was created by Antonella Cappuccio

Adriana Roncella • Christian Pristipino
Editors

Psychotherapy for Ischemic Heart Disease

An Evidence-based Clinical Approach

Springer

Editors
Adriana Roncella
San Filippo Neri Hospital
Rome
Italy

Christian Pristipino
San Filippo Neri Hospital
Rome
Italy

ISBN 978-3-319-81456-8 ISBN 978-3-319-33214-7 (eBook)
DOI 10.1007/978-3-319-33214-7

Softcover reprint of the hardcover 1st edition 2016

Printed on acid-free paper

This Springer imprint is published by Springer Nature
The registered company is Springer International Publishing AG Switzerland

We would like to dedicate this book to:
My loved father, my son and my daughter, my brother and to all those scholars interested in research on "Cardiac Psychology"
(Adriana Roncella)

To my father and mother,
To professor Attilio Maseri, mentor and master in scientific innovation,
To all the persons suffering or having suffered from ischemic heart disease and their families
(Christian Pristipino)

Preface

Cardiovascular disease is the single most frequent cause of death and disability worldwide, and ischemic heart disease (IHD) accounts for approximately one-half of these events in high-income countries. Though this death rate is somewhat lower in medium- to low-income countries, current years are witnessing a steep and accelerating rise in its weight, relative to other diseases [1]. Indeed, despite a dramatic decrease in IHD incidence and mortality since the 1970s due to improvements in treatments and prevention [2], IHD still caused over 2.1 million deaths (23 % of all deaths) [3] in Europe in 2015 and resulted in over 165 million disability-adjusted life-years (DALYs) lost in 2012 (6 % of all disability claims) [4]. Moreover, while the average age at death from IHD is climbing, due to the effectiveness of primary and secondary prevention and the treatment of acute manifestations, a progressively larger population of seniors is suffering from IHD and its late complications, including heart failure.

Further improvements are expected with more effective reductions in the prevalence of key risk factors and the widespread availability of treatments proven to be more successful in the acute and chronic phases of disease. In this regard, accumulating data demonstrate the independent importance of previously underestimated factors (e.g., psychosocial), which become more ominous by interacting with other risk-predisposing factors and pathogenic processes, like lifestyle habits and inflammation, two facets that appear to intertwine in a way that is both complex and still poorly understood.

The emerging role of these previously neglected processes reveals that the still dreadful impact of IHD must be explained not only by the imperfect or incomplete way in which accepted interventions are implemented, but also by our less than comprehensive knowledge regarding the processes underlying IHD and their way of connecting reciprocally. In fact, the concept of IHD has evolved considerably over the last few decades, starting with the genesis of myocardial infarction being seen as merely the gradual occlusion of epicardial stenosis in a fixed artery, but progressing to the discovery of the dynamic properties of the epicardial coronary tree [5], the functional contribution of the endothelium [6], and the role of systemic processes of coagulation [7, 8] and and inflammation [9] during the predisposing/precipitatory phase of acute coronary events.

Nowadays, IHD is considered a heterogenous array of different syndromes, each with different presentations and underlying pathophysiological processes, which in turn connect at several organizational levels (cell, tissue, organ, and systemic) that remain at least partially unknown [10].

Shedding light on new processes and on the way such processes interact—thereby giving rise to different manifestations in different populations and individuals, but also in the same individual at different times—will certainly contribute to improving our understanding of IHD and further the therapeutic success already achieved with existing therapies and preventative strategies. The complex, dynamic network that causes IHD is, however, highly nondeterministic and requires new, multidimensional approaches, in both research and the clinical sector, to be comprehensively addressed [11].

In this textbook, via an extensive state-of-the-art overview, we focus on one of the new promising areas of interest in ischemic heart disease: the potential to modulate the psycho-neural processes relevant in ischemic heart disease using therapeutic interventions targeting patients' psychologic dimension. These interventions have several characteristics that render them both fascinating and very different from classic medical interventions, opening new avenues into interdisciplinary approaches. Particularly, some of these issues deserve attention because they imply a shift in the general therapeutic paradigms of IHD.

First, acting through pure qualitative instruments, psychological interventions act on a multidimensional scale by simultaneously affecting mood and behavioral changes (thereby influencing changes in lifestyle and augmenting drug compliance), but also through local and remote biological processes that exert direct impacts upon ischemic heart disease.

Second, psychotherapeutic interventions can only produce benefits via active involvement of the patient being treated. As such, their implementation can only be partially manualized, with adaptations and variations often necessary.

Third, psychological interventions often require the personal, emotional, and existential involvement of a caring healthcare professional as a prerequisite to therapy, a marked shift from the prevalent paradigm that considers the physician merely an objective observer.

Several issues need to be clarified in a near future, for example, which psychological interventions are more useful in which patients and at which stage of IHD, what is the optimal timing and duration of interventions, and how can different approaches be combined, including psychopharmacologic tools. Moreover, that the intervention is largely administered in a qualitative dimension (as opposed to drugs that have fixed, quantifiable doses) should not obscure the possible existence of side effects that need to be monitored and specifically studied [12].

This monograph reports on the results of different psychological interventions performed in addition to medical approaches in ischemic heart disease patients, while providing explanations and clarifications of their theoretical basis, empirical justification, and practical application. It reviews the current state of the art and extends this to incorporate the most recent approaches, as well as future applications, thereby yielding insights into practical models that integrate psychotherapy with medical practices in hospital, outpatient clinics, and rehabilitation programs, as already implemented in different settings.

The book's contributors are experts in the fields of psychotherapy, pharmacology, and clinical and interventional cardiology, forming the basis of an interdisciplinary approach to patients. Moreover, the book is written as both a textbook and practical manual targeting psychologists, psychotherapists, psychiatrists, cardiologists, internists, cardiac surgeons, general practitioners, rehabilitation doctors, nurses, students in their first or second year of PhD or MD studies, and also patients.

In the first section, the authors summarize, in an original systemic framework, some of the published empirical evidence documenting the bidirectional relationships that exist between the psycho-neural system and the biological processes underlying ischemic heart disease. This complex framework considers both risk factors and such indirect processes as those mediated via inflammation, coagulation, and hormonal changes, along with the gastrointestinal system and the function of sleep and dreams in cardiovascular pathophysiology, two facets that are seldom considered. Additionally, the role of gender in psychobiological processes is taken into account.

In the second section, psychobiological interventions are addressed via an original and up-to-date meta-analysis of psychotherapies, while providing a general integrative framework for collaboration between medicine and psychology. Furthermore, different perspectives are explored—from pharmacology to cardiac rehabilitation to psychotherapeutics, including approaches such as mind–body and cognitive-behavioral techniques, as well as a novel short-term psychotherapeutic approach derived from ontopsychological method—to provide insights into some of the principal potential interventions and how they might be integrated. Also in this second section, a number of practical issues are reviewed, including the use of psychometric and projective tests and the importance of both verbal and nonverbal modes of communication during the delivery of psychological and medical interventions. Finally, a number of real-world experiences are described, involving both hospital inpatients and clinic outpatients, along with examples of IHD patients managed with psychotherapy.

Our overall aim is to introduce readers to the roles and breadth of psychology and psychotherapeutics in the management of heart disease patients, and how the latter needs to be integrated into the now-outdated model of medical management alone. Doing so will not only lead to a better understanding of the underlying complex pathological processes that exist during the development of ischemic heart disease, it will afford clinicians with additional, complementary tools with which to augment outcomes in these patients. Given the rapidly mounting evidence demonstrating the tremendous biopsychosocial complexity of cardiac disease, both acute and chronic, the time has come to abandon the old approach of treating just the disease itself, in favor of the contemporary and much more effective and comprehensive approach of treating the patient with evidence-based personalized strategies encompassing systems medicine approaches.

Christian Pristipino
Adriana Roncella

References

1. Global Burden of Disease Study 2010 (2012) Global Burden of Disease Study 2010 (GBD 2010) Mortality Results 1970–2010. Institute for Health Metrics and Evaluation (IHME), Seattle
2. Ford ES, Ajani UA, Croft JB et al (2007) Explaining the decrease in U.S. deaths from coronary disease, 1980–2000. N Eng J Med 356(23):2388–2398
3. World Health Organization (2014) Projections of mortality and causes of death, 2015 and 2030. http://www.who.int/healthinfo/global_burden_disease/projections/en/. Accessed 20 Jan 2016
4. World Health Organization (2013) Health statistics and information systems. Disease burden. Estimates for 2000–2012 by region. http://www.who.int/healthinfo/global_burden_disease/estimates/en/index2.html. Accessed 20 Jan 2016
5. Maseri A, Pesola A, Marzilli M et al (1977) Coronary vasospasm in angina pectoris. Lancet 1 (8014):713–717
6. Furchgott RF, Zawadzki JV (1980) The obligatory role of endothelial cells in the relaxation of arterial smooth muscle by acetylcholine. Nature 288:373–376
7. Gruppo Italiano per lo Studio della Streptochinasi nell'Infarto Miocardico (GISSI) (1986) Effectiveness of intravenous thrombolytic treatment in acute myocardial infarction. Lancet 1 (8478):397–402
8. ISIS-2 (Second International Study of Infarct Survival) Collaborative Group (1988) Randomised trial of intravenous streptokinase, oral aspirin, both, or neither among 17,187 cases of suspected acute myocardial infarction: ISIS-2. Lancet 2(8607):349–360
9. Liuzzo G, Biasucci LM, Gallimore JR et al (1994) The prognostic value of C-reactive protein and serum amyloid a protein in severe unstable angina. N Eng J Med 331(7):417–424
10. Maseri A (2000) From syndromes to specific disease mechanisms. The search for the causes of myocardial infarction. Ital Heart J 1(4):253–257
11. Pristipino C (2012) Systems medicine as a scientific method for individualizing therapies in cardiology. Monaldi Arch Chest Dis 78(1):3–5
12. Berkman LF, Blumenthal J, Burg M et al. (2003) Effects of treating depression and low perceived social support on clinical events after myocardial infarction: the Enhancing Recovery in Coronary Heart Disease Patients (ENRICHD) Randomized Trial. JAMA 289 (23):3106–3116

Acknowledgments

Acknowledgments to all our colleagues who participated in and contributed to the STEP-IN-AMI trial:

Giuseppe Richichi[1]; Giulio Speciale (see footnote 1); Cinzia Cianfrocca[2]; Silvia Scorza (see footnote 1); Vincenzo Pasceri (see footnote 1); Francesco Pelliccia (see footnote 1); Johan Denollet[3]; Susanne S Pedersen[4]; Antonella Giornetti (see footnote 1); Antonino Granatelli[5]; Carlo Pignalberi (see footnote 2); Stefano Pazzelli (see footnote 1); and Diana La Rocca (see footnote 1).

Acknowledgment for their contribution to the realization of the research goes to Anna Patrizia Jesi (see footnote 2); Massimo Santini (see footnote 2); Mario Staibano[6]; Carlo Gonnella (see footnote 1); Sebastiano La Rocca[7]; Marina Vitillo (see footnote 7); Antonio Varveri (see footnote 1); Diego Irini (see footnote 1); and Andrea Bisciglia (see footnote 1).

Acknowledgment for his support during the preparation of the book goes to Dr. Marco Picichè in the Heart Surgery Unit, San Camillo Hospital, Rome, Italy.

---

[1] Interventional Cardiology Unit, San Filippo Neri Hospital, Rome, Italy.

[2] Cardiology Unit, San Filippo Neri Hospital, Rome, Italy.

[3] CoRPS—Center of Research on Psychology in Somatic Disease, Tilburg University, Tilburg, The Netherlands.

Department of Cardiology, Thorax Center, Erasmus Medical Center, Rotterdam, The Netherlands.

Department of Cardiology, University Hospital Antwerp, Antwerp, Belgium.

[4] CoRPS—Center of Research on Psychology in Somatic Disease, Tilburg University, Tilburg, The Netherlands.

Department of Cardiology, Thorax Center, Erasmus Medical Center, Rotterdam, The Netherlands).

[5] Director of the Cardiology Unit, Tivoli Hospital, Rome, Italy.

[6] Heart Surgery Unit, San Filippo Neri Hospital, Rome, Italy.

[7] Clinical Pathology Unit, San Filippo Neri Hospital, Rome, Italy.

Contents

List of Contributors

Antonio Abbate, MD, PhD Division of Cardiology, VCU Pauley Heart Center, Virginia Commonwealth University, Richmond, VA, USA

Giuseppe Biondi-Zoccai, MD, MStat Department of Medico-Surgical Sciences and Biotechnologies, Sapienza University of Rome, Latina, Italy

Department of AngioCardioNeurology, IRCCS Neuromed, Pozzilli, Italy

Maria Bonadies, PsyD Associazione Italiana di Psicologia Analitica (AIPA), Roma, Italy

Sergio Boria, MD Italian Association of Systemic Epistemology and Methodology (AIEMS), Associazione Italiana di Medicina e Sanità Sistemica (ASSIMSS), Roma, Italy

Furio Colivicchi, MD, FESC, FACC Cardiology Unit, San Filippo Neri Hospital, Rome, Italy

Oretta Di Carlo, PsyD Forma & Azione Cultural Association, Rome, Italy

Serena Dinelli, PsyD Italian Association of Systemic Epistemology and Methodology (AIEMS), Rome, Italy

Stefania Angela Di Fusco, MD Cardiology Unit, San Filippo Neri Hospital, Rome, Italy

Loreta Di Michele, MD San Camillo-Forlanini Hospital, Rome, Italy

Giacomo Frati, MD, MSc Department of Medico-Surgical Sciences and Biotechnologies, Sapienza University of Rome, Latina, Italy

Department of AngioCardioNeurology, IRCCS Neuromed, Pozzilli, Italy

Silvio Garattini, MD IRCCS Istituto di Ricerche Farmacologiche Mario Negri, Milan, Italy

Antonella Giornetti, PsyD Department of Cardiovascular Disease, San Filippo Neri Hospital, Rome, Italy

Roberto Latini, MD IRCCS Istituto di Ricerche Farmacologiche Mario Negri, Milan, Italy

David Lazzari, PsyD Servizio di Psicologia Ospedaliera, Azienda Ospedaliera "S. Maria" Terni, Terni, Italy

Ludovico Lazzari, MD UO Cardiologia, Università degli Studi di Perugia, Azienda Ospedaliera "S. Maria" Terni, Terni, Italy

Marianna Mazza, MD, PhD Institute of Psychiatry, Catholic University, Rome, Italy

Andrew B. Newberg, MD Integrative Medicine/Nuclear Medicine, Brind-Marcus Center of Integrative Medicine, Thomas Jefferson University Hospital, Villanova, PA, USA

Stephen Olex, MD Integrative Cardiology, Brind-Marcus Center of Integrative Medicine, Thomas Jefferson University Hospital, Villanova, PA, USA

Antonia Pierobon, PsyD Psychology Unit, Salvatore Maugeri Foundation, Care and Research Institute, Montescano, Pavia, Italy

Vincenzo Pasceri, MD Department of Cardiovascular Disease, San Filippo Neri Hospital, Rome, Italy

Christian Pristipino, MD Department of Cardiovascular Disease, San Filippo Neri Hospital, Rome, Italy

Marina Risi, MD Italian Society of Psychoneuroendocrinoimmunology (SIPNEI), Rome, Italy

Leonardo Roever, MHS Department of Clinical Research, Federal University of Uberlândia, Uberlândia, Brazil

Adriana Roncella, MD Department of Cardiovascular Disease, San Filippo Neri Hospital, Rome, Italy

Marco Sanges, MD Gastroenterology Unit, Federico II University of Naples, Naples, Italy

Massimo Santini, MD, FESC, FACC Regional Research Center on Cardiac Arrhythmias, San Filippo Neri Hospital, Rome, Italy

Silvia Scorza, PsyD Department of Cardiovascular Disease, San Filippo Neri Hospital, Rome, Italy

Amit J. Shah, MD, MSCR Department of Epidemiology, Emory University, Atlanta, GA, USA

Rosa Sollazzo, MD Gastroenterology Unit, Federico II University of Naples, Naples, Italy

Marinella Sommaruga, PsyD Clinical Psychology and Social Support Unit, Salvatore Maugeri Foundation, Care and Research Institute, Milan, Italy

Marinella Spaziani Department of Cardiovascular Disease, San Filippo Neri Hospital, Rome, Italy

Giulio Speciale, MD Department of Cardiovascular Disease, San Filippo Neri Hospital, Rome, Italy

Viola Vaccarino, MD Department of Epidemiology, Emory University, Atlanta, GA, USA

Jan van Dixhoorn, MD, PhD Centre for Breathing therapy, Amersfoort, The Netherlands

About the Editors

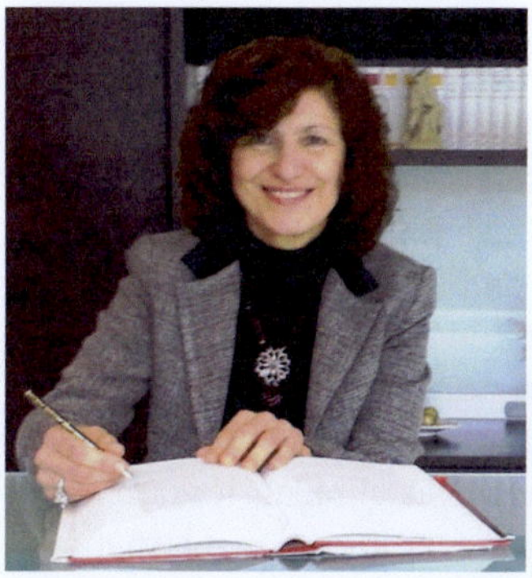

Adriana Roncella was born in Rome, where she currently lives and works. After graduating with a degree in Medicine and Surgery, she subsequently specialized in Cardiology and Psychotherapy. Since 1992, she has been working in the Cardiovascular Disease Department at San Filippo Neri Hospital in Rome. A series of fateful events and her own innate interest in the human condition ultimately led her to incorporate psychotherapy into her clinical and interventional cardiology practice. Combining these seemingly divergent medical fields, she has succeeded in developing a more holistic and effective approach to managing her patients, particularly focusing on patients with ischemic heart disease.

She has been conducting and publishing research on psychosocial risk factors in ischemic cardiac disease since 2000. She is also one of two coprincipal investigators for the randomized clinical trial *S*hort-*TE*rm *P*sychotherapy *IN* *A*cute *M*yocardial *I*nfarction (*STEP-IN-AMI*), an ongoing study that assesses the short- and long-term effectiveness of short-term psychotherapy in patients who present with an acute myocardial infarction and undergo revascularization by primary PTCA. One-year STEP-IN-AMI results were presented at the European Congress of Cardiology in Munich, Germany, in 2012 and published in the Journal of International Cardiology in 2013. For this research, Dr. Roncella was awarded the 2014 "Antonio Meneghetti Award for Research in Medicine" from the Antonio Meneghetti Scientific and Humanistic Research Foundation.

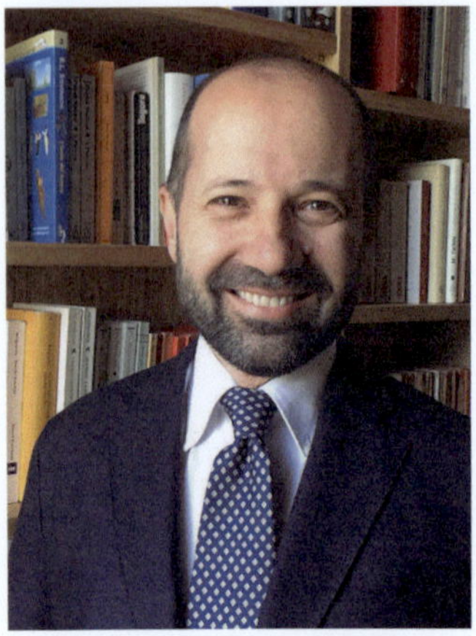

Christian Pristipino FESC, FACC, has been particularly interested in psychobiological and biopsychological relationships since 1985. He graduated in Medicine in 1992 and completed his residency in Cardiology in 1997 at Catholic University in Rome, Italy, both summa cum laude. He was appointed as Research Fellow of the European Society of Cardiology for his investigations on vasomotricity, inflammation, and endothelial activation in ischemic heart disease at the Cardiology Hospital in Lille, France, in 1998, where he also subspecialized in Interventional Cardiology in 1999. Since the year 2000, he has worked as an Interventional Cardiologist at San Filippo Neri Hospital in Rome, Italy, where he chaired research and educational activities until 2007. He was elected as a Regional President of the Italian Society of Interventional Cardiology in 2008 and founded the Personalized and Systems Medicine Unit in S. Filippo Neri Hospital in 2013. He is currently the cofounder and President of the Italian Association for Systems Medicine and Healthcare, striving to develop evidence-based interdisciplinary approaches to addressing the issue of medical management complexity at clinical, research, and administrative levels. He has presented over 100 abstracts at major international congresses in Cardiology and published over 70 papers in both national and international peer-reviewed journals. He is one of two coprincipal investigators for the STEP-IN-AMI trial.

Part I

Complex Psychoneural Processes in Ischemic Heart Disease: Evidences for a Systems Medicine Framework

1

Christian Pristipino

Simplicity does not precede complexity but follows it.
Alan J. Perlis (Perlis AJ (1982) Epigrams on programming. ACM SIGPLAN Notices 17:7–13)

1.1 Introduction

Myocardial ischemia is a dynamic mismatch between the oxygen needs of the heart and its supply through the blood. If ischemia is sufficiently prolonged and/or severe, it triggers metabolic alterations and interconnected processes at various scales of organization within the organism (from the cell to inter-apparatus level) that give rise to new dynamic pathogenic coherences, which appear in its cardinal clinical manifestations (myocardial dysfunction, pain, arrhythmias, and necrosis) (Fig. 1.1).

The variable clinical presentations have been classified as classical syndromes: acute myocardial infarction, stable and unstable angina pectoris, acute and chronic postischemic ventricular dysfunction, and sudden cardiac death. However, these syndromes also variably combine in the time domain (i.e., the lifelong history of single patients) sketching individual disease fingerprints which, surprisingly, have not yet been classified.

In this extremely intricate and dynamic mesh, emotional and mental states and their neurohumoral correlates play important roles, themselves, changing at all levels of this process (Fig.1.1). This being said, neurohumoral factors, emotions, and psychological processes are also simultaneously modulated both by ascending direct peripheral inputs originating in the affected heart and by a primary, symbolic elaboration of the disease by the subject, which may enhance psychological risk

C. Pristipino, MD (✉)
Department of Cardiovascular Disease, San Filippo Neri Hospital, Via G. Martinotti 20, 00135 Rome, Italy
e-mail: pristipino.c@gmail.com

A. Roncella, C. Pristipino (eds.), *Psychotherapy for Ischemic Heart Disease*,
DOI 10.1007/978-3-319-33214-7_1

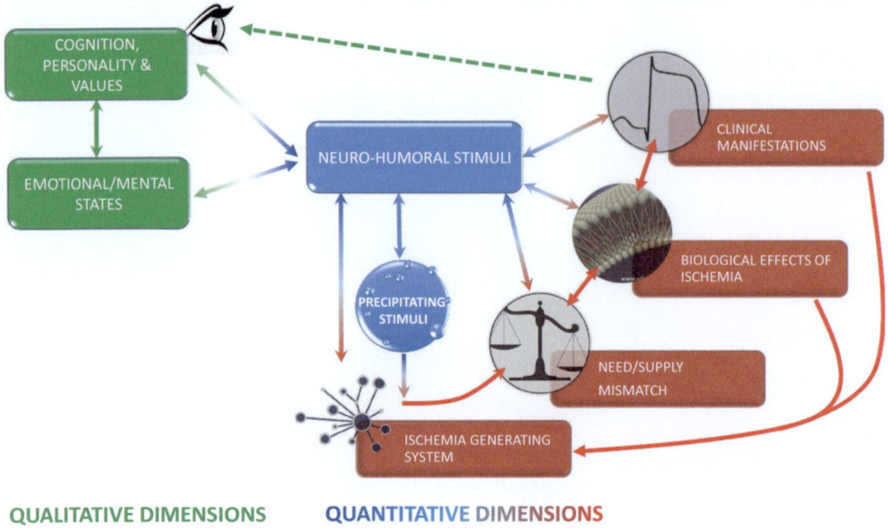

Fig. 1.1 Scheme of bidirectional psycho ↔ biologic interactions in myocardial ischemia pathophysiology. Neurohumoral factors (in *blue*) and the pathophysiology of myocardial ischemia (in *red*) reciprocally influence one another (*blue-red arrows*). The qualitative dimensions of the person, both for primary psychological processes and secondary to the elaborated perception of a heart problem (*green dotted arrow*), being in a bidirectional relationship with neurohumoral factors (*blue-green arrow*), constitute processes of pathophysiology that underlie myocardial ischemia (see text)

factors, thereby generating a vicious circle (see also Chap. 2 and Sect. 7.3) (Fig.1.1).

This recursive loop is peculiar among medical processes, because it is multidimensional, being based on classical, quantitative, neurohumoral function, as well as a merely qualitative dimension characterized by values, emotions, hopes, and meanings, features seldom considered in science because they are not reducible to any quantitative evaluation. This symbolic elaboration has a unique trait, in that it can only be self-modified via cognitive processes and can impact, more or less decisively, at the behavioral and/or neurobiological level and, hence, influence the course of disease.

To frame the pathological or healing potential of the mind in these conditions, it is therefore crucial to review how, when, and where it comes into play within the complex physiologic balance of the heart and, in particular, during the pathophysiological development of ischemic heart disease.

1.2 Coronary Blood Flow and Its Neurohumoral Control

1.2.1 Coronary Blood Flow as an Open System

The ever-changing oxygen needs of the heart are usually met by the ability of myocardial blood flow to increase to up to 500 % of its baseline level. When the coronary vascular system is dysfunctional or insufficient, myocardial ischemia is the result.

The coronary vascular system is composed of coronary arteries that control the flow into a rich capillary bed, where the diffusion of oxygen occurs in a passive way and from there into a still poorly studied venous system. Perfusion pressure in the capillaries is the main determinant of oxygen supply and is determined by an arterial autoregulating system that adapts to changes in pressure and heart metabolism. However, it is also continuously modulated by external stimuli that are primarily neural and humoral.

Flow regulation is the result of fine-tuning of the coronary arteries' caliber, due to coordinated contractions and relaxations of the vessel walls' smooth muscle cells, occurring differentially across the disparate compartments of the coronary system. The coronary arteries are the left coronary artery and the right coronary artery (Fig. 1.2), which subdivide on the surface of the heart (the epicardium) into several treelike branches of smaller and smaller arteries that penetrate deep into the heart at almost a 90° angle toward the endocardium (the inner surface of the heart chambers) (Fig. 1.2). While penetrating the heart layers, these vessels transform from muscular conductive arteries into small very dynamic vessels (pre-arterioles, arterioles, and precapillary sphincters) before opening up into the capillary compartment.

The main flow control gates are the extramyocardial pre-arterioles, which respond to pressure changes, autacoids, and neurohumoral stimuli, and the arterioles, which, being intramyocardial, are the only ones able to respond to locally diffusible metabolites downstream from neurohumoral stimuli.

Precapillary sphincters only control the topographic microdistribution of flow into capillaries.

Epicardial capacitance vessels respond to neurohumoral and local mechanical stimuli (pressure or shear stress), but they only regulate blood flow to a minor degree. Nonetheless, capillary perfusion pressure can be critically reduced if epicardial arteries are narrowed beyond the capacity of small vessels to compensate for any drop in flow via dilation.

The continuously varying response of smooth muscle cells across different coronary compartments *in series* and *in parallel* results from a dynamic integration between several correlated processes, occurring at different scales of organization: the cell level (e.g., expression of different types/densities of receptor, variable transduction of signals, different intracellular "-omics"), the tissue level (different regional presence of mechanical, autocrine, paracrine stimuli and variable mechanisms of signal diffusion between near and distant cells), and the inter-apparatus level (different endothelial, neural, endocrine effects).

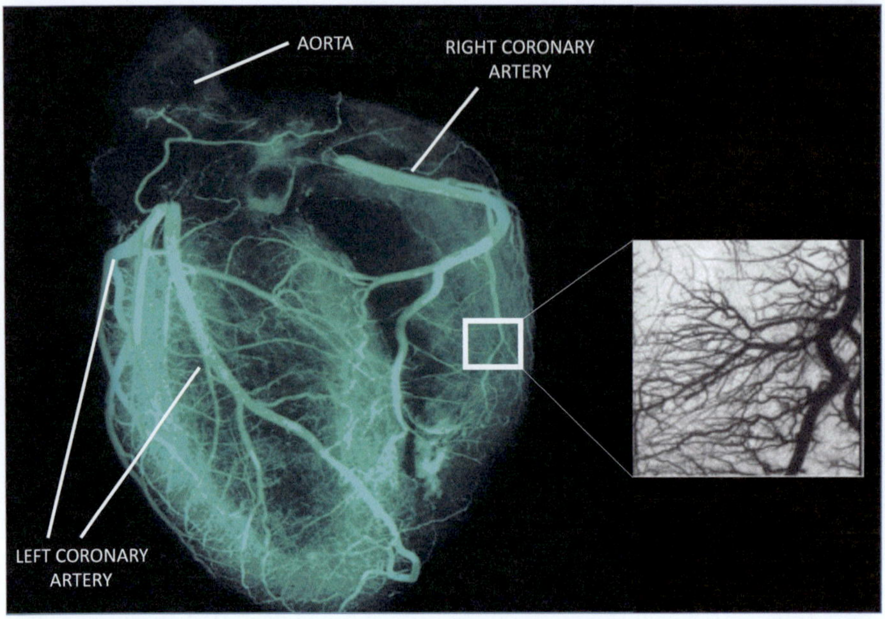

Fig. 1.2 Coronary arterial circulation. Coronary arteries subdivide in a fractal way, both at the surface of the heart and while penetrating the muscle layers. At different scales, the structural and functional properties of vessels change in series and in parallel, as does their function. The small coronary vessels represent (see magnification on the *right*) the majority of the coronary circulation, covering an area 50 times larger than the epicardial bed. At the microcirculatory level, a wide array of interconnections (anastomoses) is present between branches (Reproduced and modified with permission from AGF/Science Photo Library)

The multidimensional dynamic loops and feedback circuits of coronary flow regulation allow for it to be considered an open, complex system which is still poorly understood because it requires nonlinear and nondeterministic investigative approaches that, surprisingly, still have received little consideration [1].

1.2.2 Complex Neurohumoral Modulation of Blood Flow

The architectural complexity of coronary blood flow explains our incomplete understanding of its regulation by the autonomic nervous system. Indeed, no good deductive models yet exist that are able to describe this control using physical and physiological principles.

Experiments in animals have demonstrated a major direct influence of autonomic control of blood flow via central and peripheral influences [2–5]. In resting humans, the presence of nervous modulation of vasomotor tone is demonstrated by a 10 % increase in basal coronary blood flow with abolition of alpha adrenergic tone and by the nonpathologic changes that are observed in coronary blood flow induced by mental stress, independent of hemodynamic and heart rate changes

[6–9]. Moreover, reinnervated areas of transplanted hearts show an increase in myocardial blood flow [10], whereas mental stress-induced coronary vasoconstriction is the best predictor of daily life ischemia even in patients with coronary stenoses (see also Sect. 2.2). Furthermore, adrenergic alterations are associated with myocardial ischemia due to pure microvascular dysfunction [11], and sympathetic/parasympathetic imbalances are highly prevalent in patients with pure vasospastic angina [12, 13].

The neural modulation of flow occurs (a) directly, as a response to primary brain functions and to arch reflexes, and (b) indirectly, regulating metabolic needs, heart rate, and systemic pressure.

The indirect control is due to the extensive innervation of cardiac pacemakers, the heart conduction system, peripheral circulation, and, more scarcely, the myocardium.

The direct modulation of blood flow is made possible by the extensive innervation of coronary arteries (especially arterioles) by efferent divisions of the autonomic nervous system (sympathetic, parasympathetic, and nonadrenergic-noncholinergic). These form a tubular sheet at the border between the adventitia and media (coronary plexus) that is able to influence the vasomotor status from its outer layers, releasing a number of different mediators. To date, albeit still incompletely, study has focused mainly on sympathetic and parasympathetic mediators (norepinephrine, adrenalin, acetylcholine), while a broader list of nonadrenergic, noncholinergic mediators (adenosine triphosphate, neuropeptide Y, substance P, vasoactive intestinal peptide (VIP), endorphins, nitric oxide (NO), galanin, calcitonin gene-related peptide (CGRP), etc.) and their interactions with the former have not yet been assessed. Due to the functional complexity of the blood flow control system, each neurotransmitter has different simultaneous effects on smooth muscle cells and endothelial and heart metabolic need levels, being able to blunt or increase myocardial blood flow, depending upon the overall status of the system and of each compartment, hereby underscoring the nondeterministic behavior of the coronary blood flow system.

Reflex control is orchestrated by a complex network of neurons that extend from the cerebral cortex to the spinal cord [14], providing efferent stimuli from vagal and sympathetic neurons in the medulla in response to direct and centrally elaborated continuous sensory inputs received from different receptors (e.g., chemoreceptors from the diffuse cardiac nerve network and carotid bodies; mechanoreceptors from the diffuse cardiac nerve network, carotid sinus, aortic arch, and lungs; visceral pain receptors from all over the body; and visual, olfactory, auditory, tactile and renal, kinetosensory, and digestive nerves from what has been called "the second brain"—see Chap. 4). Additional reflexes occur in thoracic and intrinsic cardiac ganglia, enabling the heart to maintain independent reflex activity (Fig.1.3).

Central control—which is orchestrated by higher-level centers (motor, medial prefrontal, anterior cingular, and insular cortex and several other regions located in the forebrain, midbrain, medulla oblongata, and the circumventricular organs)—occurs in response to emotions, stress, cognitive and motivated activity, and both

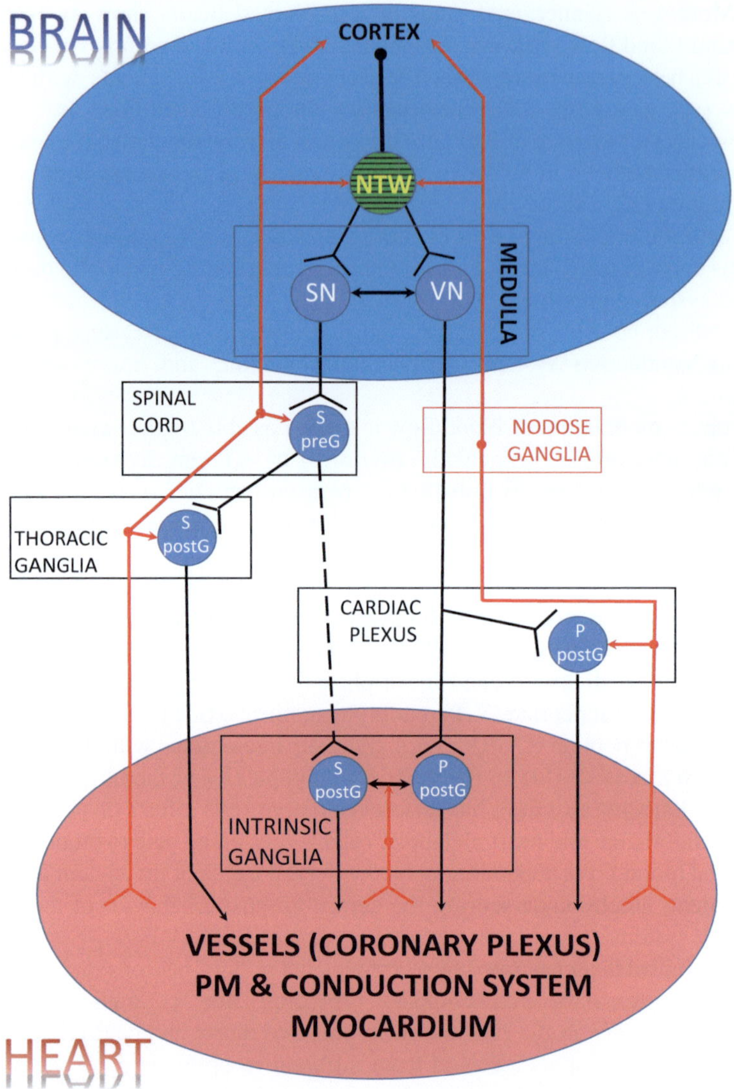

Fig. 1.3 Main heart-brain neurological connections and circuits. The neural activity of a complex cortical and subcortical network of neurons (NTW), directly and indirectly activates, in the medulla, both pre-sympathetic (cardio-excitatory, SN) and vagal (cardio-inhibitory, VN) neurons. Pre-sympathetic activity controls preganglionic neurons located in the spinal cord and is largely composed of groups of neurons located in the rostral ventrolateral medulla, paragigantocellularis nucleus, caudal raphe, A5 pons, paraventricular nucleus, and locus coeruleus. Vagal neurons give rise to preganglionic parasympathetic fibers from the dorsal motor vagal nucleus and the nucleus ambiguus. The NTW is composed of a number of connected subcortical structures, among which are the medulla (nucleus tractus solitarius and raphe magnus), the hypothalamus and pons (paraventricular nucleus, A5 cell group), the thalamus, the limbic system, basal ganglia, circumventricular organs, and higher centers such as the cortex. The efferent sympathetic post-ganglionic fibers originate mainly from paravertebral cervical and upper thoracic ganglia (S-postG), while a minority arise from intrinsic cardiac ganglia (S-postG). Efferent postganglionic parasympathetic fibers originate from the cardiac plexus (P-postG) and intrinsic cardiac ganglia

conscious and unconscious behaviors through the modulation of activity in the cardiac nuclei of the medulla (see Sect. 1.4.2) (Fig.1.3).

Different divisions work in coordination, interacting in the medulla and ganglia and at junctional terminals regulating reciprocally or synergistically [15] the release of neurotransmitters (e.g., by the activation of interneurons or by reciprocal action at nerve terminals) and modulating their time course/extent of action through catalases.

1.2.3 Other Linked Myocardial Blood Flow Controls

Situated on the inner side of the vascular wall, in direct contact with the circulation on one side and the inner muscular layers of the media on the other, the endothelium directly controls vasomotor tone, releasing vasomotor autacoids (e.g., NO, prostaglandins, endothelin, histamine, acetylcholine, kinins) which diffuse locally into the wall or downstream to other compartments through the blood. Hence, endothelium also indirectly controls blood flow through the permeability to these and other circulating factors (e.g., thrombin, thromboxane A2, leukotrienes released by granulocytes, serotonin released by platelets). Varying structural and functional properties of the endothelial system in different compartments determine its differential effect on blood flow, which in turn integrates other controls. Therefore, structural or functional alterations in the vessels, such as atherosclerosis, may interfere with the coordination that exists between the controllers, causing dysfunctional regulation of blood flow [16].

When endothelium is in a normal state, beyond its vasomotor function, it has anticoagulant properties and/or can antagonize platelet aggregation (production of NO, prostacyclin, heparin sulfate, thrombomodulin, and tissue plasminogen activator). However, when it is dysfunctional (due to neurohumoral, mechanical, inflammatory, infectious, or chemical stimuli), it has a powerful procoagulant (production of tissue factor, plasminogen activator inhibitor-1, and receptors for adhesion of platelets) and pro-inflammatory actions (via the exposition of adhesion molecules for circulating leukocytes).

In a vicious circle, thrombi can also indirectly influence blood flow due to the production of circulating substances, causing vasoconstriction and endothelial dysfunction.

Heart rate also influences myocardial blood flow, because during systole the entire volume of blood is squeezed out of the deeper vessels into the epicardial

Fig. 1.3 (continued) (P-postG). In *red*, note the non-detailed scheme of afferent sensory pathways and their sites of interaction with efferent divisions, mainly performed via the intermediation of interneurons (not displayed in the figure). *Red dots* indicate some of the main locations of sensory neurons (see Sect. 1.4.2). Overall, multiple loops and feedback circuits are present at each hierarchical level of connection, and all levels interact and are mutually influential, rendering the system both complex and nondeterministic

vessels and the aorta by muscle contraction. Therefore, whatever its autoregulation capacity, the faster the heart rate (heavily influenced by the autonomic nervous system), the lower the time for the sufficient oxygenation of muscle. For the same reason, extravascular compressive forces (i.e., muscle contracting around the vessels and the force exerted by blood pressure in heart chambers) influence coronary flow and are themselves connected to muscle metabolic activity and autonomic function within yet another recursive loop.

1.2.4 Systemic Properties of the Controls of Coronary Circulation

Coronary flow is then determined by a network of extremely complex direct and indirect, linear and nonlinear processes that occur on various scales, interdependent within and between different levels of organization (spanning the subcellular, cellular, intercellular, interorgan, and inter-apparatus levels). Any isolated or linked alterations, structural or functional, at any level of the system could engender abnormalities in the control of myocardial blood flow. However, it can also be compensated for by means of several other multiscale processes, until the limits of the whole system are reached and a critical reduction in capillary perfusion pressure emerges. Ischemia may then cause further dysfunction in the blood flow control system, thereby aggravating ischemia (see Sect. 1.4). The final effect of this complexity is that the actions of any component of the system therefore vary considerably, resulting in a physiological, compensatory, or pathological process, depending upon the system's overall coherence.

Therefore, any single component (or process) in such a complex environment can only be comprehensively understood on the basis of an iterative investigational process that takes into account the larger context in which it is playing. Fortunately, studying the systemic, nondeterministic properties of this complex system could allow for the development of new approaches and new therapeutic targets.

1.3 Psychoneural Influences on Ischemia Generation

The impossibility of confirming a critical level of atherosclerosis in up to 30 % of acute coronary syndromes [17], and evidence that overall prognosis is not improved by either the revascularization of stable syndromes [18] or using anatomy-centered approaches [19], challenge the theory of a single, initiating cause of ischemia. This conclusion should not come as a surprise, given the complexity of the coronary system, which has several aforementioned interconnected regulating mechanisms that need to be overwhelmed to result in ischemia. Indeed, myocardial ischemia is generated by a final effector system variably emerging from fluctuating interactions between the underlying dynamic networks of dysfunction and predisposing factors (Fig. 1.4).

The final effector system can be represented as composed of up to six complex processes which, interacting variably, generate a coherent ecosystem (Fig.1.5a).

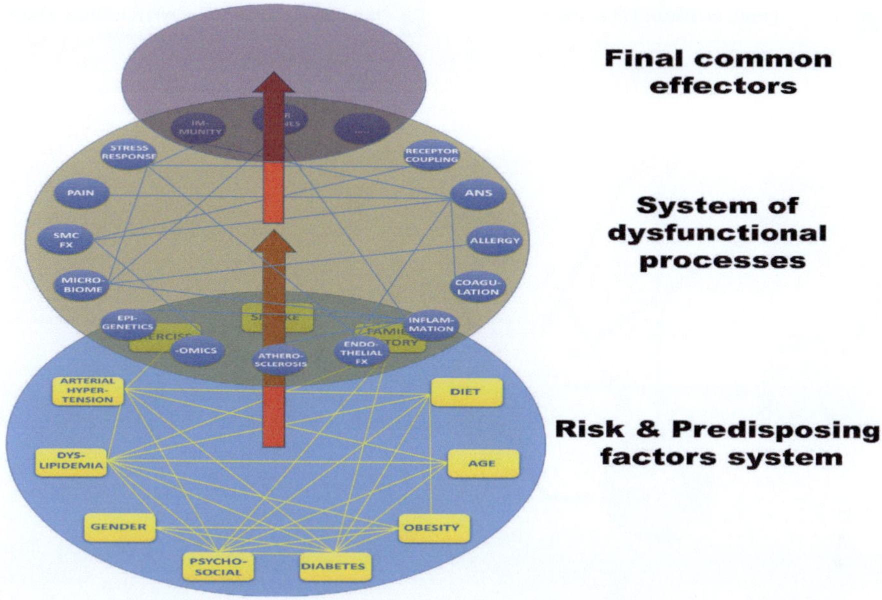

Fig. 1.4 A hierarchical systemic representation of myocardial ischemia emergence. A dynamic network of systems gives rise to myocardial ischemia: the complex system of risk and predisposing factors generates the emergence of a complex system of interconnected dysfunctional processes that, in turn, result in a system of final common effectors. The individual elements of these three networks are themselves complex systems that interact individually and collectively, either in a linear way or in nonlinear loops and feedback circuits (displayed with lines), but also among different layers of the meta-system (not displayed in the figure). *ANS* autonomic nervous system, *SMC* smooth muscle cells

The variability of these interactions is dependent on intrinsic characteristics of the final effector ecosystem, on the disparate underlying interactions of dysfunctional systems (see Sect. 1.2 and Fig. 1.4), and on the feedback effects derived both from the variable consequences of ischemia and from the underlying causative mechanisms (in turn, influenced by the emergence of ischemia) (see Sect. 1.4.1). As with any ecosystem, the effector system is nonlinear, rendering it possible that interactions between individually subcritical processes become critical when acting together, thereby precipitating ischemia (Fig. 1.5b). Linear or deterministic behaviors of this system, including isolated culprit processes, are not excluded but seen as particular cases and are less frequent.

This comprehensive perspective can explain some mechanisms behind the "false-negative" ischemia tests which, being blind to critical interactions, only reveal isolated subcritical processes without ruling out complex interacting processes. Moreover, this model is able to justify the limited success of interventions performed on isolated targets, which may or may not result in the abolition of ischemia, depending on the networking characteristics each has, which are variable case by case.

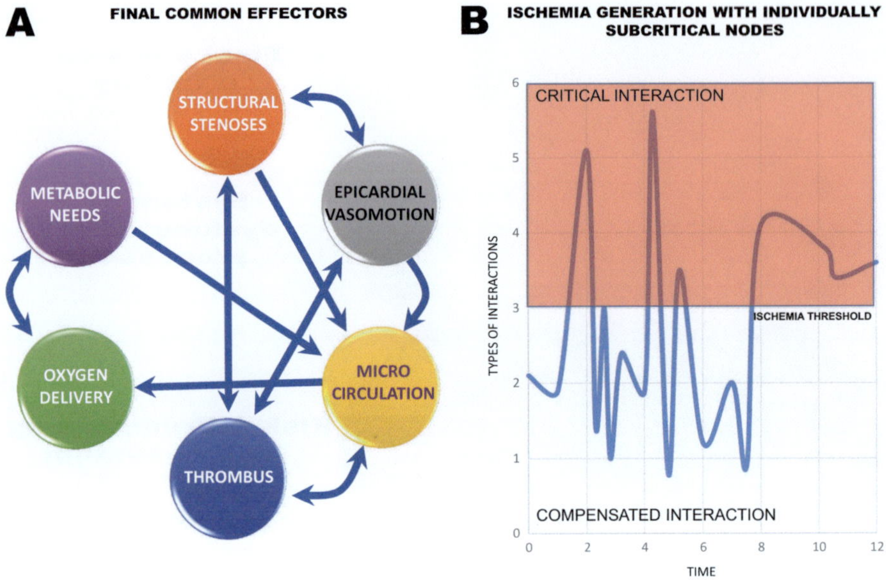

Fig. 1.5 Final common effector ecosystem. (**a**) Any ischemia can be considered the emerging property of a dynamic network composed of up to six nodes, variably intervening and interacting. (**b**) According to the type and number of interactions between the nodes, any alteration can be compensated for (*lower panel*) or cause ischemia (*upper panel*), even when the individual nodes are not sufficiently critical to trigger ischemia. When a single node becomes critical and completely predominant over the others, the system behaves linearly and becomes deterministic. Linear and nonlinear behaviors can emerge in different moments of the evolution of the same system

Therefore, an ecosystem perspective can represent the complexity of individual processes in their evolution and show that a shift in paradigm from isolated targets to comprehensive interactions could significantly advance the therapy of ischemic heart disease.

The final effectors are:

A. Structural epicardial stenosing processes

In the presence of raised metabolic needs—such as during exercise or other activities or states associated with a higher heart rate—the presence of fixed stenosis in epicardial arteries overcomes the capacity of the system to compensate when the stenosis is >70 % of the vessel's diameter. However, stable clinical pictures frequently exhibit variable combinations of the other ischemia-generating processes (see below). Subcritical stenosis (i.e., <50 % narrowing of vessel diameter), requiring additional mechanisms to cause ischemia, is often identified in acute ischemic syndromes and vasospastic angina.

Atherosclerosis is the most frequent form of structural stenosis. However, arterial dissections, intramural hemorrhages, and repetitive episodes of non-occlusive wall thrombosis, causing gradual progression of narrowing, can also be involved. Atherosclerosis is a progressive, inflammatory thickening of arteries consisting of cells, connective tissue elements, lipids, and other debris. It starts from low-density lipoprotein (LDL) cholesterol infiltration beneath the intima, which triggers a complex and prolonged process involving inflammation and immunity, primarily mediated by endothelial activation, with adhesion and penetration of leukocytes into the wall and macrophages attracted by chemokines. A possible role for infections has also been suggested. Neuropsychological factors can influence atherosclerosis in experimental models [20] and in humans [21], likely due to effects on endothelial activation and on immune and inflammatory systems (see Chap. 3).

B. Epicardial vasoconstriction

Vasomotor activity of epicardial arteries can precipitate (a) acute ischemia, when focal or diffuse occluding spasm occurs or when vasoconstriction at the site of atherosclerotic stenosis is enough to cause occlusion, and (b) effort-induced ischemia, in cases of non-occluding vasoconstriction at the site of structural stenoses.

Triggers for vasoconstriction/spasm may be, alone or in combination, psychoneural, toxic (e.g., cigarette smoking, drugs), mechanical, immunologic, thrombotic, or local inflammatory stimuli and/or abrupt changes in the cellular mechanisms of smooth muscle reactivity. Specific drugs, like nitrates and calcium antagonists, can dilate epicardial vessels. However, depending on the cause and intensity of vasoconstriction, sometimes an efficient local concentration of these drugs can only be obtained by intracoronary administration.

C. Microcirculatory dysfunction/obstruction

Isolated dysfunction of small coronary vessels can cause effort-induced ischemia (syndrome X) [22] or acute coronary syndromes (likely, at least some forms of takotsubo syndrome—see Chap. 6) [23].

More frequently, based on the multilevel vulnerability of coronary blood flow regulation (see Sect. 1.2), microcirculation dysfunction can be observed in the presence of stable epicardial stenosis, myocardial infarction (mainly due to micro-emboli and/or vasomotor substances originating from an upstream thrombus), cardiomyopathy, cardiac hypertrophy, cardiac dysfunction, and systemic diseases.

A variety of neural (e.g., neuropeptide Y) and humoral (e.g., angiotensin) stimuli, as well as autacoids produced by endothelium (e.g., leukotrienes), also directly and indirectly linked among themselves, can cause ischemia by constricting small vessels; but the site of constriction may vary between substances and specific drugs which counter small vessel dysfunction at different levels are not yet available.

D. Thrombosis

Coronary thrombosis can cause ischemia, depending upon the rapidity and severity of obstruction to flow and the release of vasoactive substances. Sudden, complete, and persistent occlusion of a coronary artery causes acute transmural ischemia and myocardial infarction and requires urgent and stable re-opening of the artery by mechanical (i.e., angioplasty) or pharmacological (i.e., thrombolysis) means. More gradual, intermittent, and/or incomplete obstruction episodes can give rise to repeated episodes of non-transmural infarction or unstable angina. Although a nonobstructing mural thrombus can induce ischemia via emboli in small vessels and/or the release of substances that induce vasoconstriction and activate the endothelium, thrombosis is observed in stable syndromes in up to 12 % of cases.

Both platelets and the humoral coagulation system are involved in intracoronary thrombus formation, in a complex spatial and time-dependent interplay that is also dependent on the triggers of coagulation. Strong thrombogenic stimuli can precipitate thrombosis even after a short period of exposure; however, prolonged weaker stimuli can also cause thrombosis in a predisposed prothrombotic milieu.

During acute infarction, coronary thrombosis is apparent in 70–80 % of cases at the site of ruptured or fissured atherosclerotic plaques, thereby exposing a highly thrombogenic necrotic core triggering acute coagulation. Rupture or a fissure can be caused by mechanical (e.g., spasm), biological (e.g., inflammatory process of atheroma, immunologic or infectious agents), or chemical stimuli. However, in 10–20 % of instances, no interruption of the plaque's cap is identified (plaque erosion or endothelial activation); and in approximately 10 % of cases of coronary thrombosis, atherosclerotic plaques are absent.

Neuropsychological factors can precipitate acute coronary thrombosis and infarction in both experimental models [24] and humans [25] (see Chap. 3).

E. Metabolic needs

The metabolic needs of heart muscle determine the threshold of flow undersupply at which ischemia will emerge. The same absolute level of blood flow can be either adequate or inadequate, depending on this threshold. Metabolic needs simultaneously depend on heart rate, myocardial contractility, blood pressure, intracardiac pressures and volume, hormonal state, heart temperature, and wall tension. All of these factors can be strongly influenced by a person's psychoneurological state.

F. Oxygen delivery

The quantity of oxygen that is delivered to heart cells over a given unit of time is determined by the oxygen content of the blood (type of hemoglobin, hemoglobin concentration, blood red cell count, lung function) and by the efficiency of oxygen extraction, which is largely dependent on local factors, like serum pH and temperature and the gradients of soluble gases (mainly PO_2 and PCO_2), in accordance with a hemoglobin dissociation curve. Oxygen extraction is 80–90 % at rest and, consequently, can only compensate against blood flow reductions to a very limited degree.

Psychoneural activity (Fig. 1.1) influences this complex system considerably via various links with the compensatory or pathogenic role of other network processes. Its effects on coagulation and platelet aggregation can prevent, facilitate, or precipitate acute thrombosis. Its effects on atherosclerosis also can vary, depending on the chronic and acute effects of the psychoneural axis on inflammation and endothelial activation (see Chap. 3). The differential effects it has on vasomotor activity in several coronary compartments may compensate critical situations, but in other networking conditions may be a chronically detrimental process or precipitating event [26]. Effects on heart rate, systemic pressure, and cardiac metabolism set the threshold for myocardial ischemia and therefore can precipitate, facilitate, blunt, or strongly antagonize any tendency toward ischemia by interfering with metabolic needs and oxygen delivery to the tissue.

Consequently, psychoneural processes within the ischemia ecosystem cannot be described in abstract terms; rather, they must be assessed relative to other processes. This implies the need for novel systemic classifications of ischemic heart disease that encompass dynamic coherences. This also generates, as a consequence, the ability of psychic and emotional activity to exert positive or detrimental effects on ischemia generation, depending on overall relationships with the complex system.

1.4 Consequences of Ischemia and Role of Psychobiological Factors

1.4.1 Nonlinear Biological Effects of Ischemia

Once blood flow is insufficient to meet the needs of the heart, the emerging effect is the initiation of coherent biological alterations in the myocardium, which reciprocally enhance the underlying causative system and determine clinical manifestations.

The first alterations caused by ischemia (within a few seconds) are at the cellular level, with profound changes in extracellular and intracellular electrolytes, causing diastolic depolarization and an early increase in intracellular Ca^{++}, which worsens with the damage of membranes. Metabolic changes that occur are inhibition of oxidative metabolism, depletion of high-energy stores (beginning usually after 1 min, with a 70 % of loss of ATP within 10 min of the start of ischemia), inhibition of protein synthesis, and the activation of anaerobic metabolism (anaerobic glycolysis, lipolysis) which is, in turn, markedly slowed as ischemia worsens because of the accumulation of end-product catabolites. Anaerobic glycolysis leads to lactate and phosphate accumulation, whereas catecholamine-dependent lipolysis of triglycerides leads to the accumulation of free fatty acids and acylcarnitine. This accumulation leads to progressive cellular edema with subsequent microvascular damage and worsened ischemia, intracellular and extracellular acidosis, the inhibition of contractility, and the intracellular activation of proteases which, in turn, contribute to membrane damage. Free radicals, produced especially if reperfusion occurs, cause severe alterations in proteins, nucleic acids, and lipids.

Activation by ischemia of sensory fibers in the myocardium causes early reflex outflow of the parasympathetic system through efferent divisions. Successively, ischemia directly causes an intense release of norepinephrine, inhibition of its reuptake from nerve terminals, and an upregulation of adrenergic receptors. Within the first few minutes of ischemia, the myocardial content of norepinephrine is moderate; whereas after approximately 20 min, it increases dramatically, reaching up to 1000 times its concentration in blood. This also causes a rise in plasma norepinephrine concentration, independently of the parallel activation of stress response (see Chap. 3). The autonomic activation that occurs during ischemia is partially cardioprotective (see the following paragraphs). However, it also causes a redistribution of coronary flow toward the epicardium (with possible increased subendocardial ischemia), direct cellular injury, an electrical excitatory effect on myocytes, and direct pro-thrombogenic and endothelial activator effects. When ischemia persists, cardiac nerve injury can develop, spanning from neural stunning to complete structural denervation of the injured area.

The presence/absence and sequence of these alterations, their relative weight, their relationships, and the ensuing clinical consequences vary considerably in their timing and extent, in accordance with the severity and duration of ischemia, local conditions in cell structures and function, genetics, -omics, cell metabolism, blood flow distribution, heart contractility, anatomic status, and several systemic conditions (including emotional status or cognitive and even cultural aspects) that precede and accompany the development of ischemia, as well as the characteristics of the underlying processes that caused the ischemia in the first place.

Therefore, also at this level, neither biological nor clinical effects of ischemia can be reduced to either a linear cause-effect relationship or a deterministic system, challenging the classic "ischemia cascade" theory with important consequences in the diagnostic process of myocardial ischemia which cannot be reduced to rigid standard manifestations [27].

1.4.2 Central Nervous System Effects

Pain is usually the reason for which ischemic patients seek medical advice, although its relationship with myocardial ischemia remains elusive. Visceral and/or somatic sensory pain is independent of ischemia extension and may be completely absent, mild, or extremely disabling, being more or less associated with a profound feeling of imminent death (affective component).

The reasons behind these variable responses reside in the reciprocal neurological traffic between the brain and heart. Myocardial ischemia metabolites excite the sensory endings of sensory afferent fibers innervating the heart through mechanical or chemical stimuli (e.g., adenosine, pH derived from lactate, serotonin histamine and thromboxane A2, free radicals, and kinins). The sympathetic unmyelinated and small myelinated fibers of the first-order neuron of upper thoracic ganglia carry pain impulses to dorsal horn neurons and upper thoracic dorsal roots (second-order neurons), where sensory somatic nerves also converge. Subsequently, through the spinothalamic tract, projections of second-order neurons reach discrete nuclei within the thalamus and from there, through third-order neurons, to the post-central cortex involved with the sensory-discriminatory component of pain.

The ascending affective component of pain is conducted by second-order neurons in the dorsal horn (expressing neurokinin 1 receptors): (a) through the spino-mesencephalic tract to the parabrachial area and periaqueductal gray matter, themselves, connected to the amygdala and hypothalamus, thereby regulating the affective dimensions of pain and, in parallel, controlling autonomic descending activity, and (b) through the spinothalamic tract to different nuclei in the thalamus, from which the message is then relayed to the anterior cingulate cortex, subserving the motivational aspects of pain and—with the lateral orbital, lateral agranular, and the dorsomedial prefrontal areas that have an important role in cognitive functions—behavioral and emotional states.

Cardiac vagal afferent fibers originate from the first-order neuron in nodose ganglia of the neck and relay impulses to second-order neurons in the vagal nuclei of the medulla (homolateral dorsal vagal nucleus, the heterolateral nucleus, cardiac nucleus adjacent to the nucleus ambiguus, and gray matter of the formatio reticularis). From there, pain impulses travel upward to higher levels in the brain stem, hypothalamus, thalamus, and cortex.

Afferent impulses may be inhibited at the spinal level by afferent somatic or visceral fibers working synergistically with descending fibers from the central nervous system, particularly via serotoninergic activation of the nucleus raphe magnus in the medulla. The nucleus raphe magnus is, in turn, modulated by several other brain structures, through descending afferents from the periaqueductal gray (analgesic functions), the paraventricular hypothalamic nucleus (involved in stress responses), the central nucleus of the amygdala (involved in conscious perceptions of emotions, memory, and the autonomic response to emotions), the lateral hypothalamic area (involved in a number of cognitive and physical responses, among which are various neuroendocrine functions, the sensitivity of bowel visceral pain, reward system), the parvocellular reticular nucleus (involved in expiration and analgesia), and the prelimbic and infralimbic (both involved in fear and memory extinction) medial and lateral (involved with movement and sensory inputs) precentral cortices.

The nucleus submedius of the thalamus also has a close relationship with ventrolateral orbital cortex and periaqueductal region that forms part of the descending inhibition system. Activation of thalamic nuclei can lead to inhibition or facilitation of nociceptive stimuli via the activation of specific on-neurons or off-neurons.

Overall, anginal nociceptive stimuli can also be modulated via the opioid system (including the pathways: cortical → periaqueductal gray → rostroventromedial medulla → spinal cord circuit and cortical → hypothalamic circuit) which can also be activated by subjective attitudes of stoicism or denial or by psychosocial stimuli. Furthermore, some data show that painful cardiac stimuli can themselves progressively modify their own central modulation with variations in susceptibility to angina during different episodes of ischemia [28], possibly via the differential genetic expression of endogenous opioids [29].

These circuits, beyond orchestrating pain perception and coronary blood flow control (summarized in Sect. 1.2.2), reveal how direct, nonsymbolic, afferent cardiac stimuli can intervene in complex functions like memory, motivation, attention, emotions, behaviors, mental associative functions, and values. Furthermore, data demonstrate that specific variations in cortical activity in ischemic heart disease may also occur independent of perceived anginal pain [30], demonstrating a broader relationship between superior cerebral functions and myocardial ischemia.

Therefore, as cortical functions simultaneously influence (see Sect. 1.2.2) and are influenced by myocardial ischemia, the psychological → biological and biological → psychological loops should be considered in unity with the myocardial ischemia ecosystem, and more than just an isolated undesirable effect, despite the scant research attention they have received to date.

1.4.3 Myocardial Dysfunction

Contractile dysfunction is one of the early (3–5 s after the onset of ischemia) and most threatening consequences of myocardial ischemia, because >80 % of resting oxygen consumption is due to contractile work. It can be worsened by reperfusion injury (mediated by free radicals). Nevertheless, it also is reversible, in proportion to the extension and duration of ischemia. Indeed, sudden massive myocardial dysfunction can cause acute cardiac failure and even death. The relationship between the reduction in blood flow and impairment of contractile function has an exponential nature. This being said, considerable heterogeneity in the response has been observed in different studies, suggesting individual susceptibility of myocardium to similar degrees of ischemia. Different susceptibility to ischemia is the result of the multidimensional characteristics and interactions of the whole system, from the genetic expression of myocytes to macroscopic interorgan communications and controls, like neurohumoral modulation and other signaling pathways. Despite the important effects of the autonomic system in myocardial dysfunction processes, the role that the brain's descending modulation of cardiac neural activity plays in this scenario has not yet been studied.

Norepinephrine (in small amounts), but principally acetylcholine released within the myocardium from efferent terminals, protects myocytes against lethal ischemia-reperfusion injury, independent of any reduction in heart rate. Exposing the myocardium to brief ischemia-reperfusion episodes protects the heart from subsequent longer periods of ischemia. This phenomenon has been called *ischemic preconditioning*. Interestingly, the myocardium is also protected by remote preconditioning, in which cycles of brief ischemia and reperfusion of another organ or tissue (e.g., the forearm by cuff occlusion) protect the heart against ischemia/reperfusion injury. Both these phenomena are mediated by autonomic pathways and by adenosine, bradykinin, and calcitonin gene-related peptide. The exact neural pathways, which also include the afferent sensory neuron and parasympathetic systems, remain unclear; but remote preconditioning could also involve interactions between multiple redundant signaling pathways.

Other forms of persistent but potentially reversible cardiac dysfunction are myocardial stunning and hibernation. The former indicates persistent myocardial dysfunction within a region with normal blood flow (usually after revascularization) due to slowly reverting modified gene expression, intracellular calcium overload, excitation-contraction uncoupling, and/or a delay in microvascular damage repair. However, the evidence documenting myocardial stunning with normal epicardial coronary arteries after a subarachnoid hemorrhage [31], and independent of myocardial blood flow variations during periods of emotional [32] or mental stress [33], indicates some role of the autonomic nervous system. Ischemia-induced neural stunning may also contribute to the delayed recovery of myocardial function.

Myocardial hibernation is a reduction in contractile function in a territory with reduced flow, but without metabolic signs of ischemia. This condition can be due to the rare case of stable stenosis >90 % over weeks or months and/or, more likely, to the inappropriate chronic contraction of pre-arteriolar vessels (on a myogenic and/or neurohumoral basis) and/or the potentially reversible resetting of the metabolic autoregulation of arterioles.

1.4.4 Electrical Alterations and Arrhythmias

Fatal arrhythmias are rare during mild and transient ischemia, but can develop as the first, immediate manifestation of transmural ischemia episodes, before any other measurable heart response. They occur more frequently during acute myocardial infarction. Fatal arrhythmias in the setting of acute myocardial infarction account for about 50 % of all deaths and generally occur within the first 2 h, independent of the size of myocardial infarction.

The underlying electrical processes are consequences of alterations that occur at the cell and tissue levels and translate into ECG alterations of the ST-T segment. The refractory period is initially shortened, but after a few minutes, it becomes longer than in adjacent nonischemic cells. Conduction of the electric impulse initially increases; but, after few minutes, it decreases until it becomes blocked or fractionated. Toxic accumulation of ischemia-driven or reperfusion-driven substances can lead to triggered activity that, in turn, may increase automaticity. It also can lead to reentry circuits, which also are facilitated by the abovementioned electrophysiologic alterations.

During an infarction, the contributions to life-threatening arrhythmias of acute ischemic heart denervation, neural stunning, tissue catecholamine content, and adrenergic stimulation are substantial, whereas any increase in vagal tone is protective, as it also is in experimental settings [34]. However, an excess in parasympathetic drive can occur with various degrees of atrioventricular block and asystole, which can be promptly reverted by atropine when they are not caused by ischemic cell damage within the conduction system.

Higher center modulation influences arrhythmogenesis in an ischemic milieu. Experimental evidence of a psychologic activation of autonomic-dependent arrhythmogenesis in myocardial ischemia is presented in Chaps. 2, 5, and 12. Moreover, also other organs can participate to autonomic-activated arrhythmogenesis in a complex network (see Chap. 4).

Also scar tissue can also constitute the substrate for reentrant circuits and threatening arrhythmias.

Similar to what was just said for myocardial dysfunction, considerable heterogeneity exists in individual's susceptibility to arrhythmias, for which the final outcome relies on a highly complex network of interactions including, as before, neurohumoral interactions. Indeed, ventricular ischemia and repair also cause deep remodeling of heart sympathetic innervation and may predispose patients to an increased risk of fatal arrhythmias [35]. The afferent spinal and supraspinal consequences of such nervous remodeling remain unknown, as do the central nervous system's descending effects.

1.4.5 Necrosis and Remodeling

Necrosis is the final outcome of ischemia: when its effects become irreversible, tissues disrupt and cells die. The time required for cell death and its extension is highly variable and again depends on a complex network of processes that include the patient's anatomy, collateral flow, duration of occlusion, metabolic activity of the tissue, individual vulnerability of myocytes, and the extent of activation of myocardial inflammatory processes.

Experimental data have demonstrated a delayed onset of necrosis with increased parasympathetic activation that lowers metabolism, slows heart rate, and probably also contributes to enhanced control of coronary blood flow. This is contrary to persistent sympathetic activity, which both accelerates and enlarges the extent of necrosis.

The extent of necrosis is the main determinant of chronic left ventricular dysfunction after a myocardial infarction, which also depends upon post-infarction repair processes. After a myocardial infarction occurs, necrotic muscular tissue is replaced by fibrosis via a complex inflammatory process (mainly driven by macrophages and granulocytes triggered by the activation of innate immunologic processes, complement activation, and reactive oxygen species release), and this may further injure myocytes and microvessels not yet irreversibly damaged by the ischemia itself [36]. Removal of necrotic tissue takes 3–6 weeks, with repair complete in 3–6 months. The complex changes that intervene in the myocardium during the repair phase may lead to ventricular remodeling, which may follow a favorable or unfavorable course, depending on the tridimensional and geometric shape changes that occur, based on the extension and depth/thickness of damage into heart muscle layers and compensatory hypertrophy of adjacent segments. When the infarction is large and transmural, the infarcted area may expand secondary to additional inflammatory processes that result from increased afterload [37]. Conversely, when it is small and subendocardial, the scar may even shrink and end up smaller than initially.

Unfavorable remodeling will increase wall tensile stress and augment intracardiac pressures, leading in turn to progressive passive and/or inflammatory enlargement of infarcted and then non-infarcted areas, in a vicious circle that can lead to heart failure and increased susceptibility to arrhythmias. In addition, a significant neurohumoral contribution to cardiac remodeling has been documented in experimental models [35]; and, as expected given this physiopathological basis, data exist to suggest that each of these processes can be influenced by descending cortical activity probably also due to its action on inflammation and stress response (see Chaps. 3 and 12; Fig. 2.2).

1.5 Clinical Role of Psychobiologic Processes and Implications for Interventions

1.5.1 Need for New Approaches to the Study of Ischemic Heart Disease

Recognizing heart physiology and the pathophysiology of myocardial ischemia as an emerging nonlinear property of auto-organization, open ecosystems are in desperate need of a new comprehensive epistemology that translates into profound consequences for taxonomy, predictability, research, and treatment. The evolution from a reductionist to a systems science framework will eventually lead to new horizons in the understanding and treatment of ischemic heart disease, where the progress and conquests achieved with the classical approach are considered adequate in some, but not all systemic conditions (i.e., when it behaves linearly).

As described in the previous paragraphs, similar clinical manifestations of myocardial ischemia can be the result of vastly different underlying functions, processes, dysfunctions, and structural alterations, with links from the genetic to the interorgan to the individual-environment interaction level. On the other hand, very different clinical pictures may share a number of pathways, alterations, and mechanisms. In fact, similar alterations (e.g., neurohumoral activation via psychological processes) taking place in different functional networks (e.g., in a complex milieu that predisposes to thrombosis versus another that is more physiological than anatomic) have very different consequences, spanning from being protective to being neutral to being key precipitating stimuli. From this perspective, no element has an absolute negative or positive role, and it is essential to address the dynamic properties of the relevant system to understand its evolving emergences and target specific processes in the correct time frame. The blindness of the classical medical approach to such complex and dynamic relationships—which altogether misses the variable value of isolated elements depending on the evolving context—might at least partially explain the puzzling mismatch between the multiplication of therapeutic targets and the paradoxical decrease in new effective therapies that have transpired in recent years.

This is particularly true for psychological or psychopharmacologic interventions for ischemic heart disease, wherein classical studies, being designed to eliminate complexity, cannot be conclusive for hard outcomes, even in typical patients (see Chaps. 9 and 10). On the contrary, focusing on the individual and time-related variability that exists within the ischemia ecosystem might generate a more precise evaluation of any intervention, as well as a more effective, personalized approach, potentially leading to further improved outcomes by overcoming the intrinsic limitations of average/typical event-based therapies.

Furthermore, the complexity of living networks is not only based upon variable links between multidimensional elements (e.g., the innumerable cause-effect loops described in previous paragraphs, rendering the system nondeterministic) but also on the fact that the basic elements (i.e., the genes and their expression, the cells, etc.) change over time in the same subject and differ between individuals. Moreover, each individual living system acquires different emergent properties at different times and levels of observation (i.e., from genes to subject-environment interactions) which warrant disparate approaches (so called *logical openness*) [38]. Specifically, as previously described, the process of myocardial ischemia includes circular processes with irreducible biologic and psychologic dimensions (Fig. 1.1) that cannot be summed up and require different models for their respective description. These characteristics oblige any observer to focus on the properties of the relationships between elements rather than merely on the characteristics of each element itself, which sometimes are even not comparable and sometimes change according to different contexts (i.e. the same molecule can regulate a process in some systems and other processes in other systems). Indeed, complex systems can be defined as those systems in which continuous processes of auto-organization and emergence take place, acquiring sequences of new properties while maintaining coherence [39]. For these reasons, myocardial ischemia systems—being incompletely, non-univocally, and non-explicitly describable in an analytic way, as well as highly nonlinear, nondeterministic, and nonreducible—are unresponsive to any explicit prescription that replace the elaboration of a perturbation by the system itself with simple orders from an external system (such as action on an electrical switch in an electrical circuit) and require specific, systems science tools [40].

The aim of any systems medicine approach is therefore to scientifically address the behaviors of connected complex systems, striving to enhance the achievable efficacy of therapies at both the individual patient and individual event level.

1.5.2 New Scientific and Clinical Tools

Changing a scientific framework allows for the development of new methods of research to integrate classic studies. In particular, randomized controlled trials (RCT) are mandatory to assess the effects of an intervention, because the process of randomization allows for at least some level of control over potential confounders. However, when performed on large populations enrolled with broad inclusion criteria, RCTs lose their ability to assess complex systems because they normalize average populations in attempts to observe a single component of the system. On the other hand, RCTs can be a valid instrument to comprehensively study complex systems when performed on samples of patients carefully characterized by homogenous, multidimensional characteristics.

This approach multiplies the study's potential when studying outliers, where it is easier to weigh single components without isolating them from their specific context and thereby be able to identify significant emerging clusters or configurations within interconnected systems [41–43].

Taking this concept to its extreme consequences, also studying single subjects can enable the assessment of dynamic changes at the individual level (i.e., not looking for similar changes, but similar dynamics of change among individuals) (called "*n* of 1 pathways"), which then could be tested in larger populations to validate the scientific transition to personalized medicine [44].

Furthermore, studies aimed at assessing the properties of networks and multidimensional processes will eventually lead to complex phenotyping in individuals. This will be made possible by the handling of huge datasets, a process that has been rendered technically feasible by recent advances in high-throughput platforms and data elaboration. Complex phenotyping stands as a major progress in medical approaches, because it combines molecular, genetic, "-omics," tissue, biochemical, clinical, psychological, social, and environmental data modeling of individual historical ecosystems. This process defines new dynamic taxonomies of health and disease, based on system structure and evolution, having the potential to complement the static syndromic classification of diseases that were construed during the pre-molecular era [45].

The label *ischemic heart disease* presently combines several disparate syndromes (myocardial infarction, stable and unstable angina, sudden cardiac death, chronic ventricular dysfunction) which are the final common clinical manifestations of the underlying dynamic system of processes summarized previously in this chapter. This classification, which is useful as a means to frame and treat immediate clinical presentations, nonetheless is time insensitive, being blind to the "longitudinal" history of the system, composed of different sequences of the abovementioned syndromes, which also are likely to be deeply influenced by the psychological perception of disease that patients have. As an example, one patient who has survived a single, unheralded, small acute myocardial infarction precipitated by exercise is obviously affected by a different underlying system of disease than another, depressed individual, who has suffered several myocardial infarctions, culminating in chronic postischemic ventricular dysfunction. However, to date, there is no taxonomic classification that provides insights into actual longitudinal heart disease profiles. Moreover, such patients are treated and followed in a standardized, syndromic way at each time point at which they present, as if they were suffering from a random sequence of different diseases that are only partially connected. Complex phenotyping is likely to more precisely predict, or at least define, similar levels of compatibility among historical transitions in health status and, from this perspective, appears to be a prominent scientific tool to aid in understanding the actual role of psychoneural influences in ischemic heart disease and ultimately achieve personalized medicine [46].

Complex phenotyping requires innovative interdisciplinary approaches, because it must link the different and irreducible dimensions of a system (e.g., the "-omics" scale, interorgan communication pathways, or symbolic dimensions of cortical function). It is particularly necessary to focus on the representative structures of coherence processes, the emergence of proprieties, and the transitions between them. The representations of these processes can rely on different tools, like the dynamic use of models (DYSAM) [47], meta-structures [48, 49], topologic properties [50], network science [51], quantum approaches [52, 53], and fuzzy inductive reasoning [54].

Certainly, at the clinical level, this approach may also have consequences. This densely meshed disease structure, encompassing an irreducible qualitative dimension that is tightly loop linked to the quantitative one, necessitates the breaking of an old taboo with the inclusion of accurate qualitative approaches to better personalize medicine on top of classical approaches (e.g., psychotherapy with its different approaches and models, various mind-body techniques, counseling, and narrative medicine). Moreover, as the symbolic, sense-derived, emotional value dimensions are irreducible to a quantitative one, the potential to include them within a therapeutic framework is only possible by means of coherent qualitative instruments (see Chaps. 14 and 17). Hence, the use of emotions and cognitive processes by both professionals and patients, far from being an obstacle to clinical reasoning [55] and therapeutic processes [56], becomes central to individualized care and involves all healthcare practitioners. One of the main challenges that cardiology, and medicine as a whole, has to face is to perform such integration while adopting a scientific approach, wherein demonstrating improved outcomes is essential.

1.6 Conclusions

Psychobiologic and biopsychological influences in ischemic heart disease are an open book and a challenge for research and therapy because of their multidimensional nature. Evidence supporting an extensive influence of psychoneural processes in heart physiology at all levels of myocardial ischemia pathophysiology is sound; but much further research remains warranted. Heart function and myocardial blood flow are extensively and directly modulated by autonomic nerves. This control is partly reflex and partly modulated by supraspinal influences that comprise cortical symbolic processes, both primary and secondary to feedback from the body. Cortical processes are thus an essential part of ischemic heart disease, all within an irreducible, coherent circuit. Moreover, several other psychoneural circuits are also pivotal in ischemic heart disease, by playing simultaneous roles in inflammation, coagulation, immune, and endocrine modulation.

Accordingly, targeting its neuropsychological aspects should be part of ischemic heart disease treatment. This being said, the complexity of the multiple and dynamic interactions of psychoneural functions with the other processes renders the whole system nondeterministic and, as such, unfit to be studied using only classical approaches which, indeed, have yielded conflicting results. Some reclassification of myocardial ischemia as complex relational phenotypes is therefore required to be able to predict which therapy is indicated for which patient and when. New methodologies of research and treatment—encompassing highly technological nondeterministic approaches of translational medicine, network analysis, big data management, systems emergence studies, and the parallel handling of qualitative aspects of care comprising symbolic, emotional, sense-related, interpersonal, and cultural features—are required to further achieve progress.

This original comprehensive framework provides the basis for testing useful, new, interdisciplinary paradigms of clinical interventions in the psycho-cardiac field to complement contemporary treatments and opens new avenues in systems medicine research as clinicians strive to attain improved outcomes, more efficient care, and more individualized approaches to care, all of which cannot be independent of the qualitative relationship that exists between health professionals and patients because it is the only dimension in which the irreducible psychic dimension can manifest itself becoming manageable for treating ischemic heart disease systems.

References

1. Goldberger AL (1996) Non-linear dynamics for clinicians: chaos theory, fractals, and complexity at the bedside. Lancet 347(9011):1312–1314
2. Kirby DA, Verrier RL (1989) Differential effects of sleep stage on coronary hemodynamic function. Am J Physiol 256(5 Pt 2):H1378–H1383
3. Billman GE, Randall DC (1981) Mechanisms mediating the coronary vascular response to behavioral stress in the dog. Circ Res 48(2):214–223
4. Klassen GA, Bramwell RS, Bromage PR et al (1980) Effect of acute sympathectomy by epidural anesthesia on the canine coronary circulation. Anesthesiology 52(1):8–15
5. Bonham AC, Gutterman DD, Arthur JM et al (1987) Electrical stimulation in perifornical lateral hypothalamus decreases coronary blood flow in cats. Am J Physiol 252(3 Pt2):H474–H484
6. Arrighi JA, Burg M, Cohen IS et al (2000) Myocardial blood-flow response during mental stress in patients with coronary artery disease. Lancet 356(9226):310–311
7. Ito H, Kanno I, Hatazawa J et al (2003) Changes in human cerebral blood flow and myocardial blood flow during mental stress measured by dual positron emission tomography. Ann Nucl Med 17(5):381–386
8. Kop WJ, Krantz DS, Howell RH et al (2001) Effects of mental stress on coronary epicardial vasomotion and flow velocity in coronary artery disease: relationship with hemodynamic stress responses. J Am Coll Cardiol 37(5):1359–1366
9. L'Abbate A, Simonetti I, Carpeggiani C et al (1991) Coronary dynamics and mental arithmetic stress in humans. Circulation 83(4 Suppl):II94–II99
10. Di Carli MF, Tobes MC, Mangner T et al (1997) Effects of cardiac sympathetic innervation on coronary blood flow. N Engl J Med 336(17):1208–1215
11. Lanza GA, Giordano A, Pristipino C et al (1997) Abnormal cardiac adrenergic nerve function in patients with syndrome X detected by [123I] metaiodobenzylguanidine myocardial scintigraphy. Circulation 96(3):821–826
12. Takusagawa M, Komori S, Umetani K et al (1999) Alterations of autonomic nervous activity in recurrence of variant angina. Heart 82(1):75–81
13. Inazumi T, Shimizu H, Mine T et al (2000) Changes in autonomic nervous activity prior to spontaneous coronary spasm in patients with variant angina. Jpn Circ J 64(3):197–201
14. Szczepanska-Sadowska E, Cudnoch-Jedrzejewska A, Ufnal M et al (2010) Brain and cardiovascular diseases: common neurogenic background of cardiovascular, metabolic and inflammatory diseases. J Physiol Pharmacol 61(5):509–521

15. Paton JF, Boscan P, Pickering AE et al (2005) The yin and yang of cardiac autonomic control: vago-sympathetic interactions revisited. Brain Res Rev 49(3):555–565
16. Yeung AC, Vekshtein VI, Krantz DS et al (1991) The effect of atherosclerosis on the vasomotor response of coronary arteries to mental stress. N Engl J Med 325(22):1551–1556
17. Ong P, Athanasiadis A, Borgulya G et al (2011) 3-Year follow-up of patients with coronary artery spasm as cause of acute coronary syndrome: the CASPAR (coronary artery spasm in patients with acute coronary syndrome) study follow-up. J Am Coll Cardiol 57(2):147–152
18. Marzilli M, Bairey Merz N, Boden WE et al (2012) Obstructive coronary atherosclerosis and ischemic heart disease: an elusive link! J Am Coll Cardiol 60(11):951–956
19. Douglas PS, Hoffmann U, Patel MR, PROMISE Investigators et al (2015) Outcomes of anatomical versus functional testing for coronary artery disease. N Engl J Med 372 (14):1291–1300
20. Roth L, Rombouts M, Schrijvers DM et al (2015) Chronic intermittent mental stress promotes atherosclerotic plaque vulnerability, myocardial infarction and sudden death in mice. Atherosclerosis 242(1):288–294
21. Janssen I, Powell LH, Matthews KA, SWAN Study et al (2011) Depressive symptoms are related to progression of coronary calcium in midlife women: the Study of Women's Health Across the Nation (SWAN) Heart Study. Am Heart J 161(6):1186–1191
22. Panting JR, Gatehouse PD, Yang GZ et al (2002) Abnormal subendocardial perfusion in cardiac syndrome X detected by cardiovascular magnetic resonance imaging. N Engl J Med 346(25):1948–1953
23. Crea F, Liuzzo G (2013) Pathogenesis of acute coronary syndromes. J Am Coll Cardiol 61 (1):1–11
24. Caligiuri G, Levy B, Pernow J et al (1999) Myocardial infarction mediated by endothelin receptor signaling in hypercholesterolemic mice. Proc Natl Acad Sci USA 96(12):6920–6924
25. Von Känel R (2015) Acute mental stress and hemostasis: when physiology becomes vascular harm. Thromb Res 135(Suppl 1):S52–S55
26. Gutstein WH, Anversa P, Beghi C et al (1984) Coronary artery spasm in the rat induced by hypothalamic stimulation. Atherosclerosis 51(1):135–142
27. Maznyczka A, Sen S, Cook C et al (2015) The ischaemic constellation: an alternative to the ischaemic cascade—implications for the validation of new ischaemic tests. Open Heart. doi:10.1136/openhrt-2014-000178
28. Droste C, Roskamm H (1990) Pain perception and endogenous pain modulation in angina pectoris. Adv Cardiol 37:142–164
29. Millan MJ, Członkowski A, Pilcher CW et al (1987) A model of chronic pain in the rat: functional correlates of alterations in the activity of opioid systems. J Neurosci 7(1):77–87
30. Soufer R, Bremner JD, Arrighi JA et al (1998) Cerebral cortical hyperactivation in response to mental stress in patients with coronary artery disease. Proc Natl Acad Sci USA 95 (11):6454–6459
31. Murthy SB, Shah S, Venkatasubba Rao CP et al (2014) Clinical characteristics of myocardial stunning in acute stroke. J Clin Neurosci 21(8):1279–1282
32. Wittstein IS, Thiemann DR, Lima JA et al (2005) Neurohumoral features of myocardial stunning due to sudden emotional stress. N Engl J Med 352(6):539–548
33. Arrighi JA, Burg M, Cohen IS et al (2003) Simultaneous assessment of myocardial perfusion and function during mental stress in patients with chronic coronary artery disease. J Nucl Cardiol 10(3):267–274
34. Malliani A, Schwartz PJ, Zanchetti A (1980) Neural mechanisms in life-threatening arrhythmias. Am Heart J 100(5):705–715
35. Ajijola OA, Yagishita D, Patel KJ et al (2013) Focal myocardial infarction induces global remodeling of cardiac sympathetic innervation: neural remodeling in a spatial context. Am J Physiol Heart Circ Physiol 305(7):H1031–H1040
36. Frangogiannis NG (2012) Regulation of the inflammatory response in cardiac repair. Circ Res 110(1):159–173

37. Oka T, Hikoso S, Yamaguchi O et al (2012) Mitochondrial DNA that escapes from autophagy causes inflammation and heart failure. Nature 485(7397):251–255
38. Licata I (2008) Logical openness in cognitive models. Epistemologia 31:177–192
39. Minati G (2016) General system(s) theory 2.0: a brief outline. In: Minati G, Abram M, Pessa E (eds) Towards a post-bertalanffy systemics. Springer, New York, NY, pp 211–218
40. Minati G, Penna MP, Pessa E (1998) Thermodynamic and logical openness in general systems. Syst Res 15:131–145
41. Merlanti B, De Chiara B, Maggioni AP, VAR Study Group et al (2015) Rationale and design of GISSI OUTLIERS VAR Study in bicuspid aortic valve patients: Prospective longitudinal, multicenter study to investigate correlation between surgical, echo distinctive features, histologic and genetic findings in phenotypically homogeneous outlier cases. Int J Cardiol 199:180–185
42. Boccaletti S, Bianconi G, Criado R et al (2014) The structure and dynamics of multilayer networks. Phys Rep 544(1):1–122
43. Lewis TG (2009) Network science: theory and applications. Wiley, Hoboken, NJ
44. Schissler AG, Gardeux V, Li Q et al (2015) Dynamic changes of RNA-sequencing expression for precision medicine: N-of-1-pathways Mahalanobis distance within pathways of single subjects predicts breast cancer survival. Bioinformatics 31(12):i293–i302
45. Chan SY, Loscalzo J (2012) The emerging paradigm of network medicine in the study of human disease. Circ Res 111(3):359–374
46. Auffray C, Chen Z, Hood L (2009) Systems medicine: the future of medical genomics and healthcare. Genome Med 1(1):2
47. Minati G, Brahms S (2002) The dynamic usage of models (DYSAM). In: Minati G, Pessa E (eds) Emergence in complex cognitive, social and biological systems. Kluwer, New York, p 41
48. Minati G, Licata I (2012) Meta-structural properties in collective behaviours. Int J Gen Syst 41:289–311
49. Minati G, Licata I (2015) Meta-Structures as multidynamics systems approach. Some introductory outlines. J Syst Cybern Inform 13(4):35–38
50. Motter AE, Albert R (2012) Networks in motion. Phys Today 65:43–48
51. Gao J, Liu YY, D'Souza RM et al (2014) Target control of complex networks. Nat Commun 5:5415
52. Del Giudice E (2010) Una via quantistica alla teoria dei sistemi. In: Urbani Ulivi L (ed) Strutture di mondo. Il pensiero sistemico come specchio di una realtà complessa, vol 1. Il Mulino, Bologna
53. Blasone M, Jizba P, Vitiello G (2011) Quantum field theory and its macroscopic manifestations. Imperial College Press, London
54. Nebot A, Cellier FE, Vallverdú M (1998) Mixed quantitative/qualitative modeling and simulation of the cardiovascular system. Comput Methods Programs Biomed 55(2):127–155
55. Moss H, Damasio AR (2001) Emotion, cognition, and the human brain. Ann N Y Acad Sci 935:98–100
56. Carlino E, Frisaldi E, Benedetti F (2014) Pain and the context. Nat Rev Rheumatol 10 (6):348–355

Psychosocial Risk Factors and Coronary Artery Disease

2

Amit J. Shah and Viola Vaccarino

> *People who are lonely and depressed are three to 10 times more likely to get sick and die prematurely than those who have a strong sense of love and community. I don't know any other single factor that affects our health for better and for worse to such a strong degree.*
>
> Dean Ornish (Ornish D (2010). Dr. Dean Ornish's program for reversing heart disease. Ivy books)

2.1 Studies on Animals

Animal research has provided significant insights into the relationship between the heart and brain. Although generalizability to humans cannot be proven, studies on animals have offered compelling experimental evidence of a connection between psychosocial factors and coronary atherosclerosis. In this section, we focus on insights gleaned from research on nonhuman primates regarding the relationship between psychosocial stress and CAD.

Cynomolgus monkeys (*Macaca fascicularis*) have been well studied with regard to psychosocial stress and heart disease. In experimental models, these animals can develop atherosclerosis with diets rich in saturated fat and cholesterol; and this process can be exacerbated by experimental exposure to psychological stress. Much of the previous research on psychosocial stress in nonhuman primates has taken advantage of the animals' social hierarchy based on established positions of dominance and subordination. Stress can then be created in groups by introducing new animals that are subjected to aggression from dominant monkeys. Over time, the effects of chronic stress can be studied. The stress exposure is highest especially in those animals prone to aggression when subjected to strangers. Studies have

A.J. Shah, MD, MSCR • V. Vaccarino, MD (✉)
Department of Epidemiology, Emory University, 1518 Clifton Road NE, Atlanta, GA 30322, USA
e-mail: ajshah3@emory.edu; lvaccar@emory.edu

A. Roncella, C. Pristipino (eds.), *Psychotherapy for Ischemic Heart Disease*,
DOI 10.1007/978-3-319-33214-7_2

shown that this reorganization can increase the average risk of atherosclerosis across the entire group, relative to those in which this type of social manipulation did not occur [1]. It has also been noted that changes in traditional risk factors, such as hyperlipidemia and hypertension, fail to explain these differences.

Animal studies have also shown that reactivity to acute mental stress predicts the development of atherosclerosis. In one experiment in which cynomolgus monkeys were fed an atherogenic diet and exposed to stress (threatened capture), those with a higher heart rate response to stress had more coronary atherosclerosis (on necropsy) than those who were not high heart rate responders. Additionally, the high heart rate responders were more aggressive and had a greater cardiac mass [2]. This study suggested, but could not prove, that high heart rate reactivity leads to accelerated atherosclerosis, perhaps due to enhanced sympathetic activity. In another study, socially stressed monkeys randomized to receive propranolol exhibited less atherosclerosis than those who were randomized to placebo. The effects of propranolol were especially pronounced among dominant monkeys, in whom the most atherosclerosis was noted [3]. These results suggest that sympathetic nervous system activation plays a role in the link between stress and atherosclerosis, at least in this animal model.

Gender differences have also been noted with regard to psychosocial stress and atherosclerosis in monkeys. In female cynomolgus monkeys, evidence has shown that atherosclerosis occurs, in part, through stress-induced ovarian dysfunction [4]. Social hierarchy also has gender-specific effects. Whereas dominant males are at higher risk of developing CAD than their subordinate counterparts, especially if placed in an unstable environment, among female monkeys the reverse is true; it is the subordinate individuals that have accelerated atherosclerosis. Subordinate females also have impaired ovarian function, dyslipidemia, and increased visceral obesity. They also exhibit behavioral features of depression. However, the relationship between social status and atherosclerosis is altered if the females have their ovaries resected; in these cases, dominant female monkeys exhibit more atherosclerosis, suggesting a protective role of their estrogen-producing ovaries. Estrogen therapy was also shown to reduce the increased CAD risk of subordinate monkeys [5]. Such studies support the role of female sex hormones in protecting against the stress-induced increased risk of atherosclerosis.

2.2 Experimental Research

2.2.1 Mental Stress Testing

One type of experimental research that can be conducted on humans in the laboratory is to assess physiological responses to mental stress after an adverse stimulus; examples include mental arithmetic, color naming, public speeches, anger recall, and similar tasks. While the stress response is externally induced compared to a more natural home or work setting, the laboratory setting is advantageous because it allows for the simultaneous measurement of blood biomarkers, heart–brain imaging, hemodynamic measures, vascular measures, and electrocardiography. Additionally, confounders can be eliminated because the patient serves as his or her own control in the comparison of stress versus rest physiology. As with the previously mentioned monkey studies, increased reactivity has been linked to adverse cardiac outcomes. However, blunted reactivity has also been found to predict adverse cardiac events [6]. Additionally, poor recovery from stress (defined as sustained cardiovascular activation above baseline levels during the posttask period) predicts adverse cardiovascular outcomes, including elevations in blood pressure and increased cardiovascular events [6].

2.2.2 Mental Stress-Induced Myocardial Ischemia

Mental stress-induced myocardial ischemia (MSIMI) reflects a supply and demand mismatch that occurs in the heart during acute mental stress. One of the first studies that demonstrated MSIMI was published by Rozanski et al. in 1998, in which 39 patients with coronary artery disease (CAD) underwent mental and exercise stress testing. In 23 of the 39 patients, they identified wall-motion abnormalities (via radionuclide ventriculography) while patients were undergoing a mental stress challenge. Subjects who were instructed to deliver an emotionally arousing speech experienced more mental stress-induced ischemia than those administered a cognitive challenge (Stroop task). The ischemia was "silent" (no chest pain) in 80 % of cases and occurred at lower heart rates than exercise-induced ischemia. Since then, MSIMI has also been discovered to predict an increased risk of future events independently of other risk factors, including exercise-induced ischemia [7].

While the prevalence of MSIMI varies depending upon the population and methodology used to measure it, approximately half of patients with exercise ischemia have been found to exhibit MSIMI [8]. As opposed to exercise-induced ischemia, MSIMI is generally not related to the severity of CAD and instead is considered to be more microvascular or vasoconstrictive in nature [9]. Coronary flow has been found to be most reduced by mental stress in areas with nonobstructive CAD; meanwhile, in areas with obstructive CAD, the flow may paradoxically increase with mental stress [10]. Mental but not exercise stress-induced myocardial ischemia correlates with ischemia measured in daily life. Although induction of MSIMI in the laboratory is not typically accompanied by chest pain, patients with MSIMI have been found to have more anginal symptoms in daily life [11].

2.2.3 Mental Stress and Arrhythmias

Acute stress is an increasingly recognized trigger of fatal arrhythmias and sudden cardiac death (SCD), which account for over 300,000 deaths per year in the United States (USA) [12, 13]. Acute severe stress is suspected as the etiology behind SCD spikes observed after earthquakes and other major life events, although a direct cause–effect relationship is difficult to prove because SCD patients cannot be interviewed [14]. Analysis of electrocardiographic changes during acute mental stress have revealed increased repolarization heterogeneity, measured by microvolt T-wave alternans (TWA), which is a risk marker for ventricular arrhythmias and SCD. Indeed, heart failure patients with implantable cardiac defibrillators who had elevated TWA during mental stress testing have been found to have an increased risk of arrhythmia or death [15].

The mechanisms by which acute mental stress may lead to arrhythmia involve the heart's autonomic nervous system [16] (also see Chap. 1). Detailed physiology studies in dogs have shown that both sympathetic activation, particularly within the left stellate ganglion [17], and parasympathetic withdrawal can stimulate arrhythmias and lower the threshold for ventricular fibrillation [18]. Ischemia with mental stress may also be arrhythmogenic, although the evidence for this is limited. Taggart et al. found that mental stress induced pathological changes in the electrical stability of CAD patients, but that pretreatment with nitroglycerin reversed the direction of the changes [19]. This implies that the changes are due to ischemia during mental stress.

2.2.4 Mental Stress, Inflammation, and Immunity

Psychological stress is well known to activate an immune system response [20]. Both sympathetic and parasympathetic branches have been found to innervate the organs that are involved in the immune response, including the spleen and bone marrow [21, 22]. This can lead to the activation of macrophages and other lymphocytes that produce cytokines and antibodies, among other behaviors. Sympathetic stimulation during stress activates the transcription factor nuclear factor kB in circulating monocytes, resulting in initiation of the inflammatory cascade. This includes increases in circulating inflammatory biomarkers, in particular interleukin-6 and interleukin-1β [5, 23], both of which are biomarkers of increased CAD risk. Additionally, when mental stress recovery is delayed, the inflammatory response can be prolonged [24], although likely it is still unproven whether higher and/or more-sustained inflammatory responses to an acute stress challenge increase the risk of future CAD events. Further details are discussed in Chap. 3.

2.2.5 Mental Stress and the Coagulation System

Mental stress has been found in several studies to impact the coagulation system [25]. In healthy individuals, mental stress activates both procoagulant and anticoagulant pathways. In individuals with CAD, however, the balance is tipped in favor of coagulation, and mental stress has a more prothrombotic effect. As an explanation, endothelial dysfunction in CAD patients may lead to the impaired secretion of anticoagulant factors [26]. Additionally, there is evidence that the procoagulant effects are mediated by the sympathetic nervous system, as adrenaline infusion has thrombotic effects that are similar to those observed during an acute mental stress challenge [27]. In one study involving 16 healthy volunteers, platelet aggregability was increased by mental stress induction through a color word conflict test, as well as via epinephrine infusion [28]. Gender differences might also exist. In one recent study, women were discovered to have more collagen-stimulated platelet aggregation during mental stress than men [29]. For further details refer to Chap. 3.

2.3 Epidemiological and Cohort-Based Research

A majority of the data that have been published on psychological risk factors and heart disease in humans was attained via observational studies, including ecological, cross-sectional, and longitudinal investigations. Although these types of study cannot prove causality, and are subject to unmeasured confounding factors, they are generally translatable to humans in real-life circumstances.

2.3.1 Acute Stress

Several ecological studies have documented the relationship between psychological factors and acute coronary syndromes [30]. One of the most famous examples involved the earthquake that occurred at 4:31 on the morning of January 17, 1994—centered in the Los Angeles, California, suburb of Northridge and rated 6.8 on the Richter scale. Over the week following the quake, a 35 % increase in hospital admissions for acute myocardial infarction (MI) was documented, relative to the week before [31]. A nearly fivefold increase in the number of cardiac deaths was also observed during that week, while no increases were evident among noncoronary deaths. On the actual day of the earthquake, in the surrounding area's general population, there were 24 deaths directly attributed to atherosclerotic cardiovascular disease versus an average of just 4.6 over the preceding week [32]. Sixteen of these 24 victims died within the first hour of the initial tremor, and only three of the deaths were associated with physical exertion.

After the World Trade Center attacks, the number of cardiovascular events in the surrounding area increased by 50 % over the following 2 months (compared to the 2 months prior to the attacks); and the number of defibrillator shocks for ventricular tachyarrhythmias also rose significantly [33, 34].

Another, more common source of acute mental stress is related to athletic events. Cardiac events in the community have been found to increase in the 2 h after the start of a sports match and are more pronounced in male than female spectators [35, 36].

Unfortunately, information on individual circumstances regarding these above-noted cardiac events is often not available, and possible alternative explanations include physical exertion (e.g., running away from a natural disaster), environmental pollutants (e.g., release of particles during an earthquake), and behavioral factors (e.g., binge drinking or eating during a sporting event).

To address these limitations, one research design that has been adopted to evaluate the emotional triggers of acute coronary events is the case-crossover design. With this design, a subject's status immediately prior to the coronary event is compared to their status during a fixed period of time prior to the event (usually 24 h beforehand). Patients are interviewed as close to the event as possible (e.g., on their way to the emergency room) so that recall bias is minimized. In the *Determinants of Myocardial Infarction Onset* study, 2.4 % of patients reported severe anger during the 2 h immediately preceding the event. This was then compared to their status 24 h earlier, and it was estimated that acute anger increased the odds of an acute MI fourfold. Similar studies have found that acute bouts of anger prior to an MI occur in from 1 to 17 % of patients, depending on how an "anger episode" is defined [30, 37].

Other types of acute emotional stressful events include work-related distress or sudden sadness; for example, bereavement over the loss of a loved one. Having a high-pressure deadline at work has been associated with a sixfold increase in acute MI [38]. For acute emotional stress, the odds ratio for unstable angina or MI is 2.5 [37]. Other generally stressful life events have been linked to takotsubo cardiomyopathy: "stunned" apical myocardium associated with severe, reversible left ventricular dysfunction that primarily affects older women.

Various possible mechanisms have been postulated for the relationship between acute stress and MI, although the exact pathophysiology is difficult to prove directly. The typical paradigm involves the erosion or rupture of a vulnerable plaque, which can then lead to sudden thrombus formation and acute occlusion of the coronary vessel. A variety of intermediate mechanisms have also been postulated [30], including a sudden increase in sheer stress on the blood vessel walls and increased hypercoagulability of the blood. Plaque ruptures are more likely to occur in patients with a significant CAD burden; consequently, this phenomenon is unlikely to be seen in patients without significant underlying atherosclerosis [39]. Certain patients who report emotional triggers for their acute coronary syndrome may also have pathological stress reactions. This includes more prolonged systolic blood pressure responses and enhanced platelet activation after acute mental stress [24]. The reasons behind some individuals having such pronounced reactions to acute psychological stress are not entirely clear; but exposure to emotional trauma at a young age and genetic factors have been implicated [40, 41]. For further details on pathophysiology of acute and chronic stress response, refer to Chap. 3.

2.3.2 Chronobiologic Stress

Stress levels vary naturally over time; and, as such, myocardial infarctions and arrhythmias are more likely to occur during certain periods of time, as well as during certain seasons of the year. In one study of 54,249 patients with recent myocardial infarctions (ARIAM), the highest risk of MI was observed at 10:07 A.M., while the lowest risk was at 4:46 A.M. [42]. In another study involving patients with a recent MI, the incidence rate increased during the winter and was lower during the summer [43]. This had more to do with colder temperatures than the actual season, however, since the authors found that, when stratified by temperature, the season was no longer predictive. As such, it is likely that circulating catecholamines increased in response to cold weather.

For a review of other chronobiologic triggers, refer to Chap. 5.

2.3.3 Chronic Stress

Repeated acute stressors during everyday life may lead to a state of chronic distress, which can be embodied by certain mental conditions like anxiety disorders and post-traumatic stress disorder (PTSD). Chronic stress may also result from sustained stressful environments like the workplace, family instability, social conditions, caregiving burden, and the neighborhood environment. Chronic stress is associated with sedentary behaviors, lack of sleep, unhealthy dietary habits, cigarette smoking, and medication nonadherence, all of which contribute further to cardiovascular risk. Chronic stress can be indirectly measured by assessing stressful conditions like job demands, financial difficulties, or the chronic illness of a loved one; however, susceptibility to or resilience against health problems varies greatly with these exposures. Some individuals suffer from mental or physical health consequences after a single traumatic event, while others remain healthy in the face of chronic or recurrent severe stress. It should also be mentioned that these stressful exposures are often interconnected; for example, individuals from low socioeconomic backgrounds may also suffer from repeated exposure to trauma, family instability, and financial stress. Therefore, studies of individual stress-related factors must be interpreted in light of the fact that they could also be markers for other exposures that might be more directly involved in cardiovascular pathogenesis. We will now review certain key risk factors.

2.3.4 Post-Traumatic Stress Disorder

PTSD is, by definition, triggered by a traumatic event, accompanied by avoidance, negative changes in cognitions and mood, and alterations in arousal and reactivity [44]. More specifically, PTSD victims may have recurrent intrusions of their traumatic memories, nightmares, increased startle responses, hypervigilance, and avoidance of situations that might trigger traumatic memories. PTSD has a lifetime prevalence of 10–12 % in women and 5–6 % in men. The lifetime prevalence of PTSD in combat veterans is 15–19 % [45]. In about half of cases, PTSD becomes a chronic condition that can last for years.

PTSD is also associated with more than a twofold increased risk of CAD and myocardial ischemia, even after adjusting for traditional risk factors, as well as depression [46]. The reasons are likely multifactorial and overlap with the pathophysiology of depression, involving autonomic and hormonal dysregulation, such as sympathetic overdrive and increased cortisol sensitivity [47]. Persons with PTSD may also have difficulties with employment, relationships, and increased rates of depression and substance abuse, which likely explain part of the relationship.

2.3.5 Work-Related Stress

Work stress has been conceptualized as "job strain" or "effort imbalance" [48]. In the job strain model, high work demands in combination with a low level of control generate stress. The highest risk situation includes a combination of these factors plus low social support at work. According to the effort–reward imbalance model, high workload is paired with low payback, including low income, low job security, and/or low job status. Job strain has been associated with a 40 % increased risk of CVD, while imbalance between effort and reward has been associated with a 60 % increase [49].

2.3.6 Marital Stress

Marital stress is another form of chronic stress that appears to be associated with an increased risk of CAD. Many previous studies have included women. In the *Stockholm Female Coronary Risk Study,* women with an MI who reported marital stress had an almost threefold higher adjusted risk of recurrent cardiac events than women with less marital stress [12, 50]. It has also been linked to atherosclerosis progression in women [51]. Unfortunately, few studies have been performed in men.

2.3.7 Caregiver Stress

Significant caregiver responsibilities can be a substantial source of chronic stress, especially among working adults. Approximately 12 % of Americans who are more than 45 years old report having caregiving responsibilities. Excessive caregiving stress has been linked to increases in blood pressure, coagulation factors, and inflammatory cytokines [52]. In the *Nurses' Health Study*, providing care to an ill or disabled spouse $\geq$9 h per week, but not to a parent or others, was associated with an 82 % increased risk of coronary events after multivariate adjustment. The risks of caregiver stress appear to be heightened when the activity is reported as subjectively stressful.

2.3.8 Low Socioeconomic Status

The relationship between low socioeconomic status and CAD is well established. The *Whitehall Study of British Civil Servants* is one of the earliest and best-known studies to examine this relationship. One of the key findings was that low social status was associated with increased cardiovascular risk, independent of income, and access to healthcare. In another study of diabetic patients referred for coronary angiography in Canada, where there is universal access to healthcare, lower household income was associated with a significantly greater severity of coronary atherosclerosis [53]. Potential reasons for these associations include poorer health habits, financial strain, adverse working conditions, and social discrimination. In the United States, an additional problem is reduced access to preventative medical care, since healthcare services are not equally accessible to all.

2.3.9 General Stress

One of the best-known and largest studies to evaluate the relationship between a combined number of stress factors and CAD is the *INTERHEART* study, an international case–control study involving 52 countries worldwide, including 11,119 patients with a past MI and 13,648 controls [54]. The study performed brief assessments of depression, locus of control, perceived stress at home or work, financial stress, and adverse life events. General stress was defined as the sum of stress at work and home, and permanent general stress was significantly associated with over a twofold increased odds of MI, adjusted for geographic region, age, sex, and smoking. This estimate was similar between regions, ethnic groups and the two genders. Each individual stress factor was significantly associated with an increased risk of MI as well. Assuming a reversible, cause–effect relationship, the authors estimated that eliminating these sources of stress would reduce the incidence of MI by 33 %. This population-attributable risk, in fact, was as high as that of traditional risk factors.

2.3.10 Adverse Childhood Experiences

Adverse childhood experiences, or "early life stresses," can be categorized as verbal, physical, and sexual abuse. Approximately one quarter (26 %) of US adults have reported verbal abuse, 15 % physical abuse, and 12 % sexual abuse during childhood [55]. Early adverse life experiences are associated with dramatic increases in anxiety, substance abuse, obesity, and smoking and predict CAD in adulthood independent of these factors [56]. Those with seven or more (out of 10) types of adverse childhood event had an adjusted 3.6-fold increased risk of CAD. Although recall bias is possible in these studies, the association with adverse outcomes is seen both when abuse is measured by self-report and when measured objectively. Adverse childhood experiences may lead to enduring changes in the nervous, endocrine, and immune systems [57]. A history of childhood maltreatment has been associated with adverse changes in brain function, greater activation of the hypothalamic–pituitary–adrenal axis during stress, and elevated inflammation [58]. These changes persist into adulthood, providing evidence of an enduring effect of early life stress on physical health. Maltreated children have exhibited higher degrees of inflammation 20 years later, which persisted after accounting for other childhood exposures and health behaviors [59].

2.3.11 Personality Traits

Anger and Hostility

Hostility is a personality trait generally described as a negative attitude toward others. Anger is an emotion that spans from mild irritation to intense fury or rage. Results regarding the association between anger–hostility and CAD have been mixed [60]. A recent meta-analysis identified the combined risk estimate for anger and hostility to be only modestly elevated, albeit still significant. Community-dwelling adults with significant anger or hostility had a 19 % increase in CAD events, and those with preexisting CAD had a 24 % increase in recurrent CAD events. The excess risk is higher in men than women and is largely explained by lifestyle factors like smoking and reduced physical activity [60]. Whether or not chronic anger or hostility can explain excess psychosocial risk above and beyond other factors remains in question.

Type D Personality

Type D (or "distressed") personality combines negative mood and social inhibitions [61]. It describes individuals who tend to experience dysphoria, tension, and worry and also are socially inhibited from expressing their emotions, thoughts, and behaviors. A recent meta-analysis linked type D personality to an over twofold increased risk of cardiovascular events [62]. Since type D personality is related to other psychosocial characteristics (hostility, anger, depression, and social isolation), its interconnection with and independence from these other factors warrants further evaluation.

2.3.12 Mood Disorders

Depression

Major depressive disorder (MDD) is a clinical psychiatric disorder that affects over 350 million people worldwide. MDD and depressive symptoms, in general, are well-recognized risk factors for CAD and associated with an approximately twofold increased risk of CAD [63, 64]. The risk of CAD death may be higher than of nonfatal CAD events; furthermore, adjusting for possible confounders, on average, reduces the effect by about 21 % [65]. Depression is also the leading cause of disability in high-income countries [66] and is characterized by some or all of the following symptoms: depressed mood, anhedonia (inability to experience pleasure), sleep disturbance, difficulty concentrating, psychomotor retardation, guilt, and, in particularly severe cases, suicide ideations and attempts. As opposed to other psychological traits like hostility, it is a clinical diagnosis and amenable to drug treatment, for example.

The etiology of depression can be multifactorial; and, in patients with significant CAD, depressive symptoms may also be rooted in chronic medical illness [67]. In fact, 15–30 % of cardiac patients have clinically significant depression, a rate that is approximately triple its prevalence in the general population. It is likely that a certain percentage of the CAD population have depression that stems from their physical illness, and others that have depression rooted in previous traumatic experiences. One line of reasoning, based mostly upon animal studies, is that depression causes an acute inflammatory response with effects on the blood–brain barrier and that this may have psychological consequences [68]. The paraventricular nucleus of the hypothalamus is potentially one of the most important regions involved, as it contributes to sympathetic activation [69]. Depression and CAD may have a common genetic cause as well [70].

Gender differences are well documented in depression. The prevalence of depression is higher in women than men, and younger women (<60 years of age) with CAD have a particularly high prevalence of depression. In one study, 40 % of women surveyed after an MI were found to have moderate to severe depression [71, 72]. Depression might also be more cardiotoxic in young women than other sociodemographic profiles and could predict an increased risk of CAD and major adverse cardiovascular events [73]. The gender-based differences in the prevalence and risk of depression form an area of active research. The gender issue in ischemic heart disease is more deeply considered in Chap. 6.

Depression likely increases the risk of CAD via several pathways [74]. The most intuitive mechanisms involve lifestyle behaviors secondary to the cognitive symptoms and motivational withdrawal associated with depression, which may result in poor decisions with regard to healthy diet, exercise, and substance abuse. Depression is also a major contributor to medication nonadherence [75].

In addition to depression's effect on lifestyle behaviors, there are several biologically plausible mechanisms that may help to explain the increased CAD risk in individuals who are depressed. Depressed patients may exhibit abnormal function in their hypothalamic–pituitary–adrenal axis and sympathoadrenal system, which may be secondary to chronic distress related to the persistent negative thinking that is characteristic of depression, or to whatever adverse life events that have contributed to depression. These abnormalities may lead to circadian disruption and adversely affect cardiovascular health, in part through effects on blood pressure, heart rate, plasma lipid, and glucose abnormalities [76]. Autonomic dysregulation, as reflected by lower 24-h heart rate variability, is also observed [77]. Depressed patients may also display evidence of hypercoagulability associated with enhanced platelet activity and exhibit an impaired ability to vasodilate under various circumstances because of endothelial dysfunction [78]. Moreover, depressed patients have higher levels of inflammation [79] and this issue is reviewed in Chap. 3.

Anxiety Disorders

Anxiety disorders are numerous and common and include generalized anxiety disorder (GAD), panic disorder, and obsessive–compulsive disorder (OCD). Common symptoms among these disorders include rumination and fear about future real or imagined events. As many as 18 % of Americans are affected by one or more anxiety disorders; but anxiety is not as strongly linked to CAD as depression. For example, a recent meta-analysis revealed a 26 % increased risk (after multivariable adjustment) of incident CAD and a 48 % increased risk of cardiac death in those with anxiety [80]. There is substantial heterogeneity across studies, however, likely because of heterogeneity in anxiety measurements.

2.4 Conclusions

The relationships between psychosocial risk factors and CAD have been investigated in a variety of laboratory and epidemiologic studies. Both acute and chronic stress exposure and depression can increase the risk of CAD. A variety of mechanisms have been investigated, including hormonal, autonomic, and hematologic. Nonetheless, data are conflicting on whether CAD risk can be ameliorated with interventions to reduce stress and depression or other therapies targeting psychosocial factors. For this reason, this remains an area of active investigation.

References

1. Manuck SB, Kaplan JR, Clarkson TB (1983) Social instability and coronary artery atherosclerosis in cynomolgus monkeys. Neurosci Biobehav Rev 7(4):485–491
2. Manuck SB, Kaplan JR, Clarkson TB (1983) Behaviorally induced heart rate reactivity and atherosclerosis in cynomolgus monkeys. Psychosom Med 45(2):95–108
3. Kaplan JR, Manuck SB, Adams MR et al (1987) Inhibition of coronary atherosclerosis by propranolol in behaviorally predisposed monkeys fed an atherogenic diet. Circulation 76 (6):1364–1372
4. Kaplan JR, Manuck SB (2008) Ovarian dysfunction and the premenopausal origins of coronary heart disease. Menopause 15(4 Pt 1):768–776
5. Kaplan JR, Manuck SB, Anthony MS et al. (2002) Premenopausal social status and hormone exposure predict postmenopausal atherosclerosis in female monkeys. Obstet Gynecol 99 (3):381–388. doi:S0029784401016593 [pii]
6. Chida Y, Steptoe A (2010) Greater cardiovascular responses to laboratory mental stress are associated with poor subsequent cardiovascular risk status: a meta-analysis of prospective evidence. Hypertension 55(4):1026–1032. doi:10.1161/HYPERTENSIONAHA.109.146621
7. Wei J, Rooks C, Ramadan R et al (2014) Meta-analysis of mental stress-induced myocardial ischemia and subsequent cardiac events in patients with coronary artery disease. Am J Cardiol 114(2):187–192. doi:10.1016/j.amjcard.2014.04.022
8. Stone PH, Krantz DS, McMahon RP et al (1999) Relationship among mental stress-induced ischemia and ischemia during daily life and during exercise: the psychophysiologic Investigations of myocardial ischemia (PIMI) study. J Am Coll Cardiol 33(6):1476–1484

9. Ramadan R, Sheps D, Esteves F et al (2013) Myocardial ischemia during mental stress: role of coronary artery disease burden and vasomotion. J Am Heart Assoc 2(5):e000321. doi:10.1161/jaha.113.000321
10. Arrighi JA, Burg M, Cohen IS et al (2000) Myocardial blood-flow response during mental stress in patients with coronary artery disease. Lancet 356(9226):310–311. doi:10.1016/s0140-6736(00)02510-1
11. Pimple P, Shah AJ, Rooks C et al (2015) Angina and mental stress-induced myocardial ischemia. J Psychosom Res 78(5):433–437. doi:10.1016/j.jpsychores.2015.02.007
12. Zipes DP, Wellens HJ (1998) Sudden cardiac death. Circulation 98(21):2334–2351
13. Strike PC, Magid K, Whitehead DL et al (2006) Pathophysiological processes underlying emotional triggering of acute cardiac events. Proc Natl Acad Sci USA 103(11):4322–4327
14. Strike PC, Steptoe A (2005) Behavioral and emotional triggers of acute coronary syndromes: a systematic review and critique. Psychosom Med 67(2):179–186
15. Lampert R (2009) Emotion and sudden cardiac death. Expert Rev Cardiovasc Ther 7(7):723–725. doi:10.1586/erc.09.75
16. Lown B, Verrier RL, Rabinowitz SH (1977) Neural and psychologic mechanisms and the problem of sudden cardiac death. Am J Cardiol 39(6):890–902
17. Zhou S, Jung B-C, Tan AY et al (2008) Spontaneous stellate ganglion nerve activity and ventricular arrhythmia in a canine model of sudden death. Heart Rhythm 5(1):131–139. doi:10.1016/j.hrthm.2007.09.007
18. Lown B (1979) Sudden cardiac death: the major challenge confronting contemporary cardiology. J Am Coll Cardiol 43(2):313–328. doi:10.1016/S0002-9149(79)80021-1
19. Taggart P, Batchvarov VN, Sutton P et al (2009) Repolarization changes induced by mental stress in normal subjects and patients with coronary artery disease: effect of nitroglycerine. Psychosom Med 71(1):23–29. doi:10.1097/PSY.0b013e31818a1d56
20. Segerstrom SC, Miller GE (2004) Psychological stress and the human immune system: a meta-analytic study of 30 years of inquiry. Psychol Bull 130(4):601
21. Borovikova LV, Ivanova S, Zhang M et al (2000) Vagus nerve stimulation attenuates the systemic inflammatory response to endotoxin. Nature 405(6785):458–462. doi:10.1038/35013070
22. Elenkov IJ, Wilder RL, Chrousos GP et al (2000) The sympathetic nerve—an integrative interface between two supersystems: the brain and the immune system. Pharmacol Rev 52(4):595–638
23. Steptoe A, Hamer M, Chida Y (2007) The effects of acute psychological stress on circulating inflammatory factors in humans: a review and meta-analysis. Brain Behav Immun 21(7):901–912
24. Steptoe A, Marmot M (2006) Psychosocial, hemostatic, and inflammatory correlates of delayed poststress blood pressure recovery. Psychosom Med 68(4):531–537. doi:10.1097/01.psy.0000227751.82103.65
25. von Kanel R, Mills PJ, Fainman C et al (2001) Effects of psychological stress and psychiatric disorders on blood coagulation and fibrinolysis: a biobehavioral pathway to coronary artery disease? Psychosom Med 63(4):531–544
26. Bombeli T, Mueller M, Haeberli A (1997) Anticoagulant properties of the vascular endothelium. Thromb Haemost 77(3):408–423
27. Jern C, Eriksson E, Tengborn L et al (1989) Changes of plasma coagulation and fibrinolysis in response to mental stress. Thromb Haemost 62(2):767–771
28. Larsson PT, Hjemdahl P, Olsson G et al (1989) Altered platelet function during mental stress and adrenaline infusion in humans: evidence for an increased aggregability in vivo as measured by filtragometry. Clin Sci (Lond) 76(4):369–376
29. Samad Z, Boyle S, Ersboll M et al (2014) Sex differences in platelet reactivity and cardiovascular and psychological response to mental stress in patients with stable ischemic heart disease. J Am Coll Cardiol 64(16):1669–1678. doi:10.1016/j.jacc.2014.04.087

30. Steptoe A, Brydon L (2009) Emotional triggering of cardiac events. Neurosci Biobehav Rev 33 (2):63–70
31. Kloner RA (2006) Natural and unnatural triggers of myocardial infarction. Prog Cardiovasc Dis 48(4):285–300
32. Leor J, Poole WK, Kloner RA (1996) Sudden cardiac death triggered by an earthquake. N Eng J Med 334(7):413–419. doi:10.1056/NEJM199602153340701
33. Allegra JR, Mostashari F, Rothman J et al (2005) Cardiac events in New Jersey after the September 11, 2001, terrorist attack. J Urban Health 82(3):358–363. doi:10.1093/jurban/jti087
34. Steinberg JS, Arshad A, Kowalski M et al (2004) Increased incidence of life-threatening ventricular arrhythmias in implantable defibrillator patients after the world trade center attack. J Am Coll Cardiol 44(6):1261–1264. doi:10.1016/j.jacc.2004.06.032
35. Kloner RA, McDonald S, Leeka J et al (2009) Comparison of total and cardiovascular death rates in the same city during a losing versus winning super bowl championship. Am J Cardiol 103(12):1647–1650. doi:10.1016/j.amjcard.2009.02.012
36. Wilbert-Lampen U, Leistner D, Greven S et al (2008) Cardiovascular events during world cup soccer. N Eng J Med 358(5):475–483. doi:10.1056/NEJMoa0707427
37. Steptoe A, Strike PC, Perkins-Porras L et al (2006) Acute depressed mood as a trigger of acute coronary syndromes. Biol Psychiatry 60(8):837–842. doi:10.1016/j.biopsych.2006.03.041
38. Moller J, Theorell T, de Faire U et al (2005) Work related stressful life events and the risk of myocardial infarction. Case-control and case-crossover analyses within the Stockholm heart epidemiology programme (SHEEP). J Epidemiol Community Health 59(1):23–30. doi:10.1136/jech.2003.019349
39. Steptoe A, Kivimaki M (2012) Stress and cardiovascular disease. Nat Rev Cardiol 9 (6):360–370. doi:10.1038/nrcardio.2012.45
40. Heim C, Nemeroff CB (2002) Neurobiology of early life stress: clinical studies. Semin Clin Neuropsychiatry 7(2):147–159
41. Wu T, Snieder H, de Geus E (2010) Genetic influences on cardiovascular stress reactivity. Neurosci Biobehav Rev 35(1):58–68. doi:10.1016/j.neubiorev.2009.12.001
42. Lopez Messa JB, Garmendia Leiza JR, Aguilar Garcia MD et al (2004) Cardiovascular risk factors in the circadian rhythm of acute myocardial infarction. Rev Esp Cardiol 57(9):850–858
43. Marchant B, Ranjadayalan K, Stevenson R et al (1993) Circadian and seasonal factors in the pathogenesis of acute myocardial infarction: the influence of environmental temperature. Br Heart J 69(5):385–387
44. American Psychiatric Association, Force DSMT (2013) Diagnostic and statistical manual of mental disorders: DSM-5. American Psychiatric Publishing, Arlington, VA
45. Dohrenwend BP, Turner JB, Turse NA et al (2006) The psychological risks of Vietnam for U.S. veterans: a revisit with new data and methods. Science 313(5789):979–982
46. Vaccarino V, Goldberg J, Rooks C et al (2013) Post-traumatic stress disorder and incidence of coronary heart disease: a twin study. J Am Coll Cardiol 62(11):970–978. doi:10.1016/j.jacc.2013.04.085
47. Bremner JD, Charney DS (2010) Neural circuits in fear and anxiety. In: Stein DJ, Hollander E, Rothbaum BO (eds) Textbook of anxiety disorders. American Psychiatric Publishing, Arlington, VA, pp 55–71
48. Backe EM, Seidler A, Latza U et al (2012) The role of psychosocial stress at work for the development of cardiovascular diseases: a systematic review. Int Arch Occup Environ Health 85(1):67–79. doi:10.1007/s00420-011-0643-6
49. Laszlo KD, Ahnve S, Hallqvist J et al (2010) Job strain predicts recurrent events after a first acute myocardial infarction: the Stockholm heart epidemiology program. J Int Med 267 (6):599–611. doi:10.1111/j.1365-2796.2009.02196.x
50. Orth-Gomer K (2007) Psychosocial and behavioral aspects of cardiovascular disease prevention in men and women. Curr Opin Psychiatry 20(2):147–151
51. Wang HX, Leineweber C, Kirkeeide R et al (2007) Psychosocial stress and atherosclerosis: family and work stress accelerate progression of coronary disease in women. The Stockholm

female coronary angiography study. J Int Med 261(3):245–254. doi:10.1111/j.1365-2796.2006.01759.x, JIM1759 [pii]
52. Dimsdale JE (2008) Psychological stress and cardiovascular disease. J Am Coll Cardiol 51 (13):1237–1246
53. Rabi DM, Edwards AL, Svenson LW et al (2010) Association of median household income with burden of coronary artery disease among individuals with diabetes. Circ Cardiovasc Qual Outcomes 3(1):48–53. doi:10.1161/CIRCOUTCOMES.108.840611
54. Rosengren A, Hawken S, Ôunpuu S et al (2004) Association of psychosocial risk factors with risk of acute myocardial infarction in 11 119 cases and 13 648 controls from 52 countries (the INTERHEART study): case-control study. Lancet 364(9438):953–962
55. Centers for Disease Control and Prevention (2010) Adverse Childhood Experiences Reported by Adults—Five States, 2009. MMWR Morb Mortal Wkly Rep 59(49):1609–1613
56. Anda RF, Felitti VJ, Bremner JD et al (2006) The enduring effects of abuse and related adverse experiences in childhood: a convergence of evidence from neurobiology and epidemiology. Eur Arch Psychiatry Clin Neurosci 256(3):174–186
57. Danese A, McEwen BS (2012) Adverse childhood experiences, allostasis, allostatic load, and age-related disease. Physiol Behav 106(1):29–39. doi:10.1016/j.physbeh.2011.08.019
58. Bremner JD (2012) Brain and trauma. In: Figley CR (ed) Encyclopedia of trauma: an interdisciplinary guide. Sage, Los Angeles
59. Danese A, Pariante CM, Caspi A et al (2007) Childhood maltreatment predicts adult inflammation in a life-course study. Proc Natl Acad Sci USA 104(4):1319–1324. doi:10.1073/pnas.0610362104, 0610362104 [pii]
60. Chida Y, Steptoe A (2009) The association of anger and hostility with future coronary heart disease: a meta-analytic review of prospective evidence. J Am Coll Cardiol 53(11):936–946
61. Denollet J, Schiffer AA, Spek V (2010) A general propensity to psychological distress affects cardiovascular outcomes: evidence from research on the type D (distressed) personality profile. Circ Cardiovasc Qual Outcomes 3(5):546–557. doi:10.1161/CIRCOUTCOMES.109.934406
62. Grande G, Romppel M, Barth J (2012) Association between type D personality and prognosis in patients with cardiovascular diseases: a systematic review and meta-analysis. Ann Behav Med 43(3):299–310. doi:10.1007/s12160-011-9339-0
63. Lichtman JH, Froelicher ES, Blumenthal JA et al (2014) Depression as a risk factor for poor prognosis among patients with acute coronary syndrome: systematic review and recommendations: a scientific statement from the American Heart Association. Circulation 129(12):1350–1369. doi:10.1161/CIR.0000000000000019
64. Nicholson A, Kuper H, Hemingway H (2006) Depression as an aetiologic and prognostic factor in coronary heart disease: a meta-analysis of 6362 events among 146 538 participants in 54 observational studies. Eur Heart J 27(23):2763–2774. doi:10.1093/eurheartj/ehl338, ehl338 [pii]
65. Meijer A, Conradi HJ, Bos EH et al (2011) Prognostic association of depression following myocardial infarction with mortality and cardiovascular events: a meta-analysis of 25 years of research. Gen Hosp Psychiatry 33(3):203–216. doi:10.1016/j.genhosppsych.2011.02.007
66. Mathers CD, Loncar D (2006) Projections of global mortality and burden of disease from 2002 to 2030. PLoS Med 3(11), e442. doi:10.1371/journal.pmed.0030442, 06-PLME-RA-0071R2 [pii]
67. Rackley S, Bostwick JM (2012) Depression in medically ill patients. Psychiatr Clin North Am 35(1):231–247. doi:10.1016/j.psc.2011.11.001
68. Liu H, Luiten PG, Eisel UL et al (2013) Depression after myocardial infarction: TNF-alpha-induced alterations of the blood-brain barrier and its putative therapeutic implications. Neurosci Biobehav Rev 37(4):561–572. doi:10.1016/j.neubiorev.2013.02.004
69. Li YF, Patel KP (2003) Paraventricular nucleus of the hypothalamus and elevated sympathetic activity in heart failure: the altered inhibitory mechanisms. Acta Physiol Scand 177(1):17–26. doi:10.1046/j.1365-201X.2003.01043.x

70. Vaccarino V, Votaw J, Faber T et al (2009) Major depression and coronary flow reserve detected by positron emission tomography. Arch Intern Med 169(18):1668–1676. doi:10.1001/archinternmed.2009.330
71. Mallik S, Spertus JA, Reid KJ et al (2006) Depressive symptoms after acute myocardial infarction: evidence for highest rates in younger women. Arch Intern Med 166(8):876–883
72. Smolderen KG, Strait KM, Dreyer RP et al (2015) Depressive symptoms in younger women and men with acute myocardial infarction: insights from the VIRGO study. J Am Heart Assoc 4(4). doi:10.1161/jaha.114.001424
73. Shah AJ, Ghasemzadeh N, Zaragoza-Macias E et al (2014) Sex and age differences in the association of depression with obstructive coronary artery disease and adverse cardiovascular events. J Am Heart Assoc 3(3):e000741. doi:10.1161/jaha.113.000741
74. Skala JA, Freedland KE, Carney RM (2006) Coronary heart disease and depression: a review of recent mechanistic research. Can J Psychiatry 51(12):738–745
75. Whooley MA, de Jonge P, Vittinghoff E et al (2008) Depressive symptoms, health behaviors, and risk of cardiovascular events in patients with coronary heart disease. JAMA 300 (20):2379–2388. doi:10.1001/jama.2008.711
76. Kent LK, Shapiro PA (2009) Depression and related psychological factors in heart disease. Harv Rev Psychiatry 17(6):377–388. doi:10.3109/10673220903463333
77. Carney RM, Freedland KE (2009) Depression and heart rate variability in patients with coronary heart disease. Cleve Clin J Med 76(2):S13–S17. doi:10.3949/ccjm.76.s2.03
78. Sherwood A, Hinderliter AL, Watkins LL et al (2005) Impaired endothelial function in coronary heart disease patients with depressive symptomatology. J Am Coll Cardiol 46 (4):656–659
79. Vaccarino V, Johnson BD, Sheps DS et al (2007) Depression, inflammation, and incident cardiovascular disease in women with suspected coronary ischemia: the National Heart, Lung, and Blood Institute-sponsored WISE study. J Am Coll Cardiol 50(21):2044–2050
80. Roest AM, Martens EJ, de Jonge P et al (2010) Anxiety and risk of incident coronary heart disease: a meta-analysis. J Am Coll Cardiol 56(1):38–46

Psychological Stress, Inflammation, Immunity, and Coagulation Intertwining in Ischemic Heart Disease

3

Christian Pristipino

I say that your chief aim in the building up of Man is... to lift his eyes and point to those higher levels on which there are no more things-in-themselves, but only aspects of that divine bond which binds all things together.

A. De Saint Exupery (1948), Cittadelle, n.187

3.1 Introduction

Myocardial ischemia and its biological and clinical consequences are a dynamic result of a complex interplay between several underlying processes that continuously auto-organize and emerge at different scales of observation, acquiring sequences of new properties while maintaining coherence (see Chaps. 1 and 2).

In this framework, some of the connections between the brain and myocardial ischemia pathophysiology have already been summarized in Chaps. 1 and 2. This chapter zooms in on certain specific key interacting circuits. These networks are discussed separately for practical reasons. However, their reciprocal interconnections and those with all the other underlying and derived processes can be understood only in a dynamic relational context that evolves over time.

C. Pristipino, MD (✉)
Department of Cardiovascular Disease, San Filippo Neri Hospital, Via G. Martinotti 20, 00135 Rome, Italy
e-mail: pristipino.c@gmail.com

A. Roncella, C. Pristipino (eds.), *Psychotherapy for Ischemic Heart Disease*,
DOI 10.1007/978-3-319-33214-7_3

3.2 The Stress Response and Its Implications in Ischemic Heart Disease

3.2.1 Stress Response and Ischemic Heart Disease Phenotypes from a Complex Perspective

Acute mental or emotional stressors can precipitate ischemia in up to 90 % of patients with stable angina [1]; they are reported to be trigger of acute coronary syndrome (ACS) in up to 18 % of patients [2] and can double the risk of an acute coronary event in asymptomatic patients [3].

Despite how frequently the word "stress" is used in everyday speech, no general agreement on a definition currently exists. Nonetheless, most researchers would agree that stress is a complex biological and psychological response that a person has to strenuous demands or pressures that can be environmental/social and/or internal. Whatever the stressor, the stress response has biological, behavioral, and emotional components that are intended to increase the host's survival chances within a hostile environment, at least in the short term. From this perspective, it is a network of adaptive homeostatic responses to external stimuli (a process called *allostasis*), in which the net final dynamic equilibrium and its consequences are a complex relational result of the intrinsic characteristics of both the stimuli and the host (genetic, behavioral, and developmental). Once the variable triggering threshold has been reached, the stress system is more or less activated, according to the host's capacity to adapt to specific stressors and become accustomed to them [4]. Determined by the extent and duration of the stress response, the end result is a range of possible clinical phenotypes, within a continuum that ranges from a normal physiological regulatory response, to a chronic or repeated wear-and-tear phase (*allostatic load*), to a frankly pathogenic result (*allostatic overload*) [5]. However, intrinsic to the relational concept of stress, regardless of the variable stress responses per se, the pathogenic potential of the adaptation process also relies upon the simultaneous general balance of whole organism. Indeed, even the normal stress response that occurs during early morning awakening can trigger an ACS and sudden death, if associated with other simultaneous dysfunctional factors within the pathogenic meta-system [6].

The consequence of these considerations is that it is necessary to address and reclassify the whole complex phenotype if you seek to study the role of acute and chronic responses to stressors in ischemic heart disease (see Chap. 1).

3.2.2 Stress Processes in Ischemic Heart Disease

Stressors can be internal or external, physical (e.g., secondary to trauma, temperature, the effects of movement, chemicals), biological (e.g., infections, other inflammatory diseases), or psychological (e.g., acute emotions, mental activity, demanding tasks, social pressures). For further details on different kinds of stressors in ischemic heart disease, refer Chaps. 2, 4, and 5.

The stress response starts within the brain and extends peripherally. With weak/mild stressors, the systemic response tends to manifest a certain level of specificity and be self-limited; while for continued or strong stimuli, the response becomes nonspecific, severe, and prolonged [7]. Individual adaptation to repeated stimuli has been reported [4]. The central neurochemical circuitry responsible for the activation of the stress system forms a complex physiological system in the central nervous system (CNS), consisting of both stimulatory and inhibitory networks with multiple sites of interaction that modulate the response. The first components identified were the hypothalamic–pituitary–adrenal (HPA) axis and the sympathetic (autonomic) nervous system, which directly stimulates adrenal glands and other organs like the thymus, spleen, bone marrow, gastrointestinal tract, sensory organs, and, of course, the cardiovascular system (Fig. 3.1). The central players among the components of this system are corticotropin-releasing hormone (CRH) and vasopressin (AVP), both released by neurons in the paraventricular nucleus of the hypothalamus, as well as the central autonomic sympathetic system that originates in the locus ceruleus of the pons and elsewhere in the brainstem. Vasopressin-producing neurons have projections to several regions of the brain that house cardiovascular neurons, causing an increase in pressure and heart rate as a response to stress. This response is partially counteracted by atrial natriuretic peptide and nitric oxide. In particular, the primary brain structures engaged in emotional responses receive extensive vasopressinergic innervation [8]. An enhanced response of the blood pressure and tachycardia component of the vasopressinergic system has been identified during post-infarct cardiac failure [9].

The autonomic nervous system initially activates the immune system (see Sect. 3.3) and pro-inflammatory cytokines—like tumor necrosis factor α (TNFα) and interleukins (IL 1 and IL 6)—to back-stimulate the HPA axis, leading to control of the inflammatory reaction via glucocorticoids. As HPA activation becomes prolonged, such as in chronic stress, inflammatory cells may uncouple from any upper-level control via downregulation of the glucocorticoid effects [10].

CRH, released into the hypophyseal portal system, stimulates the pituitary gland to secrete adrenocorticotropic hormone (ACTH), which in turn stimulates the adrenal glands (synergistically with sympathetic nervous system stimulation) to secrete glucocorticoids, androgens, aldosterone, and catecholamines into the blood stream. The resulting net cardiovascular response consists of an increased heart rate, increased arterial pressure, raised myocardial metabolic needs, increased myocardial contractility, coronary vasoconstriction with redistribution and/or decreased coronary blood flow and activation of the endothelium (for details see Sects. 1.2 and 1.3), activation and blunting of inflammation and the immune system, changes in behavior and emotions (increased arousal, alertness, vigilance, and cognition; focused attention; and enhanced analgesia), and a shifted coagulation balance towards hyper-coagulation (see Sect. 3.4).

Beyond the classical pathways, recent studies have shown that the brain's stress system is much more complex, since the neuroendocrine responses to stress are under the control of neurons that project from the forebrain, midbrain, and brainstem and produce serotonin, catecholamines, dopamine, histamine,

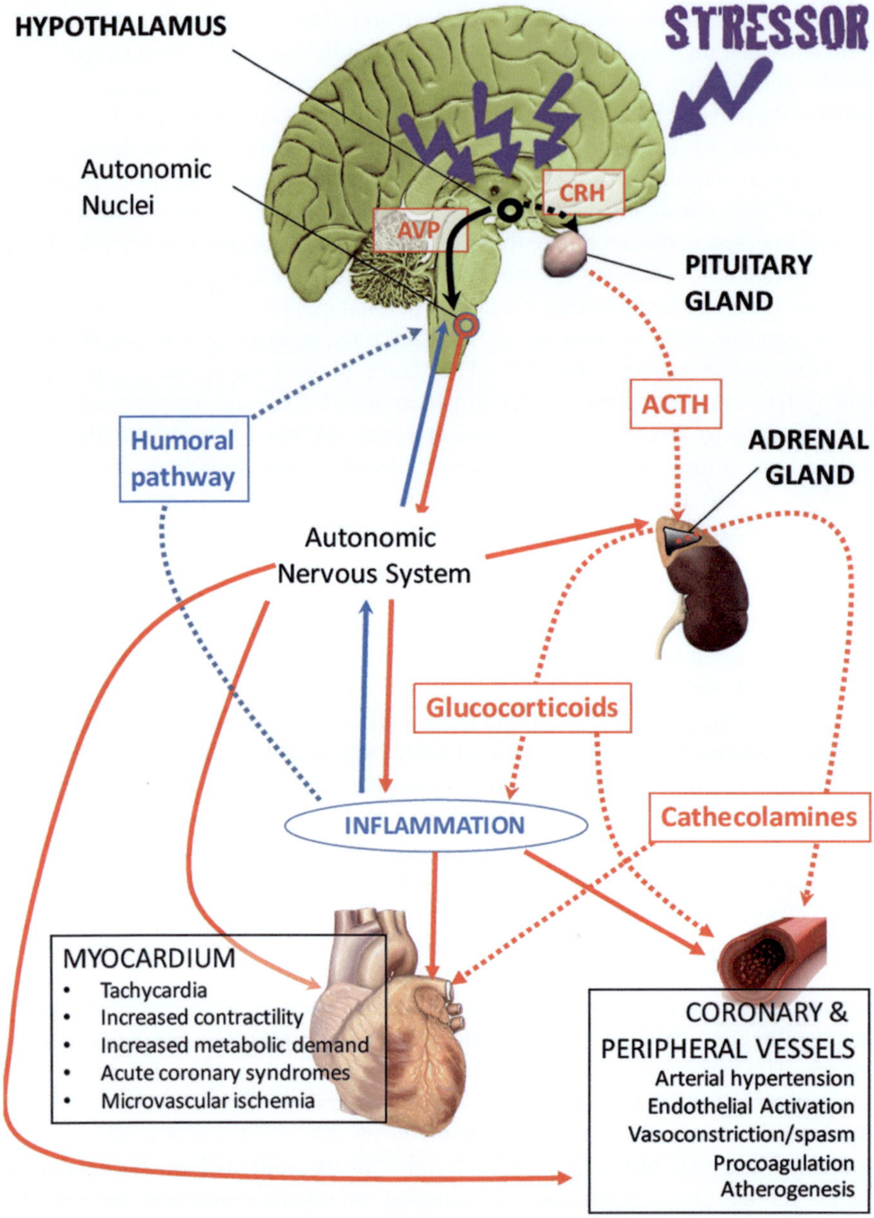

Fig. 3.1 Stress response effects on the cardiovascular system. External stressors induce a stress response when they overcome that variable's allostatic threshold (see text). Humoral (*dashed lines*) activation of a hormonal cascade involving the hypothalamus–pituitary–adrenal (HPA) axis is observed, resulting in the final secretion of glucocorticoids and cathecolamines into the blood stream. This, in turn, exerts both direct and indirect effects on ischemic heart disease. Moreover, complex simultaneous activation of the autonomic nervous system both directly and indirectly influences the pathogenesis of myocardial ischemia. Feedback consists of humoral and neural pathways. *AVP* argininvasopressin, *CRH* corticotropin-releasing hormone, *ACTH* adrenocorticotropic hormone

gammaaminobutirric acid (GABA), and several neuropeptides that are currently being investigated for their involvement in regulation of mood, behavior, and food intake. These neuropeptides include endocannabinoids, angiotensin II, IL-1, oxytocin, apelin, orexin A and B, and ghrelin [11]. Some of these aspects are more deeply discussed in Chap. 4. Specifically during the post-infarction phase [12], these neurons can act on cardiovascular nuclei in the brain stem, both directly or through interactions with other neurons [13].

As in all other processes in ischemic heart disease, the net result of these effects does not necessarily have an absolute threshold, beyond which it is intrinsically pathogenic, because it can be physiologic and may adapt to any allostatic load or predispose, trigger, and/or aggravate myocardial ischemia, depending on the specific state of the overall complex system (for details on cardiac complex systems, see Chap. 1). Indeed, HPA activation can also be both primary and/or secondary to ischemia; hence, any myocardial ischemia generated by a stress response might further enhance the stress response in a vicious, aggravating circle.

A prolonged stress response, in the presence or absence of persistent stressors, can play a pathogenic role in the myocardial ischemia meta-system through: (a) increased sympathetic-adrenal system activity, which can contribute to disturbed glucose and lipid metabolism [14, 15]; (b) behavioral changes that may affect physical activity (e.g., sedentary lifestyle) and dietary habits (e.g., increased portion size, alcohol consumption) [16]; and (c) sustained HPA activity associated with increases in visceral adiposity, insulin resistance, and the concentrations of inflammatory markers like IL-6 and C-reactive protein [17, 18]. Moreover, hyper- or hypo-sensitivity of the stress system, when associated with abnormalities in inflammatory control, may play a role in the pathogenesis of chronic inflammation and immune-related diseases that are associated with ischemic heart disease [19]. For further experimental insights, refer back to Chap. 2.

3.3 Role of Psychobiologic Processes in Inflammation and Immunity, as They Relate to Ischemic Heart Disease

3.3.1 Inflammation and Immunity in Ischemic Heart Disease

A growing body of evidence indicates that inflammation and immunity have a central role in ischemic heart disease, having been implicated at numerous levels as predisposing, precipitating, and complicating processes, but also as consequences of ischemia. Inflammatory and immune cells acting in the heart can be recruited from the circulation and spleen or can already reside within the heart, in the latter case already being highly adapted to the microenvironment [20].

Atherosclerosis itself is a vascular inflammatory process that involves a number of different molecular and cellular pathways, including the activation of innate [21] and adaptive immunity [22]. This constitutes the variable coronary background on which myocardial ischemia often develops (for details on myocardial ischemia generation, see also Sect. 1.3).

Local or widespread coronary inflammation [23] can also primarily cause plaque damage and, by controlling the thrombogenic potential of the plaque [24], trigger acute critical thrombosis, thereby giving rise to ACS or a more progressive phenomena that contributes to the evolution of chronic and stable clinical scenarios (see Sect. 1.3). An intense and systemic acute phase response is an associated trigger of acute ischemia in 60 % of cases [25] and is correlated with worse in-hospital and long-term prognosis in patients presenting with both acute and chronic disease [26]. The basis of such inflammation in ACS may at least partially reside in innate immunity, since activated monocytes, polymorphonuclear neutrophils, eosinophils, and mast cells are often found, not only at the site of plaque rupture but also throughout the entire coronary circulation of patients with these syndromes [27, 28]. Interestingly, platelets also seem to behave as innate immunity cells in acute myocardial ischemia syndromes, amplifying both inflammation and thrombosis [29]. Nonetheless, in several conditions, adaptive immunity is associated with sudden changes that lead to coronary instability as well [30], particularly some level of perturbation involving the T-cell repertoire, likely triggered by specific antigens [31, 32], which exerts a cytotoxic effect on endothelial cells [33, 34].

Microvascular alterations leading to abnormal coronary blood flow have been associated with both the remote and local effects of cytokines and inflammation [35]. On the other hand, myocardial inflammation may be secondary to ischemia, reperfusion, and necrosis, but also to hemodynamic strain, playing a pivotal detrimental role in the repair and remodeling of the myocardium after an acute myocardial infarction (see Sect. 1.4.5).

3.3.2 Psycho-neurologic Connections with Inflammation and Immunity

The inflammatory/immunologic processes in ischemic heart disease are open doors wherein psychobiologic intertwining comes into play [36].

Indeed, since the beginning of the last century, we have known that inflammatory and immune mechanisms interact profoundly with the neural system [37], and since the 1960s and 1980s, respectively, that behavior and emotions influence immunity and vice versa [38, 39]. The evidence of a more sophisticated cross talk between the inflammatory/immune and nervous systems has been observed in both animal and human studies in different clinical settings, including infections, asthma, and chronic inflammatory diseases [10]. The experimental evidences that mind–body practices improve inflammation markers show the tight relationship between mental states and inflammation/immunity and are reviewed in Chap. 12. Local pro-inflammatory mediators, like IL1 and TNFα, and the numerous neurotransmitters secreted by immune cells [40], can excite afferent nociceptive and vagal nerve terminals which, in turn, convey the stimuli to the brain, particularly the hypothalamus [41] and medulla (see Sects. 1.2.2, 1.4.2 and Fig. 3.2), thereby activating the HPA axis and/or sympathetic nervous system. In turn,

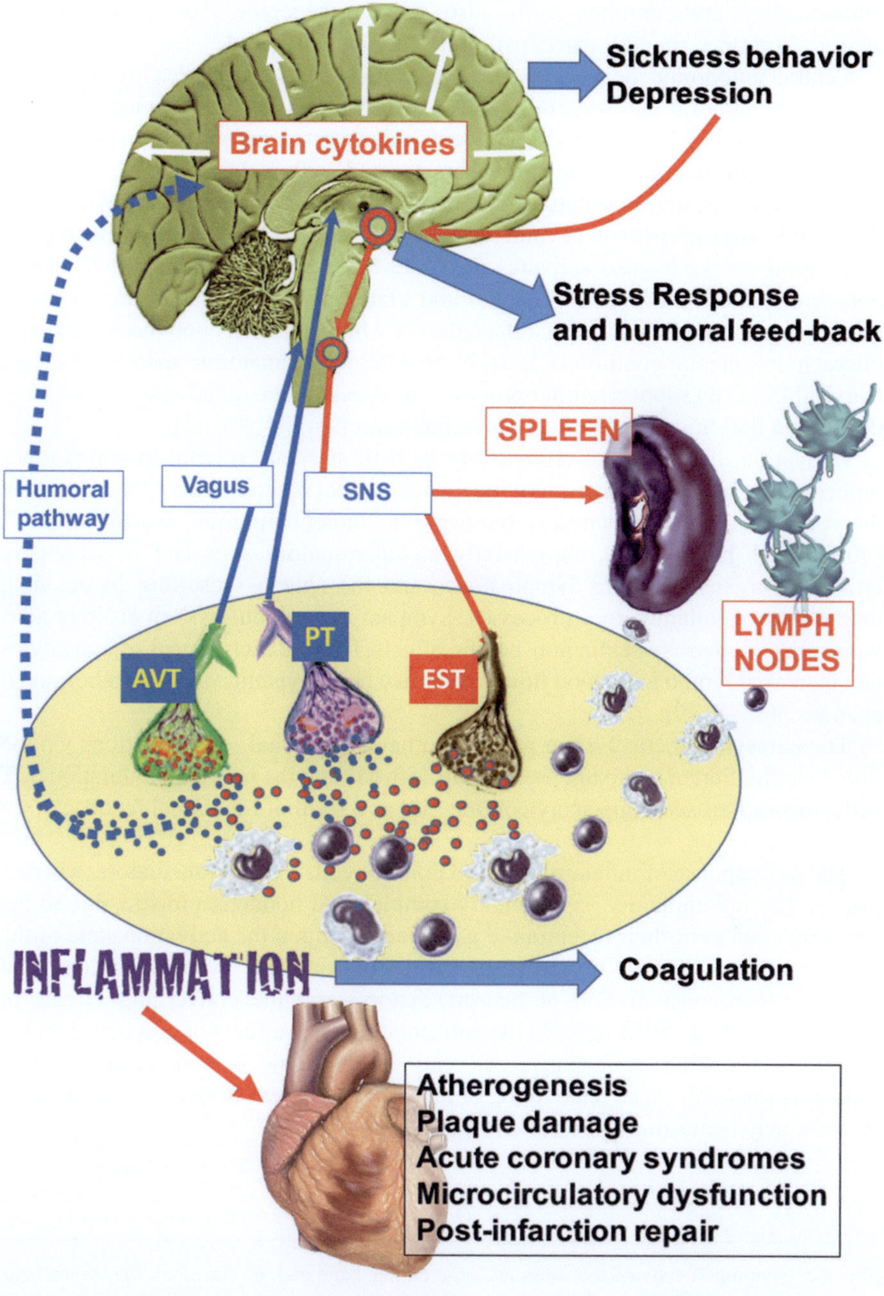

Fig. 3.2 Psycho-neural influences on ischemic heart disease through neuro-inflammatory cross talk. Inflammatory cytokines (e.g., IL-1, IL-6, TNF) (*blue dots*) stimulate afferent vagal terminals (AVT) and pain terminals (PR) that transmit the information to the brain through vagus and sensory fibers, respectively. Cytokines and other soluble inflammation byproducts also reach the brain through the circulation (humoral pathway) and locally stimulate the production of other cytokines by the microglia. The behavioral response and direct activation through neuronal paths

inflammatory and immune cells also express receptors for a number of neurotransmitters, thereby participating in a feedback loop [42].

Central autonomic nervous system activation is also triggered by a slower, convergent humoral pathway, by means of soluble and circulating mediators that enter the brain via diffusion at circumventricular organs, by active transport at the blood–brain barrier, or through receptors located within the endothelial cells of brain venules, causing microglial cells to secrete pro-inflammatory cytokynes [43]; this process may perpetuate beyond the acute phase [44]. This "mirrored secretion" of cerebral cytokines also activates disparate brain neuronal circuits and, likely, non-neuronal effects (e.g., endothelial and glial cells) that mediate the so-called "sickness behavior," the final manifestation of which depends upon the context and microenvironmental conditions, though some degree of anatomic specificity seems to exist [45]. Data support similar processes in at least some of the manifestations of depression that transpire after a myocardial infarction [44, 46, 47].

Activation of the central efferent sympathetic nervous system, in which other higher brain circuitry (as a primary independent process) comes into play, results in the release of neurotransmitters (epinephrine, norepinephrine, neuropeptide Y, substance P, nitric oxide, etc.) locally at inflammatory sites and in secondary lymphoid organs—such as lymph nodes and the spleen—resulting in the final modulation of inflammatory processes. Sympathetic nervous system efferent activation also induces systemic nonspecific effects, like the recruitment of leukocytes and increased lymph and blood flow via cardiac hemodynamic and neuro-hormonal changes [43, 48, 49].

The parasympathetic system might also have additional local functions via the direct modulation of sympathetic efferents [50, 51] and the indirect modulation of T cells, themselves secreting acetylcholine [52] as a form of functional feedback (see Chap. 12).

The net response of inflammatory and immune cells to neuro-mediators, whether pro- or anti-inflammatory, is extremely complex and nondeterministic, due to the evolving context of their receptors (e.g., depending upon the activation state of the cell, expression pattern of receptors, microenvironment, cytokine milieu, and regional microconcentration of neuromediators) and the converging effects of other systems (e.g., HPA axis via the anti-inflammatory effects of glucocorticoids). Moreover, the kind of response can vary in the same person because, while inflammation evolves, an uncoupling of the immune system from central regulating systems may occur through different mechanisms [10].

Fig. 3.2 (continued) activate the stress response on one hand and, on the other, the sympathetic nervous system (SNS) that locally modulates the inflammatory reaction by releasing a variety of neurotransmitters (*red dots*) from efferent sympathetic terminals (EST). The SNS also stimulates the release of inflammatory cells from secondary lymphatic organs. In addition, neurotransmitters are secreted by immune cells, creating a feedback loop. Inflammation and its neural regulation are thereby involved in several facets of ischemic heart disease (see text)

How these processes might be active in ischemic heart disease with specific features still remains a matter of investigation. To date, experimental data provide evidence that innervation of the heart is not only able to modulate local inflammatory activity after an acute myocardial infarction [53] and independently from it [54], but that this modulation is essential for the full expression of pro-inflammatory cytokines in the injured myocardium and circulation [55]. Additionally, enhanced cardiovascular autonomic function obtained through exercise is associated with decreased myocardial inflammation [56]. Moreover, in rats post-acute myocardial infarction, the increased production of cytokines in the hypothalamus has also been observed [55].

In a recent prospective clinical trial involving 5140 patients, inflammatory markers accounted for approximately 11 % of the rehospitalization rate for cardiovascular causes in depressed patients [57]. In addition, in a cross-sectional study involving 9258 patients, elevated C reactive levels were independently associated with comorbid myocardial infarction and depression [58]. Posttraumatic stress disorder after an acute-MI also is associated with elevated levels of inflammatory markers [59]. Generally speaking, these findings in patients with ischemic heart disease may configure a specific framework within the inflammatory model of depression, as proposed at large by several authors [60].

However, in a retrospective study on 15,634 patients with chronic inflammation (rheumatoid arthritis), the onset of depression was associated with a 40 % greater likelihood of having an acute myocardial infarction, suggesting that brain–heart interactions in ischemic heart disease are specific and go beyond general inflammatory processes, also involving other mechanisms, as suggested by other studies [61, 62]. The other possible processes coming into play in the connection between depression and ischemic heart disease are reviewed in Chaps. 2 and 4.

Taken together, these data suggest that cross talk is present between psychoneural and inflammatory processes in ischemic heart disease. However, further studies are needed to assess the weight of this cross talk, as well as its characteristics and relationships with other relevant pathophysiological processes in different stages of disease (see Chap. 1). Given the complex nature of interactions, nondeterministic and nonlinear approaches are likely to be the most appropriate to shed light on the matter. Moreover, whether new pharmacological or non-pharmacological interventions targeting each of these features can improve outcomes and ultimate prognosis is a fascinating question that still needs to be addressed in carefully selected populations, such feature including psychological and inflammatory/immunological characteristics.

3.4 Psychobiologic Effects on the Coagulation System

The coagulation system, with its thrombogenic and fibrinolytic, humoral, and cellular subsystems, plays a key role in both the stable [63] and acute manifestations of ischemic heart disease through the formation and dissolution of mural or obstructing thrombi on the vessel wall (see Sect. 1.3).

The very fact that a mental-induced stress response can precipitate acute thrombotic events like ACS highlights how psychological processes influence thrombosis [1–3]. Indeed, an acute increase in coagulation and fibrinolytic activity has been observed after an acute stress response as a physiologic adaptive response. However, when coagulation activity is exaggeratedly increased relative to increased fibrinolytic activity, a pathologic, hypercoagulable state is generated [64]. In addition to age and preexisting ischemic heart disease [65, 66], a wide array of psychosocial factors (e.g., low socioeconomic status, chronic psychosocial stress, negative affect, perceived threats, and challenges) is associated with hypercoagulation responses to stressors [67].

Extensive data show that mental-induced stress responses activate coagulation both directly (via effects on blood coagulation molecules, platelets, and fibrinolysis) and indirectly (via vasomotor actions that increase shear stress, time of flow, hemoconcentration, and inflammation) [64].

The influence of psychological processes, as effected by a stress response and/or inflammation (see previous paragraphs) on coagulation, seems to be mediated principally by sympathetic activation and catecholamine release, both of which affect the hepatic clearance of tissue-plasminogen activator (t-PA, an endogenous fibrinolytic agent) and, likely, D-dimer. Adrenergic drive also stimulates: (a) endothelial beta2-adrenergic receptors on vessels and alpha2-adrenergic receptors on platelets; (b) the release of preformed coagulation factor VIII, hemostatically active Von Willebrand factor, and t-PA from endothelial storage pools; (c) the hepatic release of factor VIII; and (d) the release of t-PA into the blood by arterial walls [64].

Also, during a mental-induced stress response, thrombin—a potent platelet activator—is formed, while platelets cross-play with inflammation, which is—in turn—tightly linked to coagulation [68], thereby underscoring the complexity of the meta-system (Fig. 3.3).

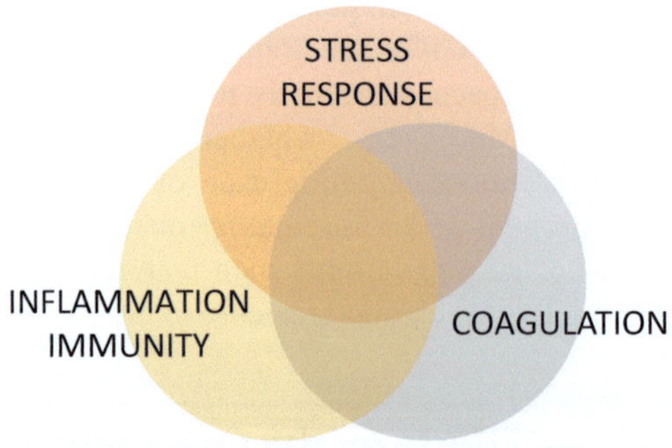

Fig. 3.3 Relationships between stress, coagulation, and inflammation. Stress, coagulation, and inflammation have varying degrees and modes of interaction, but they are tightly bound. In different patients, one of these may become more prevalent. However, their overall relationship always influences the meta-system of myocardial ischemia

The degree and rapidity of the response to thrombogenic stimuli depend upon the thrombogenic potential of the stimulus, on the time window of its activity, and on the reactivity of the coagulation system. However, in healthy individuals, hypercoagulable states, per se, do not cause vascular harm. Moreover, any hypercoagulable state that is induced by a stress response is only transient and must be prolongated by other mechanisms to cause ACS [63]. Therefore, thrombogenesis in ischemic heart disease can be explained only by taking into account the general balance of the various systems that contribute to the generation of ischemia (see Chap. 1).

3.5 Conclusions

Mental and physical stress, negative emotions, intense mental activity, and psychological processes are tightly intertwined in circular causal relationships with systems and processes that play an active role in both acute and chronic ischemic heart disease. These systems and processes include stress responses and the neurohumoral, immune, and coagulation systems. Potentially modulating these relationships is the basis of several new therapies that simultaneously act upon the patient's mind and biology. Indeed, some studies assessing therapeutic strategies to reduce stress have been shown to improve cardiovascular outcomes as well (for details, see Chap. 10–13). However, the highly interconnected nature of the networks, and their variability over time, imply that extremely heterogenous patient subpopulations exist that might "dilute" the effects of treatment if combined in a single clinical trial. This would lead to type 2 errors during statistical analysis of outcome data, failing to detect real therapeutic benefits for one or more subject subsets within the overall treatment sample, merely because other subsets are included for which the treatment holds no benefit. What this means is that, to optimize treatment outcomes and determine the most effective therapies, patients may need to be subclassified in a way that somehow encapsulates their various psychological and biological characteristics.

References

1. Strike PC, Steptoe A (2003) Systematic review of mental stress-induced myocardial ischaemia. Eur Heart J 24:690–703
2. Tofler GH, Stone PH, Maclure M et al (1990) Analysis of possible triggers of acute myocardial infarction (the MILIS study). Am J Cardiol 66:22–27
3. Wilbert-Lampen U, Leistner D, Greven S et al (2008) Cardiovascular events during World Cup soccer. N Engl J Med 358(5):475–483
4. Kirschbaum C, Prüssner JC, Stone AA et al (1995) Persistent high cortisol responses to repeated psychological stress in a subpopulation of healthy men. Psychosom Med 57 (5):468–474
5. Peters A, McEwen BS (2015) Stress habituation, body shape and cardiovascular mortality. Neurosci Biobehav Rev 56:139–150

6. Cohen MC, Rohtla KM, Lavery CE et al (1997) Meta-analysis of the morning excess of acute myocardial infarction and sudden cardiac death. Am J Cardiol 79(11):1512–1516
7. Selye H (1936) Syndrome produced by diverse nocuous agents. Nature 138:32
8. Landgraf R (2008) The vasopressin system—from antidiuresis to psychopathology. Eur J Pharmacol 583:226–242
9. Dobruch J, Cudnoch-Jedrzejewska A, Szczepanska-Sadowska E (2005) Enhanced involvement of brain vasopressin V1receptors in cardiovascular responses to stress in rats with myocardial infarction. Stress 8:273–284
10. Pongratz G, Rainer H, Straub RH (2014) The sympathetic nervous response in inflammation. Arthritis Res Ther 16:504–516
11. Szczepanska-Sadowska E, Cudnoch-Jedrzejewska A, Ufnal M et al (2010) Brain and cardiovascular diseases: common neurogenic background of cardiovascular, metabolic and inflammatory diseases. J Physiol Pharmacol 61(5):509–521
12. Cudnoch-Jedrzejewska A, Dobruch J, Puchalska L et al (2007) Interaction of AT1 receptors and V1a receptors-mediated effects in the central cardiovascular control during the post-infarct state. Regul Pept 142:86–94
13. Newson MJ, Roberts EM, Pope GR et al (2009) The effects of apelin on the hypothalamic-pituitary-adrenal axis neuroendocrine function are mediated through corticotrophin-releasing factor- and vasopressin-dependent mechanisms. J Endocrinol 202:123–139
14. Dimsdale JE (2008) Psychological stress and cardiovascular disease. J Am Coll Cardiol 51:1237–1246
15. Wirtz PH, Ehlert U, Bartschi C et al (2009) Changes in plasma lipids with psychosocial stress are related to hypertension status and the norepinephrine stress response. Metabolism 58:30–37
16. Adam TC, Epel ES (2007) Stress, eating and the reward system. Physiol Behav 91:449–458
17. Kiecolt-Glaser JK, Preacher KJ, MacCallum RC et al (2003) Chronic stress and age-related increases in the proinflammatory cytokine IL-6. Proc Natl Acad Sci USA 100(15):9090–9095
18. Rohleder N, Wolf JM, Wolf OT (2010) Glucocorticoid sensitivity of cognitive and inflammatory processes in depression and posttraumatic stress disorder. Neurosci Biobehav Rev 35:104–114
19. Elenkov IJ, Chrousos GP (2006) Stress system—organization, physiology and immunoregulation. Neuroimmunomodulation 13:257–267
20. Epelman S, Liu PP, Mann DL (2015) Role of innate and adaptive immune mechanisms in cardiac injury and repair. Nat Rev Immunol 15:117–129
21. Niessner A, Shin MS, Pryshchep O et al (2007) Synergistic proinflammatory effects of the antiviral cytokine interferon-alpha and Toll-like receptor 4 ligands in the atherosclerotic plaque. Circulation 116:2043–2052
22. Hansson GK (2005) Inflammation, atherosclerosis, and coronary artery disease. N Engl J Med 352:1685–1695
23. Mauriello A, Sangiorgi G, Fratoni S et al (2005) Diffuse and active inflammation occurs in both vulnerable and stable plaques of the entire coronary tree: a histopathologic study of patients dying of acute myocardial infarction. J Am Coll Cardiol 45:1585–1593
24. Croce K, Libby P (2007) Intertwining of thrombosis and inflammation in atherosclerosis. Curr Opin Hematol 14:55–61
25. Cristell N, Cianflone D, Durante A et al (2011) High-sensitivity C-reactive protein is within normal levels at the very onset of first ST-segment elevation acute myocardial infarction in 41% of cases a multiethnic case-control study. J Am Coll Cardiol 58:2654–2656
26. Libby P, Ridker PM, Hansson GK (2009) Inflammation in atherosclerosis: from pathophysiology to practice. J Am Coll Cardiol 54:2129–2138
27. Wyss CA, Neidhart M, Altwegg L et al (2010) Cellular actors, Toll-like receptors, and local cytokine profile in acute coronary syndromes. Eur Heart J 31:1457–1469
28. Yonekawa K, Neidhart M, Altwegg LA et al (2011) Myeloid related proteins activate Toll-like receptor 4 in human acute coronary syndromes. Atherosclerosis 218:486–492

29. Blair P, Rex S, Vitseva O et al (2009) Stimulation of Toll-like receptor 2 in human platelets induces a thromboinflammatory response through activation of phosphoinositide 3-kinase. Circ Res 104:346–354
30. Caligiuri G, Paulsson G, Nicoletti A et al (2000) Evidence for antigen-driven T-cell response in unstable angina. Circulation 102:1114–1119
31. Zal B, Kaski JC, Arno G et al (2004) Heat-shock protein 60-reactive CD4CD28null T cells in patients with acute coronary syndromes. Circulation 109:1230–1235
32. Liuzzo G, Goronzy JJ, Yang H et al (2000) Monoclonal T-cell proliferation and plaque instability in acute coronary syndromes. Circulation 101:2883–2888
33. Nakajima T, Schulte S, Warrington KJ et al (2002) T-cell-mediated lysis of endothelial cells in acute coronary syndromes. Circulation 105:570–575
34. Pryshchep S, Sato K, Goronzy JJ et al (2006) T cell recognition and killing of vascular smooth muscle cells in acute coronary syndrome. Circ Res 98:1168–1176
35. Bagi Z, Broskova Z, Feher A (2014) Obesity and coronary microvascular disease—implications for adipose tissue-mediated remote inflammatory response. Curr Vasc Pharmacol 12(3):453–461
36. Paine NJ, Bosch JA, Van Zanten JJ (2012) Inflammation and vascular responses to acute mental stress: implications for the triggering of myocardial infarction. Curr Pharm Des 18 (11):1494–1501
37. Meltzer SJ, Meltzer C (1903) On a difference in the influence upon inflammation between the section of the sympathetic nerve and the removal of the sympathetic ganglion. J Med Res 10:135–141
38. Solomon GF, Moss RH (1964) Emotions, immunity, and disease; a speculative theoretical integration. Arch Gen Psychiatry 11:657–674
39. Ader R, Cohen N (1982) Behaviorally conditioned immunosuppression and murine systemic lupus erythematosus. Science 215:1534–1536
40. Blalock JE (1989) A molecular basis for bidirectional communication between the immune and neuroendocrine systems. Physiol Rev 69:1–32
41. Besedovsky H, del Rey A, Sorkin E et al (1986) Immunoregulatory feedback between interleukin-1 and glucocorticoid hormones. Science 233:652–654
42. Carr DJJ, Blalock JE (1991) Neuropeptide hormones and receptors common to the immune and neuroendocrine systems: bidirectional pathway of intersystem communication. In: Ader R, Felten DL, Cohen N (eds) Psychoneuroimmunology, 2nd edn. Academic, San Diego, pp 573–588
43. Dantzer R, O'Connor JC, Freund GG et al (2008) From inflammation to sickness and depression: when the immune system subjugates the brain. Nat Rev Neurosci 9:46–56
44. Liu H, Luiten PG, Eisel UL et al (2013) Depression after myocardial infarction: TNF-α-induced alterations of the blood-brain barrier and its putative therapeutic implications. Neurosci Biobehav Rev 37:561–572
45. Lowry CA, Hollis JH, de Vries A et al (2007) Identification of an immune-responsive mesolimbocortical serotonergic system: potential role in regulation of emotional behavior. Neuroscience 146:756–772
46. Shang YX, Ding WQ, Qiu HY et al (2014) Association of depression with inflammation in hospitalized patients of myocardial infarction. Pak J Med Sci 30:692–697
47. Steptoe A, Wikman A, Molloy GJ et al (2013) Inflammation and symptoms of depression and anxiety in patients with acute coronary heart disease. Brain Behav Immun 31:183–188
48. Kannan H, Tanaka Y, Kunitake T et al (1996) Activation of sympathetic outflow by recombinant human interleukin-1 beta in conscious rats. Am J Physiol 270:R479–R485
49. Kimura T, Yamamoto T, Ota K et al (1993) Central effects of interleukin-1 on blood pressure, thermogenesis, and the release of vasopressin, ACTH, and atrial natriuretic peptide. Ann NY Acad Sci 689:330–345
50. Vida G, Pena G, Kanashiro A et al (2011) Beta2-Adrenoreceptors of regulatory lymphocytes are essential for vagal neuromodulation of the innate immune system. FASEB J 25:4476–4485

51. Vida G, Pena G, Deitch EA et al (2011) alpha7-cholinergic receptor mediates vagal induction of splenic norepinephrine. J Immunol 186:4340–4346
52. Rosas-Ballina M, Olofsson PS, Ochani M et al (2011) Acetylcholine-synthesizing T cells relay neural signals in a vagus nerve circuit. Science 334:98–101
53. Calvillo L, Vanoli E, Andreoli E et al (2011) Vagal stimulation, through its nicotinic action, limits infarct size and the inflammatory response to myocardial ischemia and reperfusion. J Cardiovasc Pharmacol 58:500–507
54. Levick SP, Murray DB, Janice JS et al (2010) Sympathetic nervous system modulation of inflammation and remodeling in the hypertensive heart. Hypertension 55:270–276
55. Francis J, Zhang ZH, Weiss RM et al (2004) Neural regulation of the proinflammatory cytokine response to acute myocardial infarction. Am J Physiol Heart Circ Physiol 287: H791–H797
56. Rodrigues B, Santana AA, Santamarina AB et al (2014) Role of training and detraining on inflammatory and metabolic profile in infarcted rats: influences of cardiovascular autonomic nervous system. Mediators Inflamm. doi:10.1155/2014/207131
57. Hiles SA, Baker AL, de Malmanche T et al (2015) The role of inflammatory markers in explaining the association between depression and cardiovascular hospitalisations. J Behav Med 38:609–619
58. Bjerkeset O, Romild U, Smith GD et al (2011) The associations of high levels of C-reactive protein with depression and myocardial infarction in 9258 women and men from the HUNT population study. Psychol Med 41:345–352
59. von Känel R, Begré S, Abbas CC et al (2010) Inflammatory biomarkers in patients with posttraumatic stress disorder caused by myocardial infarction and the role of depressive symptoms. Neuroimmunomodulation 17:39–46
60. Raison CL, Miller AH (2013) Malaise, melancholia and madness: the evolutionary legacy of an inflammatory bias. Brain Behav Immun 31:1–8
61. Lippi G, Montagnana M, Favaloro EJ et al (2009) Mental depression and cardiovascular disease: a multifaceted, bidirectional association. Semin Thromb Hemost 35:325–336
62. Vaccarino V, Johnson BD, Sheps DS, National Heart, Lung, and Blood Institute et al (2007) Depression, inflammation, and incident cardiovascular disease in women with suspected coronary ischemia: the National Heart, Lung, and Blood Institute-sponsored WISE study. J Am Coll Cardiol 50(21):2044–2050
63. Borissoff JI, Spronk HM, ten Cate H (2011) The hemostatic system as a modulator of atherosclerosis. N Engl J Med 364:1746–1760
64. von Kännel R (2015) Acute mental stress and hemostasis: when physiology becomes vascular harm. Thromb Res 135(Suppl 1):S52–S55
65. Strike PC, Magid K, Brydon L et al (2004) Exaggerated platelet and hemodynamic reactivity to mental stress in men with coronary artery disease. Psychosom Med 66:492–500
66. Palermo A, Bertalero P, Pizza N et al (1989) Decreased fibrinolytic response to adrenergic stimulation in hypertensive patients. J Hypertens Suppl 7:S162–S163
67. Austin AW, Wissmann T, von Känel R (2013) Stress and hemostasis: an update. Semin Thromb Hemost 39:902–912
68. von Känel R, Kudielka BM, Hanebuth D et al (2005) Different contribution of interleukin-6 and cortisol activity to total plasma fibrin concentration and to acute mental stress-induced fibrin formation. Clin Sci (Lond) 109:61–67

The Second Brain and Possible Interactions with the Heart

4

Rosa Sollazzo and Marco Sanges

Give sorrow words the grief that does not speak knits up the over wrought heart and bids it break
William Shakespeare (William Shakespeare, Macbeth: Act 4, Scene 3)

4.1 Introduction

In Europe, the anatomic dissection of the human body has progressed in an analytical and reductionist-like manner, starting with studying isolated organs, then moving to first a cellular level, and finally a molecular level. In the West, an integrated picture of the brain–gut axis only started to emerge in the nineteenth century. Conversely, the Chinese "holistic" approach has always focused on the complex interactions that exist between organs, as well as their reciprocal effects. The "discovery" of the second brain by Taoism is 2000 years old, though it was considered of little interest in the scientific community until the last century. Today it needs to be reexamined on the basis of recent scientific advances that have arisen, especially over the last 20 years.

4.2 The Second Brain

The *enteric nervous system* (ENS), which is also called the *intrinsic nervous system*, has been referred to as a second brain, given recent scientific discoveries documenting its ability to exert control over other systems. In truth, however, it really should be considered the first brain, given that it emerged evolutionarily long

R. Sollazzo, MD (✉) • M. Sanges, MD
Gastroenterology Unit, Federico II University of Naples, Naples, Italy
e-mail: sollazzo@unina.it; marcosanges1974@libero.it

A. Roncella, C. Pristipino (eds.), *Psychotherapy for Ischemic Heart Disease*,
DOI 10.1007/978-3-319-33214-7_4

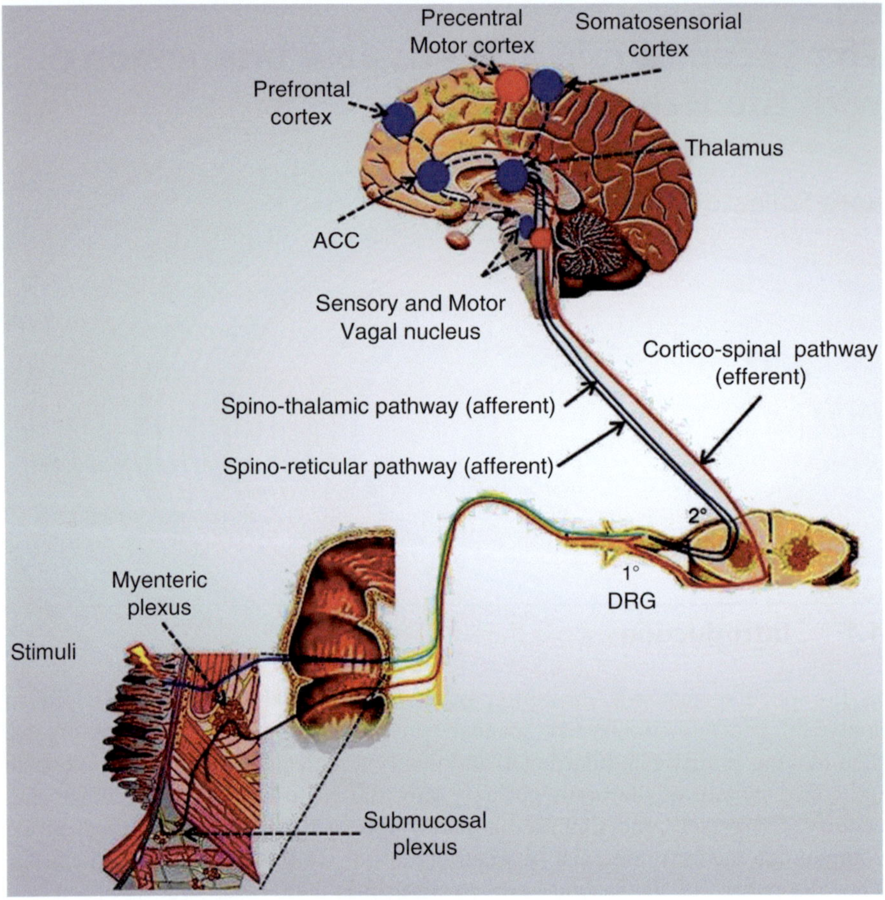

Fig. 4.1 Bidirectional brain–gut axis. Modified and adapted from *Current and Emerging Treatments—Future Medicine Ltd*

before the cerebrum. Unfortunately, the neuronal mechanisms of the gastrointestinal tract were essentially overlooked until the nineteenth century, however, when Meissner and Auerbach separately discovered its two plexuses—the myenteric and submucosal, respectively—and proposed that the gut contained its own localized regulatory functions. In 1998, roughly 100 years later, Gershon focused upon the complex neuronal functions of the long-overlooked gastrointestinal (GI) tract in his scholarly book *The Second Brain* [1]. The ENS consists of an estimated 200–600 million neurons, organized into thousands of ganglia, with the myenteric plexus functioning from the esophagus to the anus and the submucosal plexus in the small and large intestines (Fig. 4.1).

ENS neurons connect with pre- and paravertebral ganglia, as well as with the gallbladder, pancreas, and trachea. Therefore, besides the central nervous system

(CNS), it is necessary to consider this neuronal network that controls the entire digestive apparatus and is structured within the alimentary tract as a highly organized neural network intrinsic to its epithelial structure. The ENS, just like the CNS, produces neurotransmitters like acetylcholine, dopamine, and serotonin, as well as other specific neurohormones like ghrelin (also called lenomorelin). These neurohormones interact with other hormones and, in so doing, are able to modulate both the emotional and rational responses of the CNS [2]. In doing so, the integrated CNS–ENS system plays a crucial role in every stage of life, from birth to old age. Altered function of the ENS due to bowel inflammation, caused, for example, by poor eating habits, can significantly and adversely affect a person's wellness and quality of life. The main connection between the CNS and ENS occurs in the frontal lobe of the cerebral cortex, where mirror neurons are localized. This is a control area where the brain integrates and analyzes neuronal input and helps to determine appropriate response to behavioral challenge [2].

Similar to the heart–brain circuit (see Chap. 1), the GI tract communicates both ways with the CNS and ENS and constantly conveys information on its state. Consequently, every form of malfunction (even visceral pain) impacts feelings of the CNS and, in particular, may affect one's sense of hunger and satiety. In turn, the CNS provides signals to control the GI tract, signals that are mainly in reply to information generated by the ENS or alternatively to information generated within the CNS itself. For example, the sight and smell of food elicits a preparatory response from the GI tract, like salivation and the secretion of gastric juices. On the other hand, ingested food stimulates the pharynx and upper esophagus to release afferent signals, which are integrated within the encephalic trunk, followed by efferent signals to enteric neurons in the stomach to increase the secretion of gastric juice to aid in food digestion. Finally, we must take into consideration that the enteric neuronal system is also influenced by the disparate populations of intestinal bacteria that play an important role in the metabolic and immunological functions of the digestive system [3].

The first function of the ENS is to enable peristalsis and thereby propel ingested food, so that it traverses the long road from the stomach to anus, beginning with 30 cm of duodenum, followed by 5 m of jejunum and ileum, and finally 1.5 m of large intestine. The brain releases scarce information to the ENS, which is largely independent; 90 % of the information sent runs retrograde from the abdomen to the brain [4] (Fig. 4.2).

The mechanism works in the following way: neurons located within the intestinal wall sense where food is located, since they are stretched by the bolus passing through. Enterochromaffin cells secrete serotonin, an amino acid derivative that stimulates the nerve cells located in the *submucosal plexus*. In turn, these cells send signals to the muscle cells that dilate and contract the intestines. Inhibition of the peristaltic reflex, due to insufficient levels of serotonin, causes constipation, whereas prolonged stimulation, due to an overproduction of serotonin, induces diarrhea.

In humans, the intestines are one of the places where different biological systems and apparatuses interact. Within the mucosa of the epithelial intestine, billions of

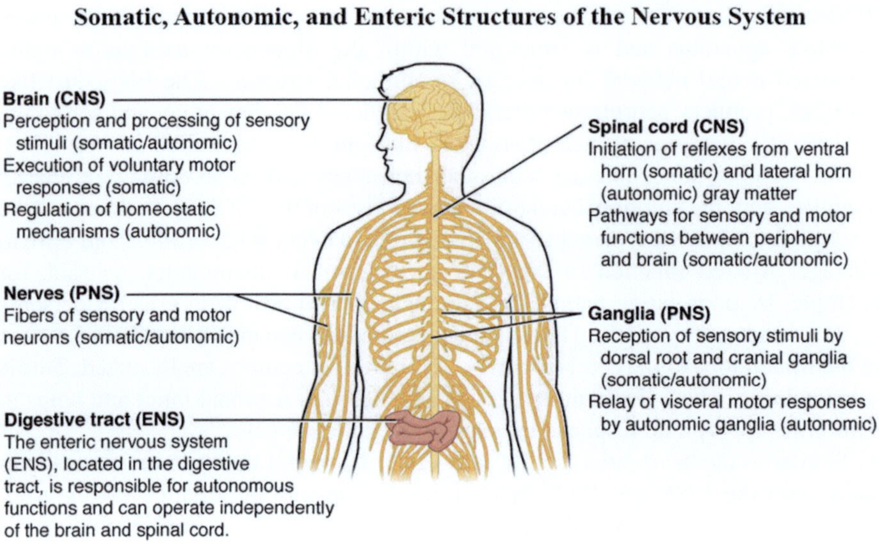

Fig. 4.2 Somatic structures include the spinal nerves, both motor and sensory fibers, as well as the sensory ganglia (posterior root ganglia and cranial nerve ganglia). Autonomic structures are found in the nerves also, but include the sympathetic and parasympathetic ganglia. The enteric nervous system includes the nervous tissue within the organs of the digestive tract. Adapted from the article "Structure and Function of Nervous System," OpenStax College produced by OpenStax QA and licensed under the Creative Commons Attribution License 3.0. *Version 1.6: Jun 28, 2013 11:37 a.m. +0000 †http://creativecommons.org/licenses/by/3.0/

eukaryotic and prokaryotic (bacterial) cells reside, side by side, with their cellular and molecular components finely tuned and responsible for prompt and effective immune responses [5].

The cellular components that cooperate to optimize the ecology of the intestinal environment are those cells involved in the immune response, located predominantly in the lamina of the GI mucosa, as well as epithelial structures that, in the digestive tract, have the dual functions of lining the intestine and being parenchymal cells.

Moreover, the daily production of IgA is greater than that of IgG. This indicates that, in intestinal mucosa, several structures and cells are responsible for the adequate immune response to antigens present in the intestinal lumen. When strongly stimulated by these antigens, cells that physiologically infiltrate the intestinal mucosa increase in number and become immunologically active and ready to initiate a local immune response, since they are primarily memory T cells. The importance of the interface between prokaryotic and eukaryotic cells is shown by the analysis of experimental models of human intestinal inflammatory diseases [6]. Such models clearly show that only two types of cell, T cells and prokaryotic cells (i.e., the bacteria that are normally present throughout the intestines), are required for the development of intestinal disease. Therefore, such an interface between the eukaryotic and prokaryotic world can be regarded as a complex organ, the function and efficiency of which are strictly regulated. Malfunction of this structure may turn a controlled physiological inflammatory state into an uncontrolled inflammatory state, i.e., intestinal disease.

Control of immunological reactivity relies on multiple mechanisms which operate at different levels: interactions between bacteria, the immune system, epithelial cells, and the ENS. Immunologically, the intestines exhibit a propensity toward either an anti-inflammatory (Th2) or regulatory response (Th3/Tr). The etiology of intestinal inflammation stems from the interplay of three elements: a genetic predisposition, some environmental factor (which is part of the normal intestinal flora), and the immune-mediated damage of tissue. Genetic factors may account for an aberrant immune response, increased intestinal permeability, or modified intestinal flora.

The connections between the brain and GI tract are clearly demonstrated by various trophic functions. Certain types of neurotransmitter—one of the families of molecule needed for brain function—are derived from essential amino acids that are consumed in dietary proteins. For instance, the amino acid tryptophan is the precursor of serotonin, whereas tyrosine is the precursor of dopamine, adrenaline, and noradrenaline. Decarboxylation of the amino acid histidine gives rise to histamine, which is then taken up by the brain. Removal of the carboxyl groups is performed by intestinal flora. Consequently, any significant change in the composition of the intestinal flora can lead to the excessive decarboxylation of tryptophan and tyrosine, with reduced uptake from the brain and then reduced synthesis of neurotransmitters. Moreover, these amino acids are in competition for access to the brain; as such, their uptake is dependent upon their plasma concentration. For example, increased decarboxylation of tryptophan raises the uptake of tyrosine. This mechanism is fundamental for survival and the basis of the so-called acute phase reaction (APR) that occurs in cases of danger. In such an instance, tryptophan uptake is reduced and, accordingly, serotonin synthesis is diminished, which leads to the anxiety that allows one to react. Indeed, low levels of tryptophan increase the uptake of tyrosine (more ability), dopamine (more discrimination capacity), noradrenaline (more muscular strength), and finally adrenaline, generating an increased ability to stand and face whatever danger there is. One important factor is the duration of the stressful event that, if prolonged, may lead to a *chronic phase reaction* (CPR), which has been defined by Bengmark as the "mother of all pathologies" [7]. As already reviewed in Chap. 3, these aspects often play a significant role in ischemic heart disease.

Tryptophan is also involved in the synthesis of neuropeptide Y (NPY), a substance that controls neurogenesis and synaptogenesis, and hence the brain's ability to repair itself. However, it is also present in the cardiac autonomic system and therefore may play a role in the neurogenic control of blood flow (for details see Chap. 1). Moreover, tryptophan controls the immune response that, in women, must cyclically diminish to avoid antibody production [6, 7]. This occurs every month at the time of ovulation and before menstruation, when the decreased amount of serotonin leads to the well-known premenstrual syndrome (PMS). For this reason, the GI tract has a greater workload in women than men: tryptophan may not return to normal levels, thus reducing the amount of NPY and the plasticity of the CNS. This may contribute to the greater incidence of neuropsychiatric disorders, like depression, in women and could have a role in gender-based differences observed in ischemic heart disease (see Chap. 6).

In addition, tryptophan controls cell death through apoptosis. Cell survival depends upon the ability of the cell to repair any damage caused by its environment (i.e., repair DNA damaged by radiation or free radicals). It is intestinal flora, with more than 50 billion cells, that supplies the "sewing" molecules that recognize and mend the DNA lesions. If this does not happen, the apoptotic response is triggered so that the cell degenerates and ultimately is eliminated by macrophages.

The daily production of lymphocytes proceeds randomly. However, the antibodies are processed during the maturation steps, and only about 3 % perform their function, the other antibodies being destroyed through apoptosis. In those individuals with greater intestinal permeability, and hence with greater antibody production, the decreased capacity to eliminate "erroneous" antibodies leads to a higher number of autoantibodies.

Moreover, it has been demonstrated that the human microbiota has a critical role in regulating host serotonin (5-hydroxytryptamine, 5H), promoting its biosynthesis from colonic enterochromaffin cells. Microbiota-dependent effects on gut serotonin levels significantly impact host physiology, modulating gastrointestinal motility [8]. Furthermore, serotonin functions as a key neurotransmitter at both terminals of the brain–gut axis. Consequently, the gut microbiota plays a critical role in regulating the normal function of this axis. The developing serotonergic system may be vulnerable to different colonization patterns in young people. In the elderly, decreased diversity may dictate serotonin-related health problems, since the enzymes involved in this pathway are immune and stress responsive. Therapeutic targeting of this gut microbiota might therefore be an effective treatment strategy for serotonin-related brain–gut axis disorders [9].

4.3 Physiology and Pathophysiology of Heart–Gut Interactions

The aforementioned, profoundly embedded nature of the gastroenteric system within the complexity of several interacting processes of the whole organism suggests some role linking the various apparatuses as part of the emergence of several diseases. In particular, increasing evidence supports some influence of the gastroenteric system on cardiovascular activity. Further to ENS and autonomic-mediated processes that regulate coronary blood flow, both directly and indirectly, other indirect mechanisms, such as inflammation and autoimmune reactions, or specific microbiota functions could play a role in ischemic heart disease (see the already-cited Chaps. 1 and 3).

One study has already demonstrated that esophageal acid stimulation can reduce coronary blood flow in patients with coronary artery disease (CAD). This reduction in coronary blood flow was associated with typical angina, in the absence of any significant change in the epicardial coronary artery diameter. It also was not associated with any significant changes in the levels of catecholamines or endothelin-1. Interestingly, coronary blood flow was not affected in a group of heart transplant recipients, suggesting a neural cardioesophageal reflex mechanism [10].

In another study, intra-esophageal acid perfusion evoked the esophago-cardiac reflex and caused subsequent coronary flow velocity reduction in 25 of 51 (49 %) of the patients evaluated. The investigators found a similar prevalence of this reflex in patients with different types of epicardial coronary artery stenosis or microvascular disease and in patients with noncardiac chest pain. This suggests that the presence of this reflex was independent of the underlying structural CAD. By contrast, patients with proven coronary spasm were significantly more liable to have acid perfusion-induced coronary flow reduction and chest pain. This may reflect sympathetic autonomic hyperreactivity in this subset of patients [11].

Since the esophago-cardiac reflex was first suspected of being a pathogenetic factor in the development of angina, a range of anatomical and physiological studies have been conducted to characterize its main features. Morphological studies in rats show that the heart receives collateral projections from nucleus ambiguus neurons. These innervate the esophagus, thereby supporting the previous physiological observation that mechanical stimulation that triggers the esophago-cardiac reflex circuit involves vagal afferents and efferent sympathetic preganglionic pathways [12, 13].

Evidence has also been published that, in humans, both electrical and mechanical stimulation of the esophagus amplify respiratory-driven cardiac vagal afferent modulation while decreasing sympathetic modulation [14, 15]. This shift in the sympatho-vagal balance toward a more parasympathetic component might lead to diminished myocardial perfusion. Furthermore, Mellow et al. were able to induce myocardial ischemia by prolonged esophageal acid stimulation [16].

Moreover, in another study, in 79 % of patients diagnosed with CAD, at least some of their symptoms were related to gastroesophageal reflux disease (GERD), implying the frequent coexistence of GERD and CAD and the necessity to take GERD into consideration in the differential diagnosis of chest pain in CAD patients. Inhibiting the secretion of gastric acid in patients with CAD also had a favorable effect on coronary reserve, estimated by the frequency of angina-like chest pain episodes and the results of electrocardiographic stress testing [17].

Several other studies have demonstrated a link between the gastroenteric and cardiovascular systems focusing on heart rhythm, a major determinant of myocardial ischemia. Some arrhythmic or ischemic episodes in cardiac-sensitive subjects might be directly linked to the functional uncoupling of GI myoelectrical activity following the consumption of particular foods or via other influences on the gut. In patients with functional GI disease, certain foods, like those containing one or more of the fermentable oligosaccharides, disaccharides, monosaccharides, and polyols (FODMAPs), tend to stimulate a quivering/tingly sensation in the mid-abdominal region within minutes to hours after they are consumed. This feeling is often followed immediately by bowel sounds and/or palpitations.

Moreover, stressful stimulation like emotional frustration or performing physical exercise after a meal may lead to heart symptoms. It is thought that the triggering process begins in the gut with the halting of a peristaltic wave contraction. This could be the result of either a slow-moving bolus creating gross distention or via neural disruption attributable to external stress. Following this functional uncoupling of the wave, the automaticity of ectopic behavior could spread to the heart, mediated by the central autonomic network [18, 19].

Studying respiratory sinus arrhythmias (RSA) while performing an electrogastrogram (EGG), a correlation between myoelectrical activity of the gut and the ANS has been further identified [20]. It was shown that the ingestion of 500 ml of water induces linearity between HRV and EGG power. An explanation for this is that whereas during fasting motor activity is modulated by the ENS, after someone is fed, vagal activity contributes to phasic motility and reflects vagal influences on the heart [21].

In fact, both autonomic and anatomical mechanisms have been postulated regarding the role of GERD as a risk factor for atrial fibrillation (AF) [22–37].

Although the actual mechanism by which GERD leads to cardiac arrhythmias remains undetermined, certain observational evidence offers possible explanations. First, GERD could induce vagal nerve stimulation. Accumulating evidence now suggests that the induction of AF may be related to afferent vagal nerve overstimulation and vagal nerve-mediated parasympathetic efferent stimulation (see Chap. 1). Second, the close anatomical relationship between the esophagus and the atria, in addition to the local inflammatory process observed in GERD, theoretically provides a mechanism by which GERD initiates AF via the close positioning of the esophagus and the atria. Third, GERD may induce an autoimmune response that contributes to AF [38–48].

Patients with irritable bowel syndrome (IBS) symptoms have also been shown to have GI sensory stimuli-mediated impaired cardiovascular autonomic responses similar to those seen in patients with GERD [49, 50]. This is likely due to the vagal irritation that occurs in both GERD and IBS. This might also explain how GI stimulation in the form of defecation, cramping, and the consumption of foods like soda, alcohol, greasy foods, and cold water appears to be an important trigger of AF in these patients. There is additional evidence of GI dysmotility after AF ablation which can further exacerbate or initiate GERD/IBS symptoms, as well as an association between esophageal hernias and sustained atrial arrhythmias that has been reported in the literature in both case reports and case series [51].

4.4 Gut–Brain Axis, Emotions, and Mood Disorders

Since the eighteenth century, with the origin of psychology and psychoanalysis, extensive research has been carried out assessing the relationships between emotions, mood disorders, and GI function. In 1909, Walter B Cannon, one of the greatest physiologists of the twentieth century, illustrated a link between psychological processes and upper abdominal symptoms of presumed gastric origin [52].

In 1950 Franz Alexander, in his fundamental book *Psychosomatic Medicine*, clearly described the influence of emotional factors on GI disturbances:

> "The alimentary process is the axis of emotional life in early infancy. The child's universe is centered in nutrition, and the strongest emotions, displeasure and gratification, become associated with various aspects of these functions. Even in later life, many phases of the alimentary process remain linked with certain emotional attitudes....The emotional attitudes which normally stimulate the gastrointestinal function are hunger, the sight and smell of food, the desire to be fed, and the less concrete desire to be helped and to relax" [53].

In the same book, Alexander outlined how "*the eliminative act becomes connected in early life with emotions of possessiveness, pride in accomplishment, the tendency to give and to retain. Certain types of hostile impulse* (*attacking, soiling*) *are also associated with these functions*."

A complete history and description of the rich psychological debate centered around this topic is beyond the scope of this chapter. Suffice it to say that contemporary medical research has taken great strides toward clarifying these relationships. In particular, tremendous progress has been made in characterizing the bidirectional interactions that exists between the CNS, the ENS, and the GI tract.

Numerous studies have demonstrated an association between functional dyspepsia and psychological traits and states or psychiatric disorders. These studies suggest an important intrinsic role of psychosocial factors and psychiatric disorders, especially anxiety and depression, in the etiopathogenesis of functional dyspepsia [54].

To elucidate the role of cerebral serotonin neurotransmission in visceral perception in functional dyspepsia (FD), Tominaga et al. examined the regional expression level of the serotonin transporter (SERT) and its correlation with clinical symptoms in nine patients relative to eight healthy controls, utilizing positron emission tomography (PET) scans of the midbrain, thalamus, caudate, putamen, amygdala, and hippocampus relative to co-registered magnetic resonance images (MRI). Clinical symptoms were assessed using the Gastrointestinal Symptoms Rating Scale (GSRS), Self-Rating Depression Scale (SDS), and State-Trait Anxiety Inventory (STAI). The investigators concluded that upregulation of the SERT level in the midbrain and thalamus may underlie the pathogenesis of FD, like abdominal and psychological symptoms, via some brain–gut interaction [55].

As reported by Bali and Jaggi [56], another important hormone implicated in the complex interactions of the brain and gut is ghrelin, which is primarily synthesized by endocrine cells in the gastric mucosa and has numerous functions that include stimulating the appetite and food intake and the regulation of growth hormone, insulin secretion, glucose and lipid metabolism, GI motility, blood pressure, heart rate, and neurogenesis. Furthermore, peripherally and centrally synthesized ghrelin in the hypothalamus regulates diverse functions in the CNS, including stress-associated behavioral functions. Exposure to stress alters ghrelin levels, and altered ghrelin levels significantly affect neuroendocrinological parameters, metabolism-related physiology, behavior, and mood. Studies have identified both an anxiolytic and anxiogenic role of ghrelin, suggesting dual roles modulating anxiety-related behaviors. However, it has been proposed that increases in ghrelin levels during stress conditions are an endogenous stress-coping behavior and that increased ghrelin levels may be required to prevent excessive anxiety. In preclinical and clinical studies, elevated ghrelin levels during depression have been correlated with its antidepressant activities. Ghrelin-induced modulation of stress and associated conditions has also been linked to alterations in the hypothalamic–pituitary–adrenal (HPA) axis and the autonomic nervous system (mainly the sympathetic nervous system and serotonergic neurotransmission). A reciprocal relationship has been reported between corticotropin-releasing hormone (CRH) and ghrelin, as ghrelin increases the release of CRH, ACTH, and corticosteroids, while CRH decreases the expression of ghrelin. Similarly, ghrelin increases serotonin turnover and, in turn, serotonin controls ghrelin signaling to modulate anxiety-related behaviors.

Moreover, there is evidence that major depression (MD) is accompanied by activation of the inflammatory response and that the inflammatory cytokines and bacterial lipopolysaccharides (LPS) released by gram-negative enterobacteria can cause depressive symptoms [57].

Vagal afferents are also an important neuronal component of the gut–brain axis, allowing bottom-up information flow from the viscera to the CNS. In addition to its role in ingesting behavior, vagal afferent signaling has been implicated as a modulator of mood and affect, including distinct forms of anxiety and fear. Studies on rats demonstrate that innate anxiety and learned fear are both subject to visceral modulation through abdominal vagal afferents, possibly by changing limbic neurotransmitter systems [58]. A series of provocative preclinical studies have suggested a prominent role of gut microbiota in these gut–brain interactions. It is notable that the majority of these studies utilized animal experiments.

In a recent review on this topic, Mayer et al. reported on data collected via studies conducted on rodents raised in a germ-free environment. These results suggest that gut microbiota might influence the development of emotional behavior, stress- and pain-modulation systems, as well as brain neurotransmitter systems. Additionally, microbiota perturbations by probiotics and antibiotics exert modulatory effects on some of these measures in adult animals. Current evidence suggests that multiple mechanisms, including endocrine and neurocrine pathways, may be involved in gut microbiota-to-brain signaling. In turn, the brain can alter microbial composition and behavior via the autonomic nervous system. Future research needs to focus on confirming that the rodent findings are translatable to human physiology and to diseases like IBS, autism, anxiety, depression, and Parkinson's disease [59].

All these observations have been combined with increasing evidence that has culminated in the concept of the brain–gut axis, which might be better referred to as the *microbiome–brain–gut axis*, where all the components are interconnected via a circuitous relationship. The debate about the directionality of the association between psychological and gut disorders is still far from settled, even today, with Cannon being the first to publically acknowledge the possibility of reciprocal interactions or a "vicious circle" [52].

While the methodologies and technologies utilized to evaluate GI function have advanced since these early days, the relationship between emotional states and gut function, both in health and disease, remains prominent in the contemporaneous research agenda.

Moreover, this model of circuitous communication underpins the biopsychosocial concept, first explicitly formulated by George Engel in the late 1970s; he postulated that all illnesses, but especially GI disorders, result from a complex reciprocal interaction between biological/genetic, psychological, and social factors [60].

Meanwhile, Wilhelmsen affirmed that we "cannot experience an emotion or think a thought without biological correlates" [61].

The described pattern becomes even more complex if we think about all the interactions that might exist within the heart–brain–gut–microbiome. In particular, related to emotional and mood disorders, research published over the past 60 years has clearly demonstrated that psychosocial risk factors—mainly depression, anxiety, and stress—can predispose individuals to ischemic heart disease in general and to atherosclerosis in particular. Moreover, they have the same impact of biological risk factors on cardiac diseases (see also Chaps. 1 and 2).

This research of the last several decades opens the way to a better understanding of human beings, who are an unfathomably complex biological system. Contrary to the old paradigm by which cognitive processes were considered an exclusive function of the brain, now we can affirm that a "second brain" also participates in emotional and cognitive processes. This being said, every other organ, but particularly the cardiovascular system, is tightly entwined in this complex set of interrelationships.

The psychophysical organization that exists in humans reaches very high states of complexity as a result of the process of "self-organization" through the balancing of two opposing processes—those involving the differentiation and connection of complex neuronal structures. This allows for harmonious biological communications between the body and the mind.

4.5 Conclusions

It is possible to conclude that gastrointestinal function in general, and the ENS in particular, plays a vital role in the overall well-being of a person. As clearly described in the current chapter, gastrointestinal function also exerts an important influence on cardiac and cardiovascular function.

In a complex paradigm that should inspire us all in our vision of modern medicine, relationships between the various parties, once understood, should generate therapeutic solutions that, to date, seem unimaginable. Health thereby becomes more and more a symphony in which all the instruments play in harmony, while the intestine plays the role of conductor to sustain health.

References

1. Gershon MD (1999) The second brain: a groundbreaking new understanding of nervous disorders of the stomach and intestine. Harper Collins, New York
2. Warden MR, Selimbeyoglu A, Mirzabekov JJ et al (2012) A prefrontal cortex-brainstem neuronal projection that controls response to behavioural challenge. Nature 492 (7429):428–432
3. Carabotti M, Scirocco A, Maselli MA, Severia C (2015) The gut-brain axis: interactions between enteric microbiota, central and enteric nervous systems. Ann Gastroenterol 28 (2):203–209
4. Janssen P, Vanden Berghe P, Verschueren et al (2011) Review article: the role of gastric motility in the control of food intake. Aliment Pharmacol Ther 33(8):880–894
5. Konturek PC, Brzozowski T, Konturek SJ (2011) Stress and gut: pathophysiology, clinical consequences, diagnostic approach and treatment options. J Physiol Pharmacol 62(6):591–599
6. Sartor B (2008) Microbial influences in inflammatory bowel disease. Gastroenterology 134:577–594
7. Bengmark S (2004) Acute and "chronic phase reaction—a mother of disease. Clin Nutr 23:1256–1266
8. Yano JM, Yu K, Donaldson GP, Shastri GG, Ann P, Ma L, Nagler CR, Ismagilov RF, Mazmanian SK, Hsiao EY (2015) Indigenous bacteria from the gut microbiota regulate host serotonin biosynthesis. Cell 161(2):264–276
9. O'Mahony SM, Clarke G, Borre YE, Dinan TG, Cryan JF (2015) Serotonin, tryptophan metabolism and the brain–gut-microbiome axis. Behav Brain Res 277:32–48
10. Chauhan A, Petch MC, Schofield PM (1996) Cardio-oesophageal reflex in humans as a mechanism for "linked angina". Eur Heart J 3:407–413
11. Rosztóczy A, Vass A, Izbéki F et al (2007) The evaluation of gastro-oesophageal reflux and oesophagocardiac reflex in patients with angina-like chest pain following cardiologic investigations. Int J Cardiol 118(1):62–68
12. Cheng SB, Hayakawa T, Kuchiiwa S et al (1999) Evidence for the collateral innervation of the esophagus and the heart from neurons in the compact formation of the nucleus ambiguus of the rat. Brain Res 832:171–174
13. Loomis CW, Yao D, Bieger D (1997) Characterization of an esophagocardiovascular reflex in the rat. Am J Physiol 272:R1783–R1791
14. Bajwa A, Hollerbach S, Kamath MV et al (1997) Neurocardiac response to esophageal electric stimulation in humans: effects of varying stimulation frequencies. Am J Physiol 272:R896–R901
15. Tougas G, Kamath M, Watteel G et al (1997) Modulation of neurocardiac function by esophageal stimulation in humans. Clin Sci 92:167–174
16. Mellow MH, Simpson AG, Watt L et al (1983) Esophageal acid perfusion in coronary artery disease. Induction of myocardial ischemia. Gastroenterology 85:306–312
17. Swiatkowski M, Budzyński J, Kłopocka M et al (2004) Suppression of gastric acid production may improve the course of angina pectoris and the results of treadmill stress test in patients with coronary artery disease. Med Sci Monit 10(9):CR524–CR529
18. Powers D (2009) Gastrointestinal influence on the electrophysiology of the heart: induction of cardiac arrhythmic episodes by myoelectrical uncoupling within the gut. J Smooth Muscle Res 45(4):139–148
19. Magge S, Lembo A (2012) Low-FODMAP diet for treatment of irritable bowel syndrome. Gastroenterol Hepatol (NY) 8(11):739–745
20. Chen CL, Kuo TBJ, Lin HH et al (2004) Transfer function analysis of heart rate variability in response to water intake: correlation with gastric myoelectrical activity. J Appl Physiol 96:2226–2230
21. Grubb BP (2005) Neurocardiogenic syncope and related disorders of Grubb orthostatic intolerance. Circulation 111(22):2997–3006

22. Gillinov AM, Rice TW (2004) Prandial atrial fibrillation: off-pump pulmonary vein isolation with hiatal hernia repair. Ann Thorac Surg 78(5):1836–1838
23. Gordon J, Saleem SM, Ngaage DL, Thorpe JA (2002) Swallow syncope associated with paroxysmal atrial fibrillation. Eur J Cardiothorac Surg 21(3):587–590
24. Nakamura H, Nakaji G, Shimazu et al (2007) Case of paroxysmal atrial fibrillation improved after the administration of proton pump inhibitor for associated reflux esophagitis. Fukuoka Igaku Zasshi 98(6):270–276
25. Stollberger C, Finsterer J (2003) Treatment of esophagitis/vagitis-induced paroxysmal atrial fibrillation by proton-pump inhibitors. J Gastroenterol 38(11):1109
26. Schilling RJ, Kaye GC (1998) Paroxysmal atrial flutter suppressed by repair of a large paraesophageal hernia. Pacing Clin Electrophysiol 21(6):1303–1305
27. Landmark K, Storstein O (1979) Ectopic atrial tachycardia on swallowing. Report on favourable effect of verapamil. Acta Med Scand 205(3):251–254
28. Spechler SJ (1992) Epidemiology and natural history of gastro-oesophageal reflux disease. Digestion 51(1):24–29
29. Dent J, El-Serag HB, Wallander MA, Johansson S (2005) Epidemiology of gastro-oesophageal reflux disease: a systematic review. Gut 54:710–717
30. Chang CS, Poon SK, Lien HC, Chen GH (1997) The incidence of reflux esophagitis among the Chinese. Am J Gastroenterol 92:668–671
31. Lee YC, Wang HP, Chiu HM et al (2006) Comparative analysis between psychological and endoscopic profiles in patients with gastroesophageal reflux disease: a prospective study based on screening endoscopy. J Gastroenterol Hepatol 21:798–804
32. Goh KL (2004) Changing epidemiology of gastroesophageal reflux disease in the Asian-Pacific region: an overview. J Gastroenterol Hepatol 19:S22–S25
33. Fock KM, Talley NJ, Fass R et al (2008) Asia-Pacific consensus on the management of gastroesophageal reflux disease: update. J Gastroenterol Hepatol 23:8–22
34. Ho KY, Cheung TK, Wong BC (2006) Gastroesophageal reflux disease in Asian countries: disorder of nature or nurture? J Gastroenterol Hepatol 21:1362–1365
35. Kunz JS, Hemann B, Edwin Atwood J et al (2009) Is there a link between gastroesophageal reflux disease and atrial fibrillation? Clin Cardiol 32:584–587
36. Bunch TJ, Packer DL, Jahangir A et al (2008) Long-term risk of atrial fibrillation with symptomatic gastroesophageal reflux disease and esophagitis. Am J Cardiol 102:1207–1211
37. Huang CC, Chan WL, Luo JC et al (2012) Gastroesophageal reflux disease and atrial fibrillation: a nationwide population-based study. PLoS One 7(10). doi: 10.1371/journal.pone.0047575
38. Kollarik M, Brozmanova M (2009) Cough and gastroesophageal reflux: insights from animal models. Pulm Pharmacol Ther 22:130–134
39. Dodds WJ, Dent J, Hogan WJ et al (1982) Mechanisms of gastroesophageal reflux in patients with reflux esophagitis. N Engl J Med 307:1547–1552
40. Schauerte P, Scherlag BJ, Pitha J et al (2000) Catheter ablation of cardiac autonomic nerves for prevention of vagal atrial fibrillation. Circulation 102:2774–2780
41. Kanoupakis EM, Manios EG, Mavrakis HE et al (2000) Relation of autonomic modulation to recurrence of atrial fibrillation following cardioversion. Am J Cardiol 86:954–958
42. Hou Y, Scherlag BJ, Lin J, Zhang Y, Lu Z et al (2007) Ganglionated plexi modulate extrinsic cardiac autonomic nerve input: effects on sinus rate, atrioventricular conduction, refractoriness, and inducibility of atrial fibrillation. J Am Coll Cardiol 50:61–68
43. Frustaci A, Chimenti C, Bellocci F et al (1997) Histological substrate of atrial biopsies in patients with lone atrial fibrillation. Circulation 96:1180–1184
44. Tsao HM, Wu MH, Higa S et al (2005) Anatomic relationship of the esophagus and left atrium: implication for catheter ablation of atrial fibrillation. Chest 128:2581–2587
45. Rieder F, Cheng L, Harnett KM et al (2007) Gastroesophageal reflux disease-associated esophagitis induces endogenous cytokine production leading to motor abnormalities. Gastroenterology 132:154–165

46. Maixent JM, Paganelli F, Scaglione J, Lévy S (1998) Antibodies against myosin in sera of patients with idiopathic paroxysmal atrial fibrillation. J Cardiovasc Electrophysiol 9:612–617
47. Chauhan A, Mullins PA, Taylor G et al (1996) Cardioesophageal reflex: a mechanism for 'linked angina' in patients with angiographically proven coronary artery disease. J Am Coll Cardiol 27:1621–1628
48. Nishida K, Qi XY, Wakili R et al (2011) Mechanisms of atrial tachyarrhythmias associated with coronary artery occlusion in a chronic canine model. Circulation 123:137–146
49. Punyabati O, Deepak KK, Sharma MP, Dwivedi SN (2000) Autonomic nervous system reactivity in irritable bowel syndrome. Indian J Gastroenterol 19(3):122–125
50. Adeyemi EO, Desai KD, Towsey M, Ghista D (1999) Characterization of autonomic dysfunction in patients with irritable bowel syndrome by means of heart rate variability studies. Am J Gastroenterol 94(3):816–823
51. Reddy YM, Singh D, Nagarajan D et al (2013) Atrial fibrillation ablation in patients with gastroesophageal reflux disease or irritable bowel syndrome-the heart to gut connection! Interv Card Electrophysiol 37(3):259–265. doi:10.1007/s10840-013-9807-5
52. Cannon WB (1909) The influence of emotional states on the functions of the alimentary canal. Am J Med Sci 137:480–486
53. Alexander F (1950) Psychosomatic medicine. Its principles and applications. W.W. Norton, New York, pp 85–86, 116
54. Van Oudenhove L, Aziz Q (2013) The role of psychosocial factors and psychiatric disorders in functional dyspepsia. Nat Rev Gastroenterol Hepatol 10(3):158–167. doi:10.1038/nrgastro.2013.10
55. Tominaga K, Tsumoto C, Ataka S et al (2015) Regional brain disorders of serotonin neurotransmission are associated with functional dyspepsia. Life Sci 137:150–157. doi:10.1016/j.lfs.2015.07.023
56. Bali A, Jaggi AS (2015) An integrative review on role and mechanisms of ghrelin in stress, anxiety and depression. Curr Drug Targets [Epub ahead of print]
57. Maes M, Kubera M, Leunis JC (2008) The gut-brain barrier in major depression: intestinal mucosal dysfunction with an increased translocation of LPS from gram negative enterobacteria (leaky gut) plays a role in the inflammatory pathophysiology of depression. Neuro Endocrinol Lett 1:117–124
58. Klarer M, Arnold M, Günther L (2014) Gut vagal afferents differentially modulate innate anxiety and learned fear. J Neurosci 34(21):7067–7076. doi:10.1523/JNEUROSCI.0252-14.2014
59. Mayer EA, Tillisch K, Gupta A (2015) Gut/brain axis and the microbiota. J Clin Invest 125 (3):926–938. doi:10.1172/JCI76304
60. Engel GL (1977) The need for a new medical model: a challenge for biomedicine. Science 196 (4286):129–136
61. Wilhelmsen I (2000) Brain-gut axis as an example of the bio-psycho-social model. Gut 47 (Suppl 4):iv5–iv7

Sleep and Dreams in Cardiovascular Pathophysiology

5

Loreta Di Michele

We are such stuff
As dreams are made on, and our little life
Is rounded with a sleep.
William Shakespeare, The Tempest

5.1 Introduction

Why do we sleep? It may appear strange, but even today neuroscientists remain unable to provide a complete answer to this question. This is probably because the field of sleep medicine is still in its relative infancy, only officially recognized in 1953 with the discovery, by Nathaniel Kleitman and Eugene Aserinsky, of rapid eye movement (REM) sleep [1]. Up until that time, sleep was considered an entirely passive state: as "the absence of wakefulness" (Lucretius) or as a "suspension of sensory faculties" (Hartley 1749–Macnish 1830) [2]. It was not until the twentieth century that sleep theories started to be based on robust scientific evaluation, the first documented research published in 1929 as Hans Berger's discovery of α waves during the first electroencephalogram (EEG) performed in a human [3]. With this capability, Loomis and collaborators first observed, in 1937, the EEG wave changes that occur as one moves through the different stages of sleep [4, 5].

Kleitman's and Aserinsky's discovery of REM sleep and its association with dreaming shook the scientific community of that time and led to intense research. EEGs performed using Rechtschaffen and Kales' technique became the fundamental tool for sleep studies all over the world [6]. The neurophysiological mechanism of REM sleep was first described in the 1960s, by Jouvet, through transection

L. Di Michele, MD (✉)
San Camillo-Forlanini Hospital, Via Portuense 332, Rome, Italy
e-mail: lorydm1965@libero.it

A. Roncella, C. Pristipino (eds.), *Psychotherapy for Ischemic Heart Disease*,
DOI 10.1007/978-3-319-33214-7_5

studies in which he discovered both the location of the pons and its role in REM sleep [7, 8].

Despite considerable evidence documenting how sleep is far from a passive state, several questions still had to be addressed. Among them were: What induces drowsiness? And what are the mechanisms that regulate the sleep/wake cycle? Kleitman believed, in accordance with the theories of his time, that wakefulness was simply maintained by means of continuous sensory afferent stimuli to the brain. This belief was based on Bremer's historical experiment, in which different levels of transection were performed on the central nervous system (CNS) of cats. For the transection called the "encephale isolé," the cut was made between the bulb and spinal cord; and the circadian patterns of rest and activity were maintained. Conversely, for the transection called "cerveau isolé," the cut was made between the brain and brain stem; after this, the experimental animal fell into a deep sleep and brain activity was characterized by continuous slow waves. Bremer hypothesized that, with the "cerveau isolé," all external stimuli were interrupted as well as all of the sensory stimuli to the cortex responsible for wakefulness [9].

In 1948, Moruzzi and Magoun invalidated Bremer's theory with their discovery of the ascending reticular activating system (RAS), located between the pons and mesencephalic tegmentum. Electrical stimulation of this area aroused the cortex, leading to wakefulness [10]. This discovery by Moruzzi and Magoun provided the physiological basis for subsequent sleep studies [11]. Also during this period, Hess postulated the existence of a "sleep center" based on the observation that electrical stimuli administered to the thalamus induced and maintained the sleep state [12]. A few years later, the importance of these areas in the active synchronization of the brain cortex was elucidated [13].

In reality, while there is a strong need to understand these mechanisms in explicit terms, sleep/wakefulness circuits should not be oversimplified. In fact, several recent studies have shown that sleep is a nervous, active, and rhythmic process ruled by a circadian pacemaker in the suprachiasmatic nucleus of the anterior hypothalamus. It is influenced by the light/dark cycle, by internal and hormonal factors, and by temperature. The thalamic reticular nucleus is the executor system that generates the synchronization and regulates different sleep stages. It is influenced by hormonal factors, previous wakefulness experiences, and various psychological and environmental factors.

5.2 Normal Sleep Architecture

Human sleep studies are conducted in accordance with the conventional method that was initially described by Rechschaffen and Kales and is based upon the visual inspection of EEG waves, submental electromyography (EMG), and eye movement detection by electrooculogram (EOG) [6]. There are two types of sleep: (a) non-REM (NREM) sleep, characterized by neuronal slowing and synchronization that determine waves of particular frequency and amplitude, and (b) REM sleep, associated with vivid dreams and intense brain activity (Table 5.1).

Table 5.1 Normal human sleep

NREM sleep (75 % of total sleep)	Stage 1	Transition from wakefulness into sleep
	Stage 2	Light sleep
	Stages 3 and 4	Slow-wave sleep–deep sleep
REM sleep (25 % of total sleep)	Tonic REM sleep	Desynchronized EEG Skeletal muscle atonia
	Phasic REM sleep	Rapid eye movements in all directions Irregular breathing Heart rate changes Variable blood pressure
Sleep cycle	Period of NREM sleep + Period of REM sleep	90–120 min
Other characteristics	Regulated by homeostatic and circadian factors	
	Modulated by environmental factors	
	Influenced by hormonal factors, previous wakefulness experience, and psychological factors	

5.2.1 NREM Sleep

Non-REM sleep is subdivided into four stages. NREM sleep stage 1 is the transition from wakefulness to sleep. Its EEG activity is characterized by diffuse theta waves (4–6 Hz) and vertex sharp waves. EMG activity decreases and the EOG exhibits slow, rolling eye movements. NREM sleep stage 2 is light sleep. Predominant theta activity exists in which sleep spindles (11–16 Hz waveforms lasting at least 0.5 s) and K complexes (triphasic slow and large waves) are inserted, especially in frontal regions. They are associated with an active synchronization process that is controlled by the thalamus, and EMG activity is reduced. NREM sleep stages 3 and 4 constitute slow-wave sleep (SWS) or deep sleep. In these last two stages of NREM sleep, the EEG is characterized by the presence of delta waves. Meanwhile, the EOG registers no eye movements and muscle tone is further diminished relative to wakefulness.

5.2.2 REM Sleep

The first REM sleep occurs 90–120 min after the onset of NREM sleep. In REM sleep, the EEG tracings are very similar to those of NREM sleep stage 1, with the exception of sawtooth waves especially over the frontal cortex. REM sleep is also called "paradoxical sleep" because the brain, unlike its state in NREM sleep, is

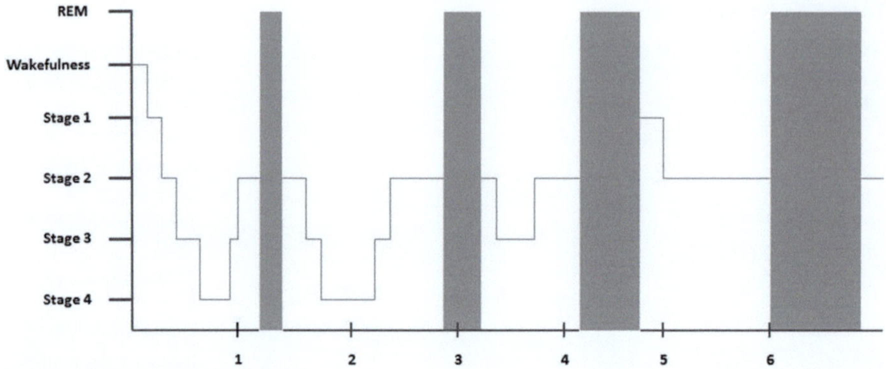

Fig. 5.1 Young adult hypnogram

metabolically, physiologically, and psychologically highly active. REM sleep is divided into two stages: tonic and phasic REM. EEG desynchronization and skeletal muscle atonia are the main features of tonic REM, while phasic REM is characterized by REMs in all directions, transient swings in blood pressure, heart rate changes, and irregular breathing due to increased sympathetic activity.

5.2.3 Sleep Cycle

The transition from wakefulness to sleep that occurs during NREM sleep becomes deeper from stage 1 through SWS. Roughly 90 min later, REM sleep begins, usually of short duration, followed by another period of NREM sleep. The sleep cycle refers to a single period of NREM sleep followed by a period of REM sleep. Each NREM to REM sleep cycle takes approximately 90–120 min and occurs four to six times each night. In general, NREM sleep is prominent over the first third of the night, while REM sleep predominates in the last third. A hypnogram (Fig. 5.1) depicts the alternating sleep phases and cycles. A normal night's sleep consists of roughly 50 % light sleep, 25 % deep sleep, and 25 % REM sleep.

5.3 Sleep and Cardiovascular Pathophysiology

In the pre-polygraphic era, scientists described "quiet" and "agitated" sleep, based upon simple visual observations. This distinction, which was due to changes in sympatho-vagal balance during sleep, was better understood only after polygraphic recordings came into existence and REM sleep was identified [14].

The autonomic nervous system (ANS) regulates vital functions related to whole-body homeostasis. Activation of the CNS, whether by external or internal stimuli, prompts a series of ANS responses, which may therefore be assimilated as a filter. The ANS consists of a sympathetic component (in essence, accelerating action) and

Table 5.2 Autonomic nervous system (ANS) activity during sleep

Sleep	Parasympathetic activity	Sympathetic activity
NREM sleep	Increased	Decreased
Tonic REM sleep Phasic REM sleep	Further increased	Further decreased Intermittent increases

a parasympathetic component (slowing action). The balance between sympathetic and parasympathetic activity is fundamental to maintaining a physiologically normal balance. Any imbalance might be unhealthy.

Sympathetic hyperactivity reduced through medicinal treatment is associated with a significant reduction in cardiovascular events. In fact, sympatho-vagal balance significantly influences the prognosis of a range of cardiovascular diseases.

In general, sympathetic activity is more evident during the day, while parasympathetic activity primarily occurs at night [15]. More specifically, during NREM sleep, parasympathetic activity increases and sympathetic activity decreases (Table 5.2). This trend progresses further during tonic REM sleep; and only in phasic REM sleep is sudden activation of the sympathetic system observed [16, 17]. Therefore, blood pressure, heart rate, cardiac output, and peripheral vascular resistance are progressively reduced, in response to increased parasympathetic activity, in NREM sleep. It is known that the heart rate slows down by 5–8 % during NREM sleep. This reduction is more evident from NREM sleep stage 1 to SWS in which parasympathetic activity is very stable, but sometimes interrupted by arousal stimuli (e.g., noise, respiratory events, position changing) during which bursts of sympathetic activity are detected. Phasic REM is characterized by great variability in sympathetic activity, resulting in phasic increases in blood pressure and heart rate. Such events often coincide with other phasic phenomena like irregular breathing, peripheral vasoconstriction, and bursts of REM.

Therefore, during phasic REM, sudden increases in heart rate and increased myocardial oxygen demand may precipitate cardiac events—ranging from nocturnal arrhythmia to myocardial ischemia and myocardial infarction—in those who are predisposed, including patients already symptomatic for ischemic heart disease (see Chap. 1). Phasic REM is then assumed to potentially provoke major cardiac events, especially in subjects with already-compromised cardiocirculatory function, due to sympathetic hyperactivity that induces increased cardiac work, enhances platelet aggregation and thrombus formation, activates the endothelium, facilitates vasospasm, might provoke the rupture of vulnerable plaques, and could cause fatal arrhythmias [18] (see Chap. 1).

Furthermore, vivid dreams with a high emotional content, which are only associated with REM sleep, can precipitate cardiac events in predisposed individuals [19]. The intensity of emotional content during the dreaming experience may be as strong as or even stronger than those experienced during wakefulness. Not coincidentally, REM sleep was defined by Jouvet as "paradoxical sleep," associated with marked muscular hypotonia to the point of near paralysis [8], yet also characterized by intense brain activity. With vivid dreams, the emotional

Table 5.3 Circadian factors that might help to precipitate myocardial infarction and stroke

Phenomena that occur upon awakening
Resumption of physical and mental activity
Potential emotional stress
Increased platelet aggregation
Increased coagulability and blood viscosity
Increased vascular tone
Increased blood pressure and heart rate
Increased serum cortisol
Increased plasma catecholamines

contents of the dream are "lived" as though the sleeper is awake. Muscular paralysis is the mechanism through which dreaming movements are prevented.

This consideration has led sleep scientists, starting in the 1960s, to suspect that REM sleep, with these particular characteristics, could be a risk factor for major cardiovascular events and even sudden death during sleep. In the 1960s, this link between REM sleep and cardiac events was documented, but did not appear to be as strong as formerly believed [20–23].

The incidence of major cardiovascular events (myocardial infarction and stroke) peaks between 6:00 A.M. and noon [24]. One explanation for this is a series of hemodynamic changes that begin during sleep and reach their peak in the morning upon awakening. With waking, platelet aggregation increases [25, 26] and, associated with a series of other phenomena that occur at this time, could lead to a major event (Table 5.3).

The sympatho-vagal balance that exists during sleep plays an important role in triggering nocturnal cardiac arrhythmias. A clear example of this is vagus-induced atrial fibrillation, which appears only during sleep and spontaneously resolves in the morning [27]. The vagal hyperactivity typical of NREM sleep can cause bradyarrhythmias even in healthy individuals. Prolonged atrioventricular (AV) conduction, Wenckebach AV block, and clinically important sinus bradycardia, which can cause pauses in sinus rhythm lasting more than 2 s, can be observed. Also in the literature are reported cases of asystole lasting up to 9 s during REM sleep in young adults with apparently normal cardiac function [20]. People with acquired or congenital Q-T interval prolongation are predisposed to nocturnal cardiac arrhythmias due to physiological variations caused by the altered sympatho-vagal balance of normal sleep. Sudden death in these individuals is not unusual, precipitated by sudden increases in sympathetic activity [28].

On its own, sympathetic hyperactivity during sleep is pro-arrhythmogenic. Nevertheless, it becomes even more pro-arrhythmogenic in the presence of ischemia, which induces myocardial alterations leading to electrical instability [29]. Obstructive sleep apnea (OSA) may be an underestimated trigger for cardiovascular events (stroke, cardiac arrhythmias, myocardial infarction) [30–38]. OSA is characterized by recurrent episodes of interrupted respiratory airflow during sleep secondary to upper airway collapse, resulting in clinically significant hemodynamic effects [30–39] due to the excessive sympathetic activity that occurs during sleep. Moreover, OSA can initiate and maintain systemic inflammation through intermittent hypoxemia [40]. Interestingly, patients with OSA appear to exhibit a different peak in sudden death incidence than otherwise generally observed, associated with a higher rate of cardiovascular events during the night, as opposed to the morning, especially in people between the ages of 30 and 49 years [41]. As such, OSA is a sleep-associated respiratory disease with neurological symptoms (e.g., excessive daytime sleepiness) that also is linked to increased mortality from cardiovascular causes [42]. Given the relatively high prevalence of OSA in the general population, especially among those who are overweight, clinicians need to remain vigilant as to its presence and treat it early in its course.

5.4 Research Perspectives

Although science is not yet able to explain all the great mysteries of sleep, considerable evidence now exists to help us to better understanding this third of our lives.

It is true that we spend nearly one third of our lives asleep; however, the pace of modern society often leads us to neglect this important and ancient biological function. Not surprisingly, the most frequent sleep disorder is voluntary sleep deprivation. Nevertheless, the need to sleep becomes irresistible at a certain point. Sleep deprivation experiments have shown how sleep is important for learning [43] and memory consolidation [44], as well as for the efficiency of our immune system [45–47]; how it is involved in controlling body weight [48]; and how it aids in the regulation of certain hormones [49, 50]. In essence, we could think of it as an essential step to achieving the proper alignment of all biological and systemic functions. Sleep deprivation increases one's risk of developing cardiovascular disease [51, 52] and extreme deprivation experiments have shown that lack of sleep leads to death. These findings have been documented in both animals [53] and humans. *Fatal familial insomnia* (FFI), a rare autosomal dominant disease of the brain, typically leads to death from exhaustion within 10 to 12 months of the onset of neurological symptoms [54]. Beyond sleep's restorative properties, recent research seems to indicate an important role of sleep in the removal of neurotoxic proteins linked to neurodegenerative diseases (e.g., β-amyloid, α-synuclein, and tau) that accumulate while we are awake [55].

Even less is known about dreams than about sleep and, in some ways, the mystery behind dreams is growing. It has become known, for example, that dream experiences may also occur during NREM sleep. Nevertheless, vivid and long-term dreams are typically REM sleep associated. Dreams and their emotional content sometimes so intense they awaken us, achieving their maximal adverse emotional impact with nightmares. Suddenly awakening from a terror-filled dream is always associated with significant increases in blood pressure and heart rate, as well as cold sweats and changes in the frequency and depth of breathing. It is therefore not so unreasonable to postulate some precipitating role of a dream's emotional content for cardiovascular events [56]. This has been reported in the literature, but further research is necessary. Establishing how the content of dreams might affect one's risk of cardiovascular disease and events has become both an intriguing and vitally important field of research.

5.5 Conclusions

Sleep is essential to life. Even though sleep researchers have been discovering numerous sleep functions that go far beyond simple mind and body restoration, the roles of dreams remain poorly understood. Freud postulated that dreams are merely the way through which our most unconscious desires are fulfilled. Consequently, since the origin of psychoanalysis, dreams have been an important area of research and application in psychology and psychotherapy.

Knowledge about the numerous physiological changes that occur in the ANS is expanding the potential role of sleep and dreams in both health and sickness. This includes the emotional content of dreams that, in themselves, might exert a further significant influence on the risk of major cardiovascular events and diseases. Further studies are clearly needed to clarify this fascinating relationship.

References

1. Aserinsky E, Kleitmann N (1953) Regularly occurring periods of eye motility and concomitant phenomena during sleep. Science 118:273–274
2. Macnish R (1830) The philosophy of sleep. E. M'Phun, Glasgow
3. Berger H (1929) Uber das elektrenkephalogram. Arch Psychiatr Nervenkrank 87:527–570
4. Loomis AL, Harvey EN, Hobart G (1935) Potential rhythms of the cerebral cortex during sleep. Science 81:597–598
5. Loomis AL, Harvey EN, Hobart G (1937) Cerebral states during sleep as studied by human brain potentials. J Exp Psychol 21:127–144
6. Rechtschaffen A, Kales A (1968) A manual of standardized terminology, techniques and scoring systems for sleep stages of human subjects. UCLA Brain Information Service/Brain Research Institute, Los Angeles
7. Jouvet M (1962) Recherches sur les structure nerveuses et les mècanismes responsables des diffèrentes phases du sommeil physiologique. Arch Ital Biol 100:125–206
8. Jouvet M (1965) Paradoxical sleep: a study of its nature and mechanism. In: Akert K, Bally C, Schadè JP (eds) Sleep mechanism. Elsevier, Amsterdam, pp 20–57
9. Bremer F (1935) Cerveau "isolè" et physiologie du sommeil. C R Soc Biol 118:1235–1241
10. Moruzzi G, Magoun HW (1949) Brain stem reticular formation and activation of the EEG. Electroencephalogr Clin Neurophysiol 1:455–473
11. Moruzzi G (1972) The sleep-waking cycle. Ergebn Physiol 64:1–163
12. Akert K, Koella WP, Hess R Jr (1952) Sleep produced by electrical stimulation of the thalamus. Am J Physiol 168(1):260–267
13. Steriade M, Dornich L, Oakson G, Dechenes M (1987) The differential reticular thalamic nucleus generates spindle rhythmicity. J Neurophysiol 57:269–273
14. Dement W, Kleitman N (1957) Cyclic variation in EEG during sleep and their relation to eye movements, body motility, and dreaming. Electroenceph Clin Neurophysiol 9:673–690

15. Cooke-Ariel H (1998) Circadian variations in cardiovascular function and their relation to the occurrence and timing of cardiac events. Am J Health Syst Pharm 55(3):S5–S11
16. Terplan M (1993) Sympathetic-nerve activity during sleep. N Engl J Med 328(25):180
17. Somers VK, Dyken ME, Mark AL, Abboud FM (1993) Sympathetic-nerve activity during sleep in normal subjects. N Engl J Med 328:303–307
18. Verrier RL, Muller JE, Hobson JA (1996) Sleep, dreams, and sudden death: the case for sleep as an autonomic stress test for the heart. Cardiovasc Res 31:181–211
19. Bassetti C, Jung HH, Hess CW (1997) Near cardiac death with onset in REM sleep: a polysomnographic case report. J Sleep Res 6(1):57–58
20. Guilleminault C, Pool P, Motta J, Gillis A (1984) Sinus arrest during REM sleep in young adults. N Engl J Med 311:1006–1010
21. Nowlin JB, Troyer WG, Collins WS et al (1965) The association of nocturnal angina pectoris with dreaming. Ann Intern Med 63:1040–1046
22. Lavery CE, Mittleman MA et al (1997) Nonuniform nighttime distribution of acute cardiac events: a possible effect of sleep states. Circulation 5:3321–3327
23. Coccagna G, Capucci A, Pierpaoli S (1999) A case of sinus arrest and vagal overactivity during REM sleep. Clin Auton Res 9:135–138
24. Muller JE, Stone PH, Turi ZG (1985) Circadian variation in the frequency of onset of acute myocardial infarction. N Engl J Med 313:1315–1322
25. Tofler GH, Brezinski D, Schafer AI (1987) Concurrent morning increase in platelet aggregability and the risk of myocardial infarction and sudden cardiac death. N Engl J Med 316:1514–1518
26. Andreotti F, Davies GJ, Hackett DR (1988) Major circadian fluctuations in fibrinolytic factors and possible relevance to time of onset of myocardial infarction, sudden cardiac death and stroke. Am J Cardiol 62:635–637
27. Singh J, Mela T, Ruskin J (2004) Images in cardiovascular medicine. Sleep (vagal)-induced atrial fibrillation. Circulation 110:32–33
28. Browne KF, Prystowsky E, Heger JJ (1983) Prolongation of the Q-T interval in man during sleep. Am J Cardiol 52:55–59
29. Bonsignore MR, Smirne S, Marrone O (1999) Myocardial ischemia during sleep. Sleep Med Rev 3:241–255
30. Bradley TD, Floras JS (2003) Sleep apnoea and heart failure. Circulation 107:1671–1678
31. Shamsuzzaman AS, Gersh BJ, Somers VK (2003) Obstructive sleep apnea: implication for cardiac and vascular disease. JAMA 290:1906–1914
32. Gami AS, Pressman G, Caples SM (2004) Association of atrial fibrillation and obstructive sleep apnea. Circulation 110:364–367
33. Harbison J, O'Reilly P, McNicholas WT (2000) Cardiac rhythm disturbances in the obstructive sleep apnea syndrome: effects of nasal continuous positive air way pressure therapy. Chest 118:591–595
34. Gami AS, Howard DE, Olson EJ (2005) Day-night pattern of sudden death in obstructive sleep apnea. N Engl J Med 352:1206–1214
35. Lavie P, Herer P, Hoffstein V (2000) Obstructive sleep apnea syndrome as a risk factor for hypertension: population study. BMJ 320:479–482
36. Mehra R, Benjamin EJ, Shahar E et al (2006) Association of nocturnal arrhythmias with sleep-disordered breathing: the sleep heart health study. Am J Respir Crit Care Med 173:910–916
37. Gami SA, Olson EJ, Shen WK et al (2013) Obstructive sleep apnea and the risk of sudden cardiac death: a longitudinal study of 10,701 adults. J Am Coll Cardiol 62(7):10–16
38. Nieto FJ, Young TB, Lind BK (2000) Association of sleep-disordered breathing, sleep apnea, and hypertension in a large community-based study. Sleep heart health study. JAMA 283:1829–1836
39. Laaban JP, Pascal-Sebaoun S, Bloch E et al (2002) Left ventricular systolic dysfunction in patients with obstructive sleep apnea syndrome. Chest 122:1133–1138

40. Foster GE, Poulin MJ, Hanly AJ (2006) Intermittent hypoxia and vascular function: implication for obstructive sleep apnoea. Exp Physiol 92:51–65
41. Lamberts M, Nielsen OW, Lip GY et al (2014) Cardiovascular risk in patients with sleep apnoea with or without continuous positive airway pressure therapy: follow-up of 4.5 million Danish adults. J Intern Med 276(6):659–666. doi:10.1111/joim.12302
42. Marin JM, Carrizo SJ, Vicente E et al (2005) Long-term cardiovascular outcomes in men with obstructive sleep apnoea-hypopnea with or without treatment with continuous positive airway pressure: an observational study. Lancet 365:1046–1053
43. Huber R (2004) Local sleep and learning. Nature 430:78–81
44. Hagewould R, Whitcomb SN, Heeringa AN (2010) A time for learning and a time for sleep: the effect of sleep deprivation on contextual fear conditioning at different times of the day. Sleep 33(10):1315–1322
45. Moldofsky H, Lue FA, Davidson JR, Gorczynski R (1989) Effect of sleep deprivation on human immune functions. FASEB J 3(8):1972–1977
46. Brown R, Pang G, Husband AJ, King MG (1989) Suppression of immunity to virus infection in the respiratory tract following sleep disturbance. Reg Immunol 2(5):321–325
47. Fondel E, Axelsson J, Franck K et al (2011) Short natural sleep is associated with higher T cell and lower NK cell activities. Brain Behav Immun 25:1367–1375
48. Seegers V, Petit D, Falissard B et al (2011) Short sleep duration and body mass index: a prospective longitudinal study in preadolescence. Am J Epidemiol 173:621–629
49. Balbo M, Leproult R, Van Cauter E (2010) Impact of sleep and its disturbances on hypothalamo-pituitary-adrenal axis activity. Int J Endocrinol 2010:759234. doi:10.1155/2010/759234
50. Spiegel K, Leproult R, Van Cauter E (1999) Impact of sleep debt on metabolic and endocrine function. Lancet 354:1435–1439
51. Meisinger C, Heier M, Lowel H et al (2007) Sleep duration and sleep complaints and risk of myocardial infarction in middle-aged men and women from the general population: the MONICA/KORA Augsburg cohort study. Sleep 30:1121–1127
52. Laugsand LE, Vatten LJ, Platou C et al (2011) Insomnia and the risk factor of acute myocardial infarction: a population study. Circulation 124:2073–2081
53. Rechtscaffen A, Gilliand MA, Bergmann MB et al (1983) Physiological correlates of prolonged sleep deprivation in rats. Science 221(4606):182–184
54. Montagna P, Gambetti P, Cortelli P et al (2003) Familial and sporadic fatal insomnia. Lancet Neurol 2(3):167–176
55. Xie L, Kang H, Xu Q et al (2013) Sleep drives metabolite clearance from the adult brain. Science 342(6156):373–377
56. Selvi Y, Aydin A, Gumrukcuoglu HA et al (2011) Dream anxiety is an emotional trigger for acute myocardial infarction. Psychosomatics 52(6):544–549

The Role of Gender in the Mind–Heart Relationship

6

Marina Risi

Listen to the woman. She is blessed with incredible intuitive power after years of hormonal cycles and after being a caretaker for her family or friends.

Vivian A Kominos [Kominos VA (2010) Cardiovascular Health. In: Maizes V, Low Dog T (Eds) *Integrative Women's Health* Oxford Press, New York, p 612]

6.1 Gender Bias in Medicine

We all "do gender" during all facets of our lives. While talking, walking, working, loving, choosing what to do next, and even thinking, we are "doing gender." And physicians are not excluded from biological and psychosocial gender influences [1], even if medical training assumes that Medical Science is neutral.

For most of history, most research in medicine was performed on male subjects only. In clinical medicine, several studies have identified differences in the diagnostic and therapeutic management of various diseases in male versus female patients [e.g., coronary artery disease (CAD), kidney disease [2], AIDS, psoriasis [3], colorectal cancer [4], and Parkinson's disease]. Most commonly, the gender bias penalizes females; but it can affect men too, prominent examples being osteoporosis, mood disorders, and migraines [5].

The terms *sex* and *gender* have often been used interchangeably; however, they do not have the same meaning. *Sex* refers to the biological differentiation of gametes and sex hormone production. We know, for example, that testosterone and estrogens have more than just hormonal functions; they also impact, in dissimilar ways, the immune and nervous systems, the magnitude of stress responses, and,

M. Risi, MD (✉)
Italian Society of Psychoneuroendocrinoimmunology (SIPNEI), Piazza Mincio 1, 00198 Rome, Italy
e-mail: paolamari.risi@tiscali.it

A. Roncella, C. Pristipino (eds.), *Psychotherapy for Ischemic Heart Disease*,
DOI 10.1007/978-3-319-33214-7_6

ultimately, one's vulnerability to various diseases. On the other hand, the term *gender* is a cultural construction that distinguishes between femininity and masculinity and, in doing so, also implies differences in role assignments, life experiences, career opportunities, ways of thinking, emotions, access to education, incomes, and, ultimately, one's personal and social identity.

Both of these factors, sex and gender, play a primary role in shaping the whole person and represent fundamental determinants of health. This being said, physicians need to pay attention to the trap of assuming the existence of gender differences where there are none, just because some stereotypes about women and men are perceived as true. The still unanswered question is: can we avoid gender bias in Medicine?

6.2 Gender Issue

CAD is a leading cause of morbidity and mortality among men and women. Since 1950, the incidence of CAD has risen among women, while it has declined among men [6]. In 1991, Bernadine Healy, the first woman director of the US National Institutes of Health (NIH), orchestrated two studies that uncovered sex bias in the management of CAD [7]. In the first study, conducted in Maryland and Massachusetts, women were less likely than men to be referred for diagnostic and therapeutic measures after being admitted for an acute coronary event [8]. In the second study, women who had been found to have significant CAD were as likely as men to undergo revascularization, but less likely to undergo the investigations typically leading to catheterization [9]. The latter study was pinpointed as an illustration of the *Yentl syndrome*: "Once a woman showed that she was just like a man, by having severe coronary artery disease . . ., then she was treated as a man would be." (Note that Yentl was the young heroine from a Jewish community in a story by Isaac Singer, who was forced to dress and act like a boy in order to be able to attend school and become educated in the Talmud.)

These publications were followed by a 'cascade' of studies examining sex and gender differences in the pathophysiology of cardiovascular disease. Numerous differences have been identified. First, women have smaller left anterior descending artery and right coronary artery diameters than men. There are also sex differences in the autonomic nervous system's control of the cardiovascular system: women have more parasympathetic activity than men, who have greater sympathetic activity [10]. The levels of lipid components vary at different ages and between the two genders. Total cholesterol and LDL cholesterol levels increase in men between 35 and 50 years of age. In general, high-density lipoprotein cholesterol levels are higher in women than in men, but decrease during the menopause transition.

Current data also suggest that, for secondary prevention, the statin drugs are equally effective in both genders; however, for primary prevention, the CV benefits of lipid-lowering therapy are less clear for women [11]. Diabetes, metabolic syndrome, hypertension, obesity, and hypertriglyceridemia are all stronger risk factors for ischemic heart disease in women than men [12]. The authors of one meta-analysis reported that women with diabetes had a 40 % greater risk of incident CAD than men with diabetes [13]. In fact, the presence of diabetes is thought to strip away any relative protection from ischemic heart disease young women have.

Gender comparisons have generally been rendered particularly difficult because the lifetime development of coronary atherosclerosis in men and women differs. Women with well-functioning ovaries and adequate circulating reproductive hormones seem to be protected against the progression of atherosclerosis until menopause. For this reason, their increase in coronary events occurs roughly 10–15 years later than in men. By the age of 70, women have as much coronary disease as men, but they also have other more complicating conditions that may cause cardiologists to refrain from enacting aggressive therapeutic procedures. Debate over whether women are underdiagnosed and undertreated has, at times, become overheated, such as in the news magazine *Der Spiegel* when it accused German cardiologists of "sexism" [14]. This debate, however, has had one positive effect: to raise public consciousness of the fact that women have virtually the same prevalence of CAD as men, only at an older age.

One explanation for the delay in the recognition of women's cardiac risk may be differences in the clinical presentation of heart disease, as perceived by physicians. Among other differences, their chest pain is more often associated with less typical symptoms like fatigue, shortness of breath, sleep disturbance, back pain, nausea, and weakness [15]. In one historical study [16], 44 internists were randomized to three different groups: two groups viewed videotapes of the same actress performing the role of a patient in a scripted physician–patient interview, but using two distinct approaches. The first physician group observed a "histrionic" characterization, the second a "businesslike" portrayal. Meanwhile, the third group of physicians read a transcript of the interview. The results were that the initial diagnostic impressions differed dramatically: whereas a cardiac cause was suspected by 50 % of physicians within the second and third groups, only 13 % of those viewing the histrionic portrayal suspected heart disease. Twenty years after its initial description, the Yentl syndrome seemed to still be "alive and well" [17].

To date, CAD is still seen as a male disease. It follows that disease prevention policies aim to protect women especially from the risk of breast cancer, neglecting epidemiological data on females' cardiac vulnerability. Currently, the probability of having an acute myocardial infarction at the age of 60 is greater for men than for women (60.6 vs. 33 %). On the other hand, CAD accounts for more deaths in women at the age of 35 years than breast cancer [18]. The female cardiovascular system is protected by estrogens, which enhance vascular function and promote cardiac myocyte survival. However, after menopause the risk of CAD rises 10-fold, compared to 4.6-fold increase in men at the same age. This has been known for several decades; so much that, over the last 30 years of the past century, cardiologists, gynecologists, and family practitioners tended to prescribe hormonal replacement therapy in menopausal women to prevent CAD. Later, epidemiological evidence demonstrated that the remedy was worse than the disease [19]. Consequently, almost magically, physicians suddenly seemed to forget that middle-aged women had a significant and rapidly rising cardiac risk. Apparently, a mechanistic model of medicine struggles to take into account the complex issue of the progressive probability of CAD in women and that more than just a drug is required.

Prevention should start early, during a woman's fertile period, because multiple pregnancies are correlated with an increase in cardiovascular risk [20], particularly if associated with preeclampsia, gestational diabetes, or pregnancy-induced hypertension. Polycystic ovary syndrome is an endocrine/metabolic syndrome that significantly increases the risk of CAD in young women [21]. Recent studies have also shown that women undergoing radiotherapy for breast cancer have an increased risk of cardiac disease and that the magnitude of cardiovascular risk is significantly correlated with the ionizing radiation dose; hence, reducing the ionizing radiation dose and changing a patient's position during radiotherapy might save her from breast cancer, without increasing her risk of death from cardiovascular disease [22]. It may seem incredible, but there is often no exchange of fundamental clinical information between gynecologists, cardiologists, endocrinologist, and radiologists. However, such a multifaceted management team could be fundamental to the correct prevention and treatment of CAD.

Another gender difference is that women very often have a lower burden of atherosclerosis and obstructive CAD relative to the degree of their angina. However, even though they present with less severe CAD symptoms, they still have a worse prognosis than men. Their management is further complicated by women's marked underrepresentation in clinical trials [23], in which they typically account for just 15–30 % of subjects. As a result, women suffering from CAD are handled using a diagnostic and therapeutic protocol based upon conclusions drawn almost exclusively from research on males.

In clinical trials, it is necessary to consider that pharmacokinetics and pharmacodynamics depend on various factors that differ between men and women, like body composition (with women generally having more body fat than men of equal weight), plasma volume, plasma binding proteins, and enzymatic patterns, all of crucial importance in metabolism and consistently different in the two sexes [24].

Therefore, women, who account for 51 % of the human beings on Earth, continue to represent a clinical challenge for cardiologists. Since it is no longer a matter of misogyny or sexism, the recognition of biological sex-based differences should be widespread, so that women can be preventively treated according to their own "real" risk. It must be recognized that the American Heart Association elaborated guidelines for the prevention of cardiovascular disease in women in 2011 [25]. Nevertheless, considerable work still needs to be done to insert a gender-aware perspective into doctors' training.

6.3 Stress and Gender

The assessment of psychosocial influences requires a gender perspective: men and women certainly both undergo life adversities; but stressor patterns, the ways in which personal psychological discomfort presents, and allostatic strategies may differ considerably.

The term *stress* describes an organism's state under the influence of either external or internal stressors that threaten to alter its dynamic equilibrium (see Chaps. 2 and 3). Adaptive changes that occur in response to stressors are both behavioral and physical. Once a certain threshold has been exceeded, a systemic reaction takes place that involves the stress system in the brain, along with its peripheral components, the hypothalamic–pituitary–adrenal (HPA) axis, and the autonomic sympathetic system. Central players among the components of this system are corticotropin-releasing hormone (CRH) and vasopressin (AVP), both released by neurons in the paraventricular nucleus of the hypothalamus, and norepinephrine, which is released from the locus coeruleus within the brain stem as part of an autonomic (sympathetic) response.

Glucocorticoids act upon the immune system, and, in turn, pro-inflammatory cytokines—like tumor necrosis factor-α, interleukin 1, and interleukin 6—stimulate hypothalamic CRH and/or AVP secretion leading indirectly, via glucocorticoid secretion, to limiting the inflammatory reaction.

Since the pioneering studies of Hans Selye [26], it has become clear that the response to stress is nonspecific, but that the biological effects are the same, independent of the pattern of stimulus.

Several other studies have demonstrated that psychosocial stress is a risk factor for cardiovascular disease in both patients with previously established and nonestablished disease [27–29], suggesting that psychosocial support is not only important in the prevention but also in the progression of CAD.

Despite the controversial results of pioneering studies, currently the link between life adversities, stress perception, socioeconomic status, social support, and cardiovascular risk is widely accepted. A broad array of scientific literature describes the steps that lead to maladaptive responses under conditions of chronic stress, consisting of biological factors like increased blood pressure and cholesterol, insulin resistance, atherosclerosis and thrombus formation, endothelial and arterial vasomotor dysfunction, and oxidative stress, in others words, direct enhancement of the inflammatory response. Maladaptive responses during chronic stress may also act indirectly, facilitating dangerous behaviors like smoking, physical inactivity, excessive eating, and sleep deprivation. Unfortunately, males were either the only subjects or a disproportionate majority of subjects in most of these studies. For a review of gender influence on the bidirectional relationships between stress and gastrointestinal function, refer to Chap. 4.

One of the first exceptions was the *Stockholm Female Coronary Risk Study* [30], which has made numerous significant contributions to current knowledge regarding psychosocial risk factors in women. In this study, 292 female patients between the ages of 30 and 65 years who had been hospitalized for either an acute myocardial infarction or unstable angina pectoris were followed for 5 years. The investigators highlighted the role of family and partnership troubles, as well as the double burden of holding a job and caring for the family. And all of these factors were associated with increased cardiovascular risk. Among women who were married or cohabiting with a male partner, those who complained about stress in their relationship had a 2.9-fold increased risk of recurrent events, after adjusting for age, estrogen status, educational level, smoking, diabetes mellitus, triglyceride and LDL cholesterol levels, and left ventricular dysfunction. These findings differed from previous results detected in men.

More recent research confirms the connection between increased cardiovascular risk and a poor-quality marriage in women, but not in men, and mostly at older ages [31]. Termination of a long-term relationship due to the death of a partner is another risk factor, but more so for men than women [32].

One can recognize how a gender perspective is relevant, observing that women have been included on a large scale only over the last two decades in studies examining the relationship between multiple social conflicts or trait personality [33] and health-related outcomes. Not only marital status but competitive events, job-related stress, loneliness, lack of social support, and negative social exchanges with close others can influence systemic well-being, in men as well as in women. Moreover, this is through the same biological mechanism: a heightened inflammatory response. However, both the biological and behavioral adaptive response could be different in men and women. In particular, the following main differences between men and women can be highlighted:

- In the preclinical literature, sex differences in the stress responsiveness of the HPA axis have been known for a long time [34], and sex differences have been reported in response to prenatal stress and resilience [35].
- Many brain regions involved in the stress response (hypothalamus, amygdala, hippocampus, anterior cingulated cortex) are sexually dimorphic, both morphologically and functionally [36].
- In a recent survey involving a total of 33,425 participants, women exhibited a greater tendency than men to gain weight under chronic exposure to stressful life events [37].
- In a clinical trial, lipopolysaccharide-induced production of pro-inflammatory cytokines after acute mental stress was examined in a healthy sample of 28 men and 34 women, with men showing a significant decrease in their production of cytokines from baseline to post-task and then an increase during the recovery period, whereas premenopausal women exhibited an increase in cytokines just during recovery. Interestingly, postmenopausal women had a continuously increased inflammatory response from the time of the task through the recovery period, which implies a greater susceptibility of middle-aged women to stress-related inflammatory responses [38].

The mechanism underlying sex differences in the HPA axis can be tied to either organizational or activational responses to steroid hormones. Seale [39] demonstrated that neonatal females treated within 24 h of birth with testosterone had, in adulthood, an HPA axis phenotype similar to males, which consists of a reduced corticosterone response to chronic stress and lower levels of CRH.

Psychologists Shelley Taylor and Laura Cousino Klein provided an important contribution to understanding the gender-dissimilar strategies of responses and adaptations to stress. Starting from the well-known mechanism "fight or flight" and its neuroendocrine correlates, they suggested that human females have developed another way of responding to challenges: a so-called *tend-and-befriend* response that is more protective of themselves and their offspring. The fight or flight response, first described by W. Cannon in 1932, is characterized by activation of the sympathetic nervous system that, in turn, stimulates the adrenal medulla to increase the production of catecholamines, particularly epinephrine and norepinephrine. However, studies examining the fight or flight response were conducted mainly on males. Taylor and Cousino Klein proposed a more evolutionary point of view, in particular, that

> ". . .high maternal investment should lead to the selection of female stress responses that do not jeopardize the health of the mother and her offspring and that maximize the likelihood that they will survive. Tending, that is quieting and caring for the offspring and blending into the environment, may be effective for addressing a broad array of threats. Befriending process is the creation of networks of associations that provide resources and protection for the female and her offspring under conditions of stress. In contrast, fight responses on the part of females may put themselves and their offspring in jeopardy, and flight behavior on the part of females may be compromised by pregnancy or the need to care for immature offspring. Thus, alternative behavioral responses are likely to have evolved in females" [40].

In fact, female aggression (the fight response) is not mediated by sympathetic arousal and the release of testosterone, as in men, given that women enact their aggressive behavior in a more indirect way [41]. The female neuroendocrine correlate is oxytocin, a pituitary hormone that is involved in many functions—such as labor, breastfeeding, orgasms, and maternal and social bonding. Due to these functions, oxytocin has been called "the love hormone." It also reduces perceptions of stress and anxiety. Under stress conditions, women release more oxytocin than men, and this response is sex steroid mediated, since estrogens enhance oxytocin secretion and androgens decrease it. This explains how loneliness and social isolation can be especially dangerous for women and how housework and family responsibilities could be viewed as a rewarding experience as opposed to merely a burden.

Moreover, we can speculate that women and men, according to their cultural conditioning, allow themselves to perceive stress in a way more suitable to their specific gender. For example, women who are tired often express this by saying that they "feel sad and depressed"; meanwhile, men who are heartbroken often claim that they "feel tired and too busy."

Lastly, women, mostly in industrialized countries, have increasingly been exposed to new stressors for which they have not been culturally prepared, so that their innate biological and behavioral protective mechanisms now may be less effective.

6.4 The Broken Heart: Takotsubo Cardiomyopathy

In the 1990s, Japanese authors reported the first cases of takotsubo cardiomyopathy (TTC), a reversible form of cardiac failure precipitated by acute and severe emotional stress in five postmenopausal women [42]. This stress-related clinical entity was clinically characterized as having an onset similar to a myocardial infarction, associated with specific and reversible apical and wall motion abnormalities in the absence of any atherosclerotic CAD. The term *takotsubo* comes from the Japanese name for an octopus trap, which mimics the ballooning aspect of the left ventricle during systole. Otherwise called *apical ballooning syndrome* and *broken heart disease*, it has been acknowledged by the American Heart Association [43] and the American College of Cardiology as a form of reversible cardiomyopathy. Presently, it is recognized that this form of acute reversible cardiomyopathy may present with other different kinetic patterns associated with alterations in the left ventricular wall, and it seems to be more common than initially believed. Recent estimates are that it accounts for 2 % of all cases of suspected coronary syndrome overall, but for 10 % when the patient is female [44]. Chronic elevation of catecholamines, as a maladaptive response to chronic stress in vulnerable individuals, could be the pathogenic mechanism underlying TTC (see Chap. 1). In a recent Japanese study [45], gender differences were assessed in 284 women and 84 men with TTC; and while previous psychological stress was more evident in women, prior physical exertion was more often reported by men. Another gender-related finding observed in the aforementioned Japanese study was the worse prognosis in men, despite the higher female incidence, with composite cardiac events—including severe pump failure, serious ventricular arrhythmias, and cardiovascular death—significantly more common in male than female patients.

6.5 Conclusions

In summary, understanding sex and gender differences should elicit a better and more comprehensive clinical understanding of the strengths and weaknesses of those who are ill. At this time in medical history, it should be considered urgent to create a new model of care that takes into account the biological, psychological, and narrative characteristics of each patient, wherein gender is a key component of determining the specificity and identity of each person as a whole.

References

1. Risberg G, Johansson EE, Hamberg K (2009) A theoretical model for analysing gender bias in medicine. Int J Equity Health 8:28–35
2. Jindal RM, Ryan JJ, Sajjad I et al (2005) Kidney transplantation and gender disparity. Am J Nephrol 25:474–483
3. Nyberg F, Osika I, Evengård B (2008) "The Laundry Bag Project"—unequal distribution of dermatological healthcare resources for male and female psoriatic patients in Sweden. Int J Dermatol 47:144–149
4. Kotake K, Asano M, Ozawa H et al (2016) Gender differences in colorectal cancer survival in Japan. Int J Clin Oncol 21(1):194–203. doi:10.1007/s10147-015-0868-6
5. Kempner J (2006) Gendering the migraine market: do representations of illness matter? Soc Sci Med 63:1986–1987
6. Elveback LR, Connolly DC, Melton LJ 3rd (1986) Coronary artery disease in residents of Rochester. Incidence 1950 through 1982. Mayo Clin Proc 61(11):896–900
7. Healy B (1991) The Yentl syndrome. N Engl J Med 325:274–275
8. Ayanian JZ, Epstein AM (1991) Differences in the use of procedures between women and men hospitalized for coronary heart disease. N Engl J Med 325:221–225
9. Steingart RM, Packer M, Hamm P et al (1991) Sex differences in the management of coronary artery disease. N Engl J Med 325:226–230
10. Dart AM, Du XJ, Kingwell BA (2002) Gender, sex hormones and autonomic nervous control of the cardiovascular system. Cardiovasc Res 53(3):678–687
11. Mercuro G, Deidda M, Bina A et al (2011) Gender-specific aspects in primary and secondary prevention of cardiovascular disease. Curr Pharm Des 17(11):1082–1089
12. Kanaya AM, Grady D, Barrett-Connor E (2002) Explaining the sex difference in coronary heart disease mortality among patients with type 2 diabetes mellitus: a meta-analysis. Arch Intern Med 162(15):1737–1745
13. Peters SA, Huxley RR, Woodward M (2014) Diabetes as risk factor for incident coronary heart disease in women compared with men: a systematic review and meta-analysis of 64 cohorts including 858,507 individuals and 28,203 coronary events. Diabetologia 57(8):1542–1551
14. Die stille Epidemie (1994) Der Spiegel n. 39
15. DeVon HA, Ryan CJ, Ochs AL, Shapiro M (2008) Symptoms across the continuum of acute coronary syndromes: differences between women and men. Am J Crit Care 17:14–24
16. Birdwell BG, Herbers JE, Kroenke K (1993) Evaluating chest in pain. The patient's presentation style alters the physician's diagnostic approach. Arch Intern Med 153(17):1991–1995
17. Merz CN (2011) The Yentl syndrome is alive and well. Eur Heart J 32(11):1313–1315
18. Go AS, Mozaffarian D, Roger VL et al (2014) Heart disease and stroke statistics—2014 update: a report from the American Heart Association. Circulation 129:28–292
19. Grady D, Herrington D, Bittner V et al (2002) Cardiovascular disease outcomes during 6.8 years of hormone therapy: heart and estrogen/progestin replacement study follow-up (HERS II). JAMA 288(1):49–57
20. Parikh NI, Cnattingius S, Dickmann PV (2010) Parity and risk of later life maternal cardiovascular disease. Am Heart J 159:215–221
21. Moran LJ, Misso ML, Wild RA et al (2010) Impaired glucose tolerance, type 2 diabetes and metabolic syndrome in polycystic ovary syndrome: a systematic review and meta-analysis. Hum Reprod Update 16(4):347–363
22. Brenner DJ, Shuryak I, Jozsef G et al (2014) Risk and risk reduction of major coronary events associated with contemporary breast radiotherapy. JAMA Intern Med 174(1):158–160
23. Tsang W (2012) The impact of cardiovascular disease prevalence on women's enrollment in landmark randomized cardiovascular trials: a systematic review. J Gen Intern Med 27:93–98
24. Rosano GM, Lewis B, Agewall S et al (2015) Gender differences in the effect of cardiovascular drugs: a position document of the working group on pharmacology and drug therapy of the ESC. Eur Heart J 36(40):2677–2680

25. Mosca L, Benjamin EJ, Berra K et al (2011) Effectiveness-based guidelines for the prevention of cardiovascular disease in women—2011 update: a guideline from the American Heart Association. Circulation 123(11):1243–1262
26. Selye H (1936) Syndrome produced by diverse nocuous agents. Nature 138:32
27. Ruberman W, Weinblatt E, Goldberg JD, Chaudhary BS (1987) Psychosocial influences on mortality after myocardial infarction. N Engl J Med 311:552–559
28. Rosengren A, Tibblin G, Wilhelmsen L (1991) Self-perceived psychological stress and incidence of coronary artery disease in middle-aged men. Am J Cardiol 68:1171–1175
29. Steptoe A, Hamer M, Chida Y et al (2007) The effects of acute psychological stress on circulating inflammatory factors in humans: a review and meta-analysis. Brain Behav Immun 21:901–912
30. Orth-Gomér K, Wamala SP, Horsten M et al (2000) Marital stress worsens prognosis in women with coronary heart disease: the Stockholm female coronary risk study. JAMA 284 (23):3008–3014
31. Liu H, Waite L (2014) Bad marriage, broken heart. Age and gender link between marital quality and cardiovascular risks among older adults. J Health Soc Behav 55(4):403–423
32. Parkes CM, Benjamin B, Fitzgerald RG (1969) Broken heart: a statistical study of increased mortality among widowers. Br Med J 1(5646):740–743
33. Tindle HA, Chang YF, Kuller LH et al (2009) Optimism, cynical hostility, and incident coronary heart disease and mortality in the women's health initiative. Circulation 120 (8):656–662
34. Handa RJ, Burgess LH, Kerr JE, O'Keefe JA (1994) Gonadal steroid hormone receptors and sex differences in the hypothalamo-pituitary-adrenal axis. Horm Behav 28:464–476
35. García-Cáceres C, Lagunas N, Calmarza-Font I et al (2010) Gender differences in the long-term effects of chronic prenatal stress on the HPA axis and hypothalamic structure in rats. Psychoneuroendocrinology 35:1525–1535
36. McEwen BS (1983) Gonadal steroid influences on brain development and sexual differentiation. In: Greep R (ed) Reproductive physiology, vol 4. University Park, Baltimore, pp 99–145
37. Udo T, Grilo CM, McKee SA et al (2014) Gender differences in the impact of stressful life events on change in body mass index. Prev Med 69:49–53
38. Prather AA, Carroll JE, Fury JM (2009) Gender differences in stimulated cytokine production following acute psychological stress. Brain Behav Immun 23(5):622–628
39. Seale JV, Wood SA, Atkinson HC et al (2005) Postnatal masculinization alters the HPA axis phenotype in adult female rats. J Physiol 563:265–274
40. Taylor SE, Klein LC, Lewis BP et al (2000) Biobehavioral responses to stress in females: tend-and-befriend, not fight-or-flight. Psychol Rev 107:411–429
41. Holmstrom R (1983) Female aggression among the great apes: a psychoanalytic perspective. In: Bjorkqvist K, Niemela P (eds) Of mice and women: aspects of female aggression. Academic, San Diego, CA, pp 295–306
42. Dote K, Sato H, Tateishi H et al (1991) Myocardial stunning due to simultaneous multivessel coronary spasms: a review of 5 cases. J Cardiol 21:203–214 (in Japanese)
43. Maron BJ, Towbin JA, Thiene G et al (2006) Contemporary definitions and classification of the cardiomyopathies: an American Heart Association Scientific Statement from the Council on Clinical Cardiology, Heart Failure and Transplantation Committee; Quality of Care and Outcomes Research and Functional Genomics and Translational Biology Interdisciplinary Working Groups; and Council on Epidemiology and Prevention. Circulation 113 (14):1807–1816
44. Sharkey SW, Maron BJ (2014) Epidemiology and clinical profile of Takotsubo cardiomyopathy. Circ J 78(9):2119–2128
45. Murakami T, Yoshikawa T, Maekawa Y et al (2015) Gender differences in patients with Takotsubo cardiomyopathy: multi-center registry from Tokyo CCU network. PLoS One 10(8): e0136655. doi:10.1371/journal.pone.0136655

Part II

Integrated Approach for Cardiac Patients and Psychological Interventions

7

David Lazzari and Ludovico Lazzari

When minds are closed and the wisdom is excluded, people remain related to the disease.

Huang DI [Huangdi or The Emperor's Inner Canon (The Yellow Emperor, reign 2698–2598 B.C.)]

7.1 Introduction

Optimizing the care of the patient suffering from a disease that results from multiple pathological conditions requires the comprehension of the disease's underlying physiological and pathogenetic mechanisms. As described in Chap. 1, it is now understood that acute coronary syndromes (ACS) are the final endpoint of a complex and variable interplay between a broad array of pathophysiological factors and each patient's personal predispositional milieu [1]. These participating factors include coronary vasomotricity, coagulation, and endogenous fibrinolysis, as well as the patient's immune, neural, and inflammatory systems, all of which can vary considerably between different individuals and at different times in the same individual. Psychological risk factors (PRFs) have also been shown to be important, both predisposing to and precipitating coronary artery disease (CAD) and acute ischemic events [2–4]. However, PRFs can also be a consequence of CAD, potentially creating a vicious circle [5] (see the already-mentioned Chaps. 1–3). Indeed, PRFs co-occur with CAD at rates that significantly exceed fortuitous comorbidity.

D. Lazzari, PsyD (✉)
Servizio di Psicologia Ospedaliera, Azienda Ospedaliera "S. Maria" Terni, Viale Tristano di Joannuccio, 1, 05100 Terni, Italy
e-mail: lazzarid@aospterni.it

L. Lazzari, MD
UO Cardiologia, Università degli Studi di Perugia, Azienda Ospedaliera "S. Maria" Terni, Terni, Italy
e-mail: ludovicolazzari@alice.it

A. Roncella, C. Pristipino (eds.), *Psychotherapy for Ischemic Heart Disease*,
DOI 10.1007/978-3-319-33214-7_7

For example, whereas the prevalence of depressive disorders is estimated to be between 15 and 20 % in the ischemic heart disease (IHD) population, and clinically relevant depressive symptoms are present in up to 40 % [6], comparative rates in the general population are 5–9 % in females and 2–3 % in males [7].

In the opinion of most of the authors cited here, CAD risk is related to specific psychosocial domains: depression, anxiety, social isolation, anger, chronic life stress, and personality factors like pessimism [3, 5, 8]. Several key points emerge from the understanding of the interaction between PRFs and CAD and constitute the basis for integrated therapy that incorporates psychological interventions:

1. PRFs have an independent causative role in the development of IHD and should be identified, diagnosed, and treated in the same way as classical risk factors like hypertension, dyslipidemia, and smoking [4, 9].
2. PRFs cluster with classical risk factors; therefore, effectively treating them should also reduce classical risk factors [10–12].
3. The stress axis (predominantly chronically increased adrenergic-sympathetic axis and adrenocortical activity) represents a common pathway for the organic response to ACS (physiological response) and is enhanced by the perceived stress caused by hospitalization and the disease itself. In this context, stress management and the identification of specific patient needs that go beyond the treatment of organic disease may improve hospitalized patient outcomes.
4. A state of acute and/or chronic disease can worsen patients' prognoses by creating or worsening their anxiety and/or depression and/or self-defeating behaviors.

7.2 Primary Prevention

Almost every 4–5 years, the various cardiological societies propose new guidelines for primary prevention of CAD. At present, we focus on the messages of lifelong prevention and the use of risk scores, which help cardiologists to assess the overall cardiovascular risk in relatively healthy people, so they can then opt for an effective strategy of global prevention while neither under- nor overtreating their patients. The message is this: clinicians must estimate each individual patient's risk profile and choose what is appropriate to treat and prioritize to reduce that patient's personalized risk of cardiovascular events. The optimal approach to primary prevention of CAD should therefore be multimodal, integrating current practices preventing traditional cardiovascular risk factors with the recognition and treatment of PRFs. From this perspective, robust data like those of the INTERHEART study [9] should help experts to draw up tables of risk that might also include psychosocial risk factors, since they have been officially entered into the list of comorbidities that can increase CAD risk.

The issue of primary prevention should concern society as a whole, involving all health professions and endorsing a policy of health and university education, aiming to make it understood that PRFs must be diagnosed and treated in the same way as traditional risk factors. Wide implementation of such medical education would take time, probably a full generation, to become ingrained in routine clinical practice. Meanwhile, general practitioners and cardiologists who treat patients in the long term, given that they have the opportunity to recognize PRFs as well as canonical risk factors, should also focus on personal and environmental issues like chronic stress. The primary aim is thereby to reduce the excessive rate of undiagnosed and untreated psychological comorbidities in cardiac patients. However, routine screening for depression does not contribute to better cardiac prognosis in the absence of changes in current models of cardiovascular care [13].

To further illustrate the importance of PRF and "behavioral cardiology," one must only think of the "time is muscle" strategy current being adopted and continuing efforts to strengthen emergency networks and thereby reduce the time from symptoms to reperfusion via percutaneous revascularization in acute myocardial infarction (AMI). In the prehospital phase of an AMI, psychological factors are decisive contributors to delays in first medical contact. The reasons for the delay caused by patients' behavior are still incompletely understood, so it is difficult to create specific preventative strategies. An attitude of denial might cause patients with threatening symptoms of an imminent ongoing infarction, like long-lasting angina pectoris, to misinterpret their severity [14], delaying their access to medical care.

It is important to determine whether there are signs of negative affectivity, especially anxiety or depressed mood, and whether a patient is of low social status or has an inadequate social network. Simple initial screening methods for PRFs could be accomplished using self-rating questionnaires, like the "Patient Health Questionnaire" [15], which helps to identify depression, anxiety, and somatoform disorders, or the Hospital Anxiety and Depression Scale [16], to help identify depression and anxiety, or the simple questions suggested by the ESC guidelines on cardiovascular disease prevention [13] (see Table 7.1).

However, there is no doubt that, if a physician is unfamiliar to a patient, it may not be easy for that doctor to perform such screening. Patients should therefore be informed of their risk and provided with adequate explanations about psyche-soma relationships and the advantages of effectively coping with stress, so that psychotherapy can be offered and accepted with the same ease and mutual trust as treatment for dyslipidemia.

To actualize multimodal behavioral interventions, adequate control of all risk factors is currently recommended (IA) by the European Society Cardiology (ESC) guidelines for the prevention of heart disease [13].

7.3 Psychological Functioning Following Myocardial Infarction and Consequent Treatment Strategies

As stated previously, the physical and psychological consequences of IHD create considerable impairment in a patient's quality of life in all dimensions, both physical and mental. Moreover, PRFs that may have contributed to the genesis of

Table 7.1 Core questions for the assessment of psychosocial risk factors in clinical practice

Low socioeconomic status	What is our highest educational degree? Are you a manual worker?
Work and family stress	Do you lack control over how to meet the demands at work? Is your reward inappropriate for your effort? Do you have serious problem with your spouse?
Social isolation	Are you living alone? Do you lack a close confident?
Depression	Do you feel down, depressed, and hopeless? Have you lost interest and pleasure in life?
Anxiety	Do you frequently feel nervous, anxious, or on edge? Are you frequently unable to stop or control worrying?
Hostility	Do you frequently feel angry over little things? Do you often feel annoyed about other people's habits?
Type D personality	In general, do you often feel anxious, irritable, or depressed? Do you avoid sharing your thoughts and feelings with other people?

Modified from: Perk J, De Backer G, Gohlke H et al, European Guidelines on cardiovascular disease prevention in clinical practice (version 2012). Eur Heart J 33 (13): 1635–1701

the disease, unlike other risk factors, may be subject to acute worsening. As one example of this, patients who experience a myocardial infarction (MI) as a first clinical presentation of CAD may react with denial, refusing to accept that they have a complex, chronic disease. These patients can then be poorly adherent to both treatment and secondary prevention. They also may exhibit ineffective coping with illness; poorer self-management; a propensity for depression, isolation, and social withdrawal; self-imposed limitations in their daily activities; and frequent high levels of fear of symptom recurrence [17]. The culmination of all these effects of worsened psychological status could be further acute events, including sudden death. The serious health consequences and the necessity to introduce numerous changes into their everyday functioning are reasons why acute cardiac events are perceived by many patients as among the most serious and life-threatening experience that can occur. On the other hand, it has been shown that perceived social support can counteract the adverse effects of depression [18]. Moreover, patients who are able to take advantage of various forms of social support tend to report better quality of life in their first year following their MI [17], whereas a lack of support seems to reinforce adverse consequences of the disease [19].

Below is an overview of the main PRFs and related intervention strategies (see Fig. 7.1). For a more thorough review of these topics, refer back to Chaps. 2, 3, and 10.

- **Depression.** Fifteen to thirty percent of cardiac patients have clinically significant depression, which is approximately triple the prevalence found in the general population. In about half of these patients, depressive symptoms remit following routine cardiac treatment. In the other half, symptoms persist for months or years if specific psychotherapeutic or pharmacologic interventions

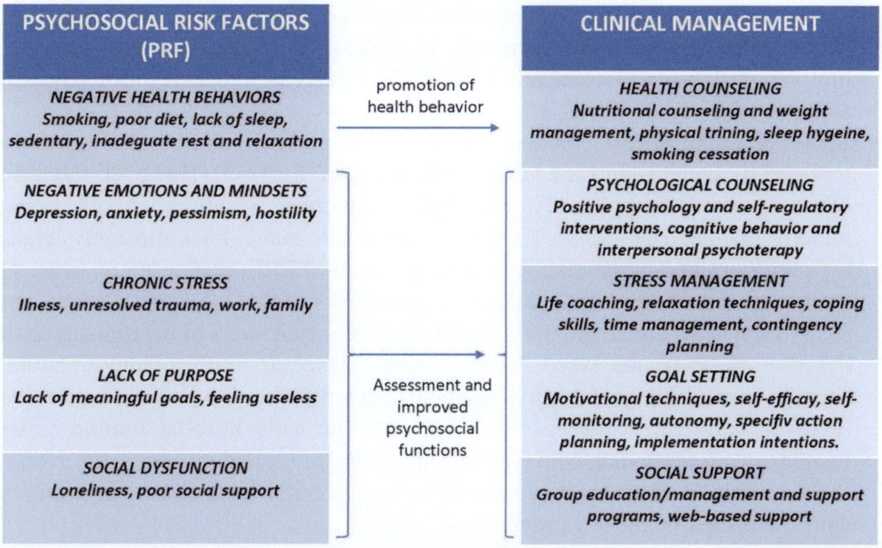

Modified from Rozanski 2014

Fig. 7.1 Psychosocial risk factors and clinical management

are not provided [20]. Difficulties in diagnosing depression in cardiac patients are at least partially due to its atypical clinical presentation. For this reason, patients need to be screened for depressive symptoms during their hospital stay, and again early in their post-discharge follow-up, to identify those who require further diagnostic measures and therapy. It is notable that different depressive symptom dimensions vary in how they affect post-MI outcomes. For example, symptoms that fall into the somatic/affective dimension (e.g., fatigue, sleep problems, and poor appetite) appear to be associated with a worse cardiac outcome than those within the cognitive/affective dimension (e.g., shame, guilt, and negative self-image), with a 1-year follow-up odds ratio (OR) of 1.49 documented for poorer hemodynamic compensation and mortality [21], probably related to unhealthy behaviors.

- **Anxiety**. Anxiety is a negative affective state that results from an individual's perception of threat. It is characterized by a perceived inability to predict, control, or achieve preferred results in a given situation. In the setting of an acute MI, it is associated with less effective disease management and reduced quality of life. Patients' beliefs about the causes of their disease may influence their receptivity to psychosocial interventions: depressed or anxious patients are more likely to endorse negative emotions as among the causes of their heart disease. This affects the possibilities of coping with the consequences of MI [22]; for example, they may become despondent enough to give up on all preventative measures and rehabilitation programs they are offered [23], without taking advantage of psychological support. Anxiety and depression frequently coexist, but the association between anxiety and a poor post-MI prognosis appears to be less than for depression. Psychological support reduces the severity of anxiety and depressive symptoms considerably. It also increases patients' motivation to participate in rehabilitation and increases their level of physical activity [24].

- **Stress**. Chronic "stress" related or not to their medical condition is frequently reported by patients and is a well-recognized PRF for CAD. However, the term often is used ambiguously in clinical practice, resulting in its being underestimated. The reasons for this ambiguity are many. First, most physicians are poorly trained in the diagnosis and treatment of PRFs and/or are unaware of their impact on the pathophysiology and prognosis of CAD. Second, stress is not easily measured, unlike the traditional risk factors, and many of the terms used to describe it—even the word "stress" itself—have no uniform interpretation. Finally, in the setting of modern medicine, in which hospitalizations tend to be relatively short, it is not easy to insert into the daily hospital routine either insights or professionals who can help in its diagnosis and management. Nonetheless, stress management programs have repeatedly been shown to improve subjective well-being and prognosis [25–27].

To clarify what we are referring to when we talk about of stress, what we think is the underlying mechanism of its genesis and the consequent correct interpretation, take for example the "balance model" (see further Chap. 21).

Demanding environmental situations are termed "external stressors," to which are added the internal demands (i.e., "internal stressors") that are influenced by a person's own perception of their life situation. The person's situational response, termed a "stress reaction," is a consequence of how these requirements are likely to outweigh potential resources to counteract the stress that also can either be external—like social support and the help of caregivers—or internal, like the patient's own innate ability to adapt to stressors. A balance between this demand and supply can result in homeostasis, while an imbalance between the amount of threat and challenges that a person perceives and their various coping resources may lead to a "maladaptive" reaction. This might be compared to the imbalance between the demand and supply of oxygen and metabolic precursors, which is at the very basis of tissue ischemia. Since this balance is influenced by external and internal factors, not all individuals are equally vulnerable to distress and harmful stress reactions during times of increased demand. The accompanying neurobiological, neuroendocrine, and autonomic activation patterns shape the stress response to elicit a wide range of adaptive cognitive, behavioral, and physiological changes in attempts to maintain or restore homeostasis (i.e., the balance between offers and requests).

However, if exaggerated or sustained, stress reactions may become maladaptive, resulting in dysfunctional cognition and biological changes pertinent to IHD [3, 28, 29].

- **Positive psychosocial functioning**. Similar to cardiovascular risk factors, which generally are continuous in their extent, ranging from normal to severely pathological, psychosocial factors can also be visualized on a spectrum, ranging from positive to negative. As already described, PRFs promote illness, both by fostering negative health behaviors and via direct pathophysiological effects [2, 3, 8]. By contrast, positive psychosocial factors are associated with more healthy behaviors and promote favorable physiological effects, including enhanced immune, endothelial, and autonomic function [8, 30, 31]. Furthermore, positive psychosocial functioning helps to promote vitality, a sense of well-being, and the ability to set appropriate goals for one's own health and pursue them consciously, consistently, and appropriately [32]. Future investigators need to examine the interaction between each chronic stressor and the sense of meaning that is associated with that stressor. For example, whereas a "good stressor" generally helps us to face the challenges of life and overcome them, "bad stressors" may become overwhelming, uncontrollable, or nonhelpful. Exposure to adverse life events typically predicts subsequent negative effects on mental health and well-being, such that more adversity predicts worse outcomes. However, adverse experiences also may foster resilience, with resulting advantages for both mental health and well-being. This concept might help to explain the interesting U-shaped relationship that exists between the magnitude of experiential stress and clinical outcomes shown in a recent longitudinal study in which a history of some lifetime adversity predicted relatively lower global distress, lower self-rated functional impairment, fewer post-traumatic stress symptoms, and higher life satisfaction over time [33].

On the basis of what has just been stated, a variety of behavioral and psychosocial intervention trials have been implemented in cardiac patients. A discussion of the most significant and recent reviews on the subject, in addition to a review of 24 original randomized trials, is presented in Chap. 10.

Briefly, a number of meta-analyses on psychological interventions for cardiac patients in general and CAD patients more specifically were published from 2004 to 2011 [25, 26, 34–36]. They demonstrated that a range of psychotherapies improve psychological outcomes; however, conflicting results were observed for cardiovascular outcomes. On the other hand, in their umbrella and updated meta-analyses, Biondi-Zoccai et al. confirmed the role of psychotherapeutic interventions in reducing the incidence of anxiety and depression, but also in improving mortality and morbidity in patients with IHD (see Chap. 10).

While these results appear inconclusive and contradictory, attention must be paid to the studies of numerous differences, including heterogeneous methodology, timing, and integration with conventional medical or behavioral treatment. Moreover, in most of the trials analyzed, placebo effects could not be discounted, and many studies were conducted before modern treatments for IHD had been introduced.

Contradictions in study results also might stem from classical research designs, which are methodologically inadequate to study complex nondeterministic systems (see Chap. 1). Indeed, to date, clear superiority has only been demonstrated for a multimodal approach, combining elements of cognitive behavioral therapy ("stress management") and changes in health behaviors, including the adoption of a regular exercise regimen.

7.4 Goals of Psychological Interventions and Operational Strategies

Several key elements of successful psychosocial intervention programs for patients with IHD have been identified. To enable the operational implementation of an integrated view and approach in people already suffering from cardiovascular disease, it appears crucial to have an integrated model of intervention. An accurate overview of possible interventions is provided in Chaps. 8 and 11–13.

The proposed model consists of several components and proposes partially differentiated paths determined by the needs that are identified for each individual patient. This model, described below, is summarized in Figs. 7.1 and 7.2. It entails the initial psychological screening of patients and the identification of their differentiated paths relative to the dynamics of their adaptation to disease, all within a framework of cooperation between psychologists, doctors, nurses, other healthcare givers, and personal caregivers.

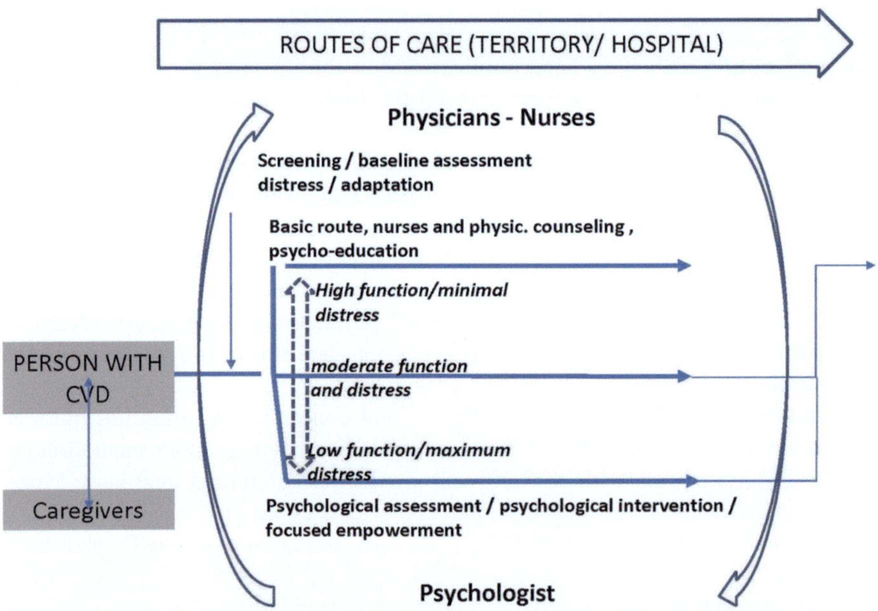

Fig. 7.2 A model of integration

It is expected that:

(a) Conducting basic screening using easy tools (e.g., Kessler Psychological Distress Scale [37], DASS 21 [38], and the Hopkins Symptom Checklist [39]) will allow for the assessment of levels of distress and adaptive balance linked to the disease.
(b) This screening, in addition to a clinical evaluation of health status by physicians and nurses, will focus also on the presence of dysfunctional elements and discomfort and should guide the future path of the patient to address his or her personal needs (i.e., a psychosocial classification of patients with cardiovascular disease).
(c) This classification will divide patients into three different levels of need: (1) those who are high functioning and have low-level distress, (2) those with moderate levels of function and distress, and (3) those who are low functioning and have high-level distress.
(d) Patients in the first category, who have generally adapted well, might be offered lifestyle counseling by either physicians or nurses and psychoeducational activities guided by psychologists.
(e) Patients in the last category, who have adapted most poorly, will be offered a much more thorough level of psychological examination, which also will guide the subsequent course of both their own course and, potentially, that of their caregivers (i.e., psychological assessment and related interventions of empowerment, whether psychotherapy). These activities would be orchestrated by psychologists and psychotherapists, but might also involve collaborations with physicians, nurses, and other healthcare professionals, when appropriate.
(f) Patients in the middle category, who fall into the intermediate range in terms of their ability to adapt and level of stress, could be offered treatment that complements standard treatment in whatever ways are deemed necessary.
(g) The therapeutic approaches just mentioned might be carried out individually, and/or in groups, and/or online.

7.5 Conclusions

Aspects of psychological interest in cardiac patients (behavior, emotions, attitudes, stress, feelings, relationships) impact either the genesis of heart disease or their course and effectiveness of care. It therefore seems necessary to extend the concept of appropriateness of interventions—both prevention and care—to include these aspects.

First, making professional psychological and psychotherapeutic support available in a cardiological context as an investment in terms of treatment effectiveness and—according to available literature—cost-benefits. Second, it is critical that, in these patients, psychological interventions are viewed in a way similar to medical interventions, in terms of their relevance to both outcomes and patient management.

This requires a specific attention to both PRFs and psychological consequences of IHD by the medical and nursing staff—specially trained in this way—and the availability of psychologists and psychotherapists. The activities carried out by psychologists, especially in care, must be provided according to criteria based on integration with the usual care and of the actual needs of patients.

References

1. Maseri A (2000) From syndromes to specific disease mechanisms. The search for the causes of myocardial infarction. Ital Heart J 1:253–257
2. Rozanski A, Blumenthal JA, Kaplan J (1999) Impact of psychological factors on the pathogenesis of cardiovascular disease and implications for therapy. Circulation 27:2192–2217
3. Rozanski A, Blumenthal JA, Davidson KW et al (2005) The epidemiology, pathophysiology, and management of psychosocial risk factors in cardiac practice. J Am Coll Cardiol 45:637–651
4. Rosengren A, Hawken S, Ounpuu S et al (2004) Association of psychosocial risk factors with risk of acute myocardial infarction in 11,119 cases and 13,648 controls from 52 countries (the INTERHEART study): case–control study. Lancet 364:953–962
5. Hamer M, Molloy GJ, Stamatakis E (2008) Psychological distress as a risk factor for cardiovascular events: pathophysiological and behavioral mechanisms. J Am Coll Cardiol 52 (25):2156–2162
6. Tully PJ, Baumeister H (2014) Collaborative care for the treatment of comorbid depression and coronary heart disease: a systematic review and meta-analysis protocol. Syst Rev 28 (3):127. doi:10.1186/2046-4053-3-127
7. American Psychiatric Association (2000) Diagnostic and statistical manual of mental disorders: DSM-IV-TR, 4th edn. American Psychiatric Publishing, Arlington, VA
8. Rozanski A (2014) Behavioral cardiology—current advances and future directions. J Am Coll Cardiol 64(1):100–110
9. Yusuf S, Hawken S, Ounpuu S, INTERHEART Study Investigators et al (2004) Effects of potentially modifiable risk factors associated with myocardial infarction in 52 countries (the INTERHEART study): case–control study. Lancet 364:937–952
10. von Känel R, Mausbach BT, Dimsdale JE et al (2011) Regular physical activity moderates cardiometabolic risk in Alzheimer's caregivers. Med Sci Sports Exerc 43(1):181–189
11. Surwit RS, Williams RB, Siegler IC et al (2002) Hostility, race, and glucose metabolism in non diabetic individuals. Diabetes Care 25(5):835–839
12. Shen BJ, Countryman AJ, Spiro A 3rd, Niaura R (2008) The prospective contribution of hostility characteristics to high fasting glucose levels: the moderating role of marital status. Diabetes Care 31(7):1293–1298
13. Perk J, De Backer G, Gohlke H, European Association for Cardiovascular Prevention and Rehabilitation (EACPR), ESC Committee for Practice Guidelines (CPG) et al (2012) European guidelines on cardiovascular disease prevention in clinical practice (version 2012). The fifth joint task force of the European society of cardiology and other societies on cardiovascular disease prevention in clinical practice (constituted by representatives of nine societies and by invited experts). Eur Heart J 33(13):1635–1701. doi:10.1093/eurheartj/ehs092
14. Ladwig KH, Gärtner C, Walz LM et al (2009) The inner barrier: how health psychology concepts contribute to the explanation of prehospital delays in acute myocardial infarction: a systematic analysis of the current state of knowledge. Psychother Psychosom Med Psychol 59 (12):440–445
15. Löwe B, Spitzer RL, Zipfel S, Herzog W. Gesundheitsfragebogen für Patienten (PHQ D). Komplettversion und Kurzform. Testmappe mit Manual, Fragebögen, Schablonen. 2. Auflage. Pfizer, Karlsruhe

16. Zigmond AS, Snaith RP (1983) The hospital anxiety and depression scale. Acta Psychiatr Scand 67(6):361–370
17. Mierzyńska A, Kowalska M, Stepnowska M, Piotrowicz R (2010) Psychological support for patients following myocardial infarction. Cardiol J 17(3):319–324
18. Frasure-Smith N, Lesperance F, Gravel G et al (2000) Social support, depression, mortality during the first year after myocardial infarction. Circulation 101:1919–1924
19. Horsten M, Mittleman MA, Wamala SP et al (2000) Depressive symptoms and lack of social integration in relation to prognosis of CHD in middle-aged women. The Stockholm female coronary risk study. Eur Heart J 21:1072–1080
20. Thombs BD, Bass EB, Ford DE et al (2006) Prevalence of depression in survivors of acute myocardial infarction. J Gen Intern Med 21(1):30–38
21. Roest AM, Thombs BD, Grace SL et al (2011) Somatic/affective symptoms, but not cognitive/affective symptoms, of depression after acute coronary syndrome are associated with 12-month all-cause mortality. J Affect Disord 131:158–163
22. Day RC, Freedland KE, Carney RM (2005) Effects of anxiety and depression on heart disease attributions. Int J Behav Med 12:24–29
23. Yohannes AM, Yalfani A, Doherty P, Bundy C (2007) Predictors of drop-out from an outpatient cardiac rehabilitation program. Clin Rehabil 21:222–229
24. Yoshida T, Kohzuki M, Yoshida K et al (1999) Physical and psychological improvements after phase II cardiac rehabilitation in patients with myocardial infarction. Nurs Health Sci 1:163–170
25. Linden W, Phillips MJ, Leclerc J (2007) Psychological treatment of cardiac patients: a meta-analysis. Eur Heart J 28:2972–2984
26. Rees K, Bennett P, West R et al (2004) Psychological interventions for coronary heart disease. Cochrane Database Syst Rev 2:CD002902
27. Gulliksson M, Burell G, Vessby B et al (2011) Randomized controlled trial of cognitive behavioral therapy vs standard treatment to prevent recurrent cardiovascular events in patients with coronary heart disease: Secondary Prevention in Uppsala Primary Health Care Project (SUPRIM). Arch Intern Med 171:134–140
28. Cacioppo JT, Berntson GG, Malarkey WB et al (1998) Autonomic, neuroendocrine, and immune responses to psychological stress: the reactivity hypothesis. Ann NY Acad Sci 840:664–673
29. McEwen BS, Gianaros PJ (2010) Central role of the brain in stress and adaptation: links to socioeconomic status, health, and disease. Ann NY Acad Sci 1186:190–222
30. Endrighi R, Hamer M, Steptoe A (2011) Associations of trait optimism with diurnal neuroendocrine activity, cortisol responses to mental stress, and subjective stress measures in healthy men and women. Psychosom Med 73:672–678
31. Ikeda A, Schwartz J, Peters JL et al (2011) Optimism in relation to inflammation and endothelial dysfunction in older men: the VA normative aging study. Psychosom Med 73:664–671
32. Kubzansky LD, Sparrow D, Vokonas P et al (2001) Is the glass half empty or half full? A prospective study of optimism and coronary heart disease in the normative aging study. Psychosom Med 63:910–916
33. Seery MD, Holman EA, Silver RC (2010) Whatever does not kill us: cumulative lifetime adversity, vulnerability, and resilience. J Pers Soc Psychol 99:1025–1041
34. van Dixhoorn J, White A (2005) Relaxation therapy for rehabilitation and prevention in ischaemic heart disease: a systematic review and meta-analysis. Eur J Cardiovasc Prev Rehabil 12:193–202
35. Whalley B, Rees K, Davies P et al (2011) Psychological interventions for coronary heart disease. Cochrane Database Syst Rev 8:CD002902
36. Baumeister H, Hutter N, Bengel J (2011) Psychological and pharmacological interventions for depression in patients with coronary artery disease. Cochrane Database Syst Rev 9:CD008012

37. Kessler RC, Andrews G, Colpe LJ et al (2002) Short screening scales to monitor population prevalences and trends in nonspecific psychological distress. Psychol Med 32(6):959–976
38. Lovibond SH, Lovibond PF (1995) Manual for the depression anxiety stress scales, 2nd edn. Psychology Foundation, Sydney
39. Derogatis LR, Lipman RS, Rickels K et al (1974) The Hopkins symptom checklist (HSCL): a self-report symptom inventory. Behav Scie 19(1):1–15

Psycho-educational Interventions and Cardiac Rehabilitation

8

Furio Colivicchi, Stefania Angela Di Fusco, and Massimo Santini

The cure of the part should not be attempted without treatment of the whole, and also no attempt should be made to cure the body without the soul, and therefore if the head or body are to be well, you must begin by curing the mind: that is the first thing ... For this is the error of our day in the treatment of the human body, that physicians separate the soul from the body.

Plato (Athens 428/427 bce–348/347 bce)

8.1 Introduction

As emphasized by Eugene Braunwald in his 1980 preface to the first edition of the textbook *Heart Disease*, cardiovascular disease is the greatest scourge afflicting industrialized nations [1]. Despite the fact that the age-adjusted mortality rate for cardiovascular disease has declined in recent years, to this day cardiovascular disease still remains one of the greatest dilemmas in both developed and developing countries.

Relevant changes in dietary and lifestyles patterns that have occurred with economic development and market globalization are significant causes of the growing morbidity linked to cardiovascular disease [2]. To date, cardiovascular disease has become increasingly linked to an unhealthy lifestyle, unbalanced diet, physical inactivity, and psychosocial stress. According to the World Health Organization recommendations, the first step towards reducing cardiovascular disease

F. Colivicchi, MD, FESC, FACC • S.A. Di Fusco, MD (✉)
Cardiology Unit, San Filippo Neri Hospital, Rome, Italy
e-mail: furio.colivicchi@asl-rme.it; doctstefania@hotmail.com

M. Santini, MD, FESC, FACC
Regional Research Centre on Cardiac Arrhythmias, San Filippo Neri Hospital, Rome, Italy
e-mail: m.santini@rmnet.it

A. Roncella, C. Pristipino (eds.), *Psychotherapy for Ischemic Heart Disease*,
DOI 10.1007/978-3-319-33214-7_8

Table 8.1 Recommendations for behavioural change according to European guidelines on cardiovascular disease prevention in clinical practice (version 2012) [6]

Recommendations	Class	Level	Grade
Established cognitive behavioural strategies (e.g. motivational interviewing) to facilitate lifestyle change are recommended	I	A	Strong
Specialized healthcare professionals (e.g. nurses, dieticians, psychologists, etc.) should be involved whenever necessary and feasible	IIa	A	Strong
In individuals at very high cardiovascular disease risk, multimodal interventions, integrating education on healthy lifestyle and medical resources, exercise training, stress management, and counselling on psychosocial risk factors, are recommended	I	A	Strong

burden is to recognize the essential role of unhealthy habits. The major lifestyle and behavioural factors that influence the incidence of ischaemic heart disease (IHD) and the progression of existing IHD are exercise, diet, and smoking. Preventative strategies should aim to provide information and education about a healthy lifestyle, as well as to raise awareness of IHD risk factors and their clinical implications.

Although the term *psycho-education* originally referred to a therapeutic approach to mental illness [3], it is now also increasingly used in the setting of cardiovascular disease to refer to a method of disease management that extends beyond traditional medical care, by providing patients with lifestyle and psychological support [4, 5]. Growing evidence indicates that psycho-education is an important component in treating a variety of medical problems. For efficient psycho-educational interventions, interdisciplinary teams composed of trained and competent professionals are necessary. In addition to the cardiologist, specialized healthcare professionals like nurses, dieticians, and psychologists are needed to support behavioural change (Table 8.1) [6]. A complete psycho-educational intervention should be carefully planned and periodically reviewed and revised to accommodate the changing needs of participants. A psycho-educational programme also must contain specific components of interventions, which include information about the disease and its clinical manifestations, management of medical treatment, nutritional education, physical activity/exercise programmes, and emotional/psychosocial support.

8.2 Counselling in Psycho-educational Interventions

Because the main purpose of psycho-educational interventions is to help empower patients to take control of their healthcare, one critical component for their efficacy is that patients understand the relevance of the proposed intervention programmes. One of the first steps is to give precise and comprehensible information about the disease. Patients must know the significance of IHD symptoms, the relevance of treatment adherence, and the key role of preventive strategies that address specific risk factors. It is essential that patients are counselled to recognize the need and relevance of lifestyle change. The aim of a psycho-educational approach is to instil in patients the knowledge of both heart-healthy and heart-unhealthy behaviours, as well as to help them to develop the skills necessary for the adoption of a healthy lifestyle. It is advisable to establish an empathic and positive relationship that will increase patient adherence to the recommended changes and prescribed drugs. Psycho-educational interventions must take into account cultural and social factors that, unavoidably, influence an individual's behaviours [7]. Programmes that consist of frequent follow-up sessions are more effective at establishing trust between the healthcare provider and patient and in reinforcing individual commitment. Indeed, with reduced contact frequency, the likelihood of behavioural change success also decreases [8]. Group-based interventions can provide added advantages for patients and families, such as the sharing and encouragement of peer support, an increased desire to succeed due to the commitment inside the group, and the opportunity to learn from the feedback of group members. Group interventions should be tailored to provide patients with practical information regarding multiple lifestyle components like diet, exercise, sleep, relaxation, and stress [9]. Educational interventions should be considered part of a comprehensive programme that includes exercise and psychological support. Below, we report recommendations regarding physical activity and a cardiovascular healthy diet that have been confirmed in the setting of IHD. We also summarize interventions aimed at smoking cessation and the management of psychological needs in IHD patients.

8.3 Physical Activity and Exercise Training

According to national and international guidelines and expert consensus on IHD prevention, it is strongly recommended that lifestyle modifications include physical activity for all patients [6, 10–13]. The expression *physical activity* refers to any bodily movement that results in energy expenditure above the basal level, whereas exercise is a planned and structured physical activity performed to improve fitness [14]. There is clear evidence that a sedentary lifestyle is one of the major risk factors for cardiovascular disease [15], whereas physical activity is associated with beneficial effects in both primary and secondary cardiovascular prevention. Physical activity counselling and exercise training should be the core components of all cardiovascular prevention programmes. The numerous biological mechanisms activated and promoted by aerobic physical activity explain its beneficial effects on the cardiovascular system and its favourable impact upon cardiovascular risk factors [16]. Overall, regular physical activity leads to an increased ability to use oxygen to derive energy for work, improving both cardiac output and peripheral oxygen extraction. Further favourable cardiovascular effects of aerobic exercise are the decreased platelet adhesiveness that is associated with improved endothelial function, suppressed pro-inflammatory cytokine production, and the promotion of fibrinolytic activity that results in an antithrombotic effect [17, 18]. Additional recognized beneficial effects are linked to a favourable modulation of autonomic balance, which leads to a reduction in arrhythmic risk [19]. Scientific evidence demonstrates that regular physical activity has significant favourable effects on many of the established risk factors for cardiovascular disease. Regular physical activity has a positive impact on glycaemic control, lipid profile, and blood pressure [20]. In patients with IHD, aerobic exercise training programmes that last at least 3 months are associated with a 30 % reduction in cardiovascular mortality [21]. A 12-month programme of regular daily exercise in patients with stable IHD has been found to result in higher event-free survival and exercise capacity, when compared with coronary angioplasty [22]. Aerobic exercise includes not only sports-related activities like running, bicycling, and swimming, but everyday activities like walking quickly, climbing stairs, and doing house and gardening work. Each exercise programme prescribed must be tailored to an individual's profile, by evaluating his or her medical history, physical examination, resting ECG, transthoracic echocardiography, and exercise stress test results. Combining exercise training with sessions of relaxation therapy has positive effects on both psychological stress and haemodynamic parameters which are superior to that of an exercise programme alone [23, 24].

8.4 Nutritional Education

Proper diet and nutritional strategy affect several risk factors for IHD, including obesity, diabetes, dyslipidaemia, and hypertension. An unhealthy diet is one of the major modifiable risk factors for cardiovascular disease. It is necessary to provide patients with clear information about the essential role of a healthy diet in primary and secondary cardiovascular disease prevention. There is clear evidence that an unhealthy diet increases one's risk of myocardial infarction and accounts for approximately 30 % of population-attributable risk [25]. Nutrients that mainly have an impact in cardiovascular disease are fatty acids, minerals, and fibre. In cardiovascular prevention, the fatty acid composition of the diet is more important than the total fat content. Dietary supplementation with 1 g/day of *n*-3 polyunsaturated fatty acids after a myocardial infarction has been found to be associated with a significant reduction in cardiovascular death [26]. It is recommended that daily saturated fatty acid intake is less than 10 % of the total energy and that saturated fatty acids are replaced by the increased intake of polyunsaturated fatty acids [6], rather than by monounsaturated fatty acids or carbohydrates [27]. However, the reduction in saturated fatty acids should not lead to the total elimination of foods like milk and dairy products, which contain other important nutrients like calcium, potassium, and vitamin D. In fact, a significantly higher rate of diabetes and hypertension has been found in patients who avoid all milk and dairy products [28]. A recent meta-analysis also supports the beneficial effects of dairy consumption on cardiovascular disease [29]. Numerous convincing data demonstrate that diets with a low glycaemic index and low glycaemic load reduce the risk of both diabetes and IHD [30]. High-fibre intake has been found to reduce postprandial glycaemia after carbohydrate-rich meals and to lower total and LDL cholesterol

Table 8.2 Main characteristic of a healthy diet, according to European guidelines on cardiovascular disease prevention in clinical practice (version 2012) [6]

• Saturated fatty acids should account for <10 % of the total energy intake
• Trans-unsaturated fatty acids: as little as possible
• <5 g/day of salt
• 30–45 g/day of fibre from whole-grain foods, fruits, and vegetables
• 200 g/day of fruit (2–3 servings)
• 200 g/day of vegetables (2–3 servings)
• Fish at least twice per week, one of which should be oily fish
• Consumption of alcoholic beverages should be limited to two glasses per day for men and one glass per day for women

levels [31]. A large body of evidence supports modest sodium intake restriction and recommends increases in dietary potassium intake to prevent cardiovascular disease [32]. Fruits and vegetables are good sources of potassium and contain high contents of fibre and antioxidants. It is likely that all these nutrients contribute to the reported protective effects of fruits and vegetables on IHD [33]. Epidemiological studies and meta-analyses appear to show that light to moderate alcohol consumption protects against IHD and improves outcomes in patients with cardiovascular disease [34, 35]. In summary, nutritional education should aim to teach patients the basis of a healthy dietary pattern, which involves reducing their intake of saturated fats, trans-fatty acids, sugar, and salt while promoting the increased intake of fresh fruits and vegetables (Table 8.2). The Mediterranean diet, which is comprised of fruits, vegetables, whole grains, legumes/nuts, fish, unsaturated fats from olive oil, and moderate alcohol consumption, largely corresponds to the previously reported recommendations for a healthy diet. Indeed, several studies have shown the benefits of the Mediterranean diet in cardiovascular disease [36, 37].

8.5 Smoking Cessation

Cigarette smoking is an established and modifiable risk factor for cardiovascular disease. In patients with IHD, smoking cessation is one of the main psycho-educational interventions. Several observational studies have detected a significantly lower mortality rate when patients with known IHD have quit smoking relative to those continue to smoke [38]. Patients who quit smoking can expect to see a reduction in their risk of cardiovascular disease within 2 years, and after 10–15 years, their risk becomes similar to that of non-smokers [39]. Despite the well-known benefits of smoking cessation, usually it is very difficult for patients to quit smoking. Tools useful for helping them to achieve this include counselling, education, and pharmacological assistance (e.g. nicotine substitutes, bupropion, varenicline). Patients should be questioned carefully about their history of tobacco use, evaluating current smoking habits, daily tobacco consumption, previous smoking cessation efforts, motivation to stop, and exposure to passive smoking. Patients reluctant to quit may be unaware of the dangerous effects of tobacco use and the substantial benefits of smoking cessation or may be demoralized because of prior failure [40]. Concise and clear information about the increased cardiovascular risk associated with tobacco use is an essential first step in smoking cessation interventions. It has been proven that brief psycho-education can affect craving patterns during smoking cessation [41]. Table 8.3 reports the key points to address during counselling on smoking cessation. One of the main points is behavioural intervention aimed at enhancing motivation and self-regulatory capacity. The journey towards smoking cessation includes a series of motivational stages (Fig. 8.1) [42]. Clinical studies evaluating the additional value of behavioural strategies tailored to each stage have generated conflicting results [43]. Therefore, it is currently not clear if a stage-based intervention is a more effective strategy for achieving permanent abstinence. Peer support has proven to be a useful strategy for reducing cardiovascular risk factors and specifically for predicting smoking cessation success.

Table 8.3 Tobacco cessation management

• Inquire about smoking history
• Warn about the cardiovascular risks of tobacco use, providing clear information
• Strongly encourage patient to quit
• Support tobacco cessation using behavioural and/or pharmacological interventions
• At follow-up visits
In case of cessation, emphasize the success
In case of relapse, consider further support interventions

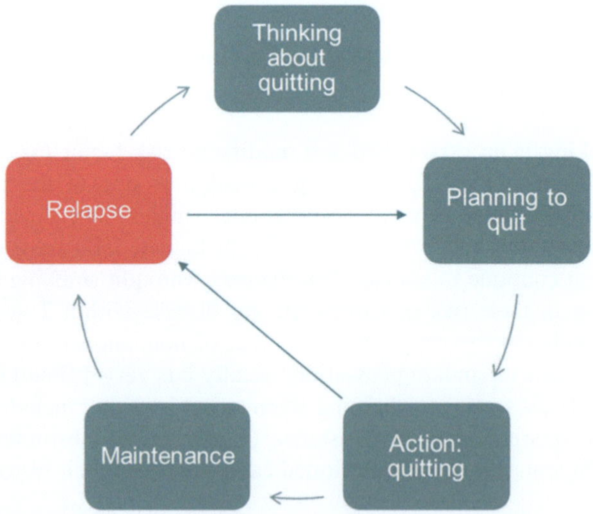

Fig. 8.1 Stages of smoking cessation, modified from Prochaska et al. [42]

8.6 Psychological Support in Ischaemic Heart Disease

Psycho-educational interventions to prevent IHD must address not only behavioural risk factors but also psychological needs. In the short-term psychotherapy in acute myocardial infarction (STEP-IN-AMI) trial, psychological treatment in addition to standard optimal therapy after an acute myocardial infarction was shown to reduce all-cause rehospitalization rates and improve quality of life at 1 year of follow-up [44]. The benefits of short-term psychotherapy, delivered with an ontopsychological approach in the STEP-IN-AMI trial [45], were found to exist irrespective of the patient's baseline depression state. The psychotherapeutic intervention that was tested initially involved individual meetings that were tailored to the specific needs of each patient and focused on the interpretation of body language and dream analysis. After 3–11 individual meetings, group sessions provided, among other interventions, educational therapy, music-guided breathing, and muscular relaxation [46]. Indeed, previous studies showed some favourable effects of supervised relaxation practice after an acute cardiac event, including a reduction in resting heart rate, anxiety, and the frequency of angina pectoris [24]. Results of these studies support the benefits of relaxation therapy in the secondary prevention of IHD.

Epidemiological research has shown that emotional disorders and psychosocial distress are associated with both a higher risk of developing IHD and poorer outcomes when clinical disease is present [47]. Patients with psychosocial distress seem to have a higher suicide risk in the 5 years following an acute cardiac event [48], the peak risk being within the first few months after discharge. AHA/ACCF guidelines on secondary prevention suggest screening for depression in patients who have had recent coronary artery bypass graft surgery or myocardial infarction [10]. Depression seems to reduce an individual's ability to modify unhealthy lifestyle habits that affect cardiovascular risk [49]. Milder forms of psychological distress—such as minor depression, job stress, and difficulty relaxing—may be appropriately managed by practical behavioural interventions [50]. Effective psycho-educational interventions to manage psychological distress include health information, nutritional counselling, exercise, and relaxation training. A growing body of evidence indicates that patients with IHD and depressive symptoms benefit from physical activity and behavioural interventions that support physical activity. In a randomized controlled trial, interventions that motivated patients' participation in physical activity after angioplasty resulted in increased physical activity and decreased depressive symptoms by 12 months of follow-up [51]. A secondary analysis of data from the same trial showed that an increase in energy expenditure in patients with high depressive symptoms was associated with reduced cardiovascular morbidity and mortality [52]. Other studies confirm that patients with depressive symptoms after a coronary event who engage in exercise have a lower mortality rate than depressed patients who do not [53, 54]. Overall, subjects with IHD and high psychosocial stress seem to have more benefits from exercise training, in terms of mortality reduction, than patients without psychosocial stress [55]. Published data represent important incentives for developing practical exercise programmes, not only after acute events but also as a primary preventative measure in patients with IHD risk factors. To improve global outcomes in patients

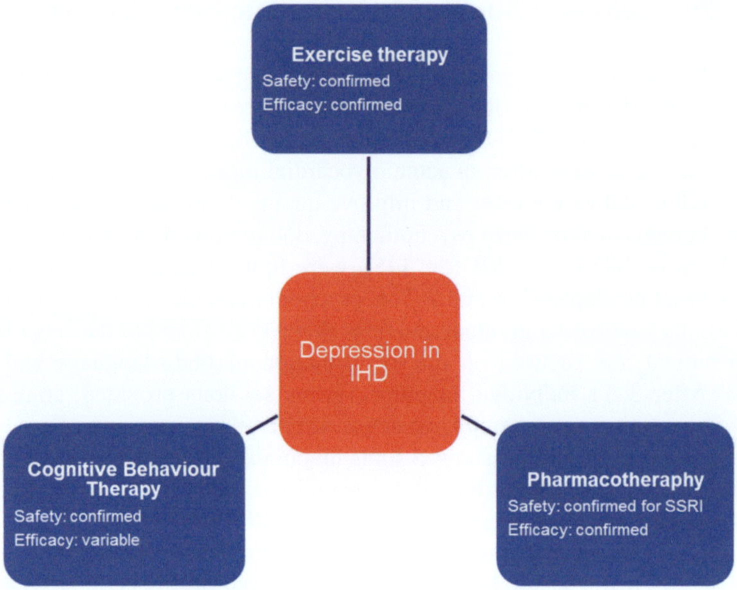

Fig. 8.2 The impact of interventional strategies on depression in patients with ischaemic heart disease, modified from Hare et al. [56]. *IHD* ischaemic heart disease, *SSRI* selective serotonin receptor reuptake inhibitor

with IHD and depression, exercise programmes should be used in association with other intervention strategies (Fig. 8.2) [56, 57]. Cognitive behavioural therapy, which is effective at improving depression symptoms, also seems to reduce cardiovascular events [58]. Additional strategies for the management of depressed patients with IHD include pharmacological treatment. It seems that patients with a previous history of major depression reap the greatest benefits from antidepressant pharmacotherapy [56]. The reduction in depressive symptoms observed in patients receiving antidepressant medication has been found to be comparable to that associated with exercise. Overall, the favourable effects of exercise training go beyond the well-documented fitness benefits. Further studies are necessary to standardize psychological interventions and to confirm that the clinical outcomes of all patients with a previous cardiac event benefit from psychological treatment.

8.7 A Comprehensive Approach to Cardiac Rehabilitation

The first cardiac rehabilitation (CR) programmes date back to more than 50 years ago [59], when the main goals after an acute event were early mobilization and the facilitation of physical recovery through physician-supervised exercise training. Although physical activity is still among the core components of CR, the aim of CR programmes has shifted from simple physical rehabilitation to more comprehensive interventions [60]. Modern CR is a secondary prevention programme that focuses

Table 8.4 Cardiac rehabilitation according to the international guideline. *Na* not available

Recommendations	Class	Level	Grade	References
All patients requiring hospitalization or invasive intervention after an acute ischaemic event should participate in a cardiac rehabilitation programme to improve prognosis by modifying lifestyle habits and increasing treatment adherence	IIa	B	Strong	[6]
All eligible patients with ACS or whose status is immediately post-coronary artery bypass surgery or post-PCI should be referred to a comprehensive outpatient cardiovascular rehabilitation programme either prior to hospital discharge or during their first follow-up office visit	I	A	Na	[10]
Attendance at cardiovascular disease secondary prevention and cardiac rehabilitation after a cardiac event decreases morbidity and mortality and improves quality of life	I	A	Na	[11]

on patient education, individually tailored exercise training, risk factor modification, and the overall well-being of the patient. The majority of current international guidelines strongly recommend CR to improve prognosis and quality of life after a cardiac event (Table 8.4) [6, 10, 11]. Cardiac rehabilitation with multifactorial interventions has been found to reduce mortality, cardiovascular events, cardiovascular risk factors, and psychosocial stress, improving psychological well-being and quality of life [55, 61, 62]. Indeed, addressing patient's psychological problems has been recommended since the first programmes for the rehabilitation of cardiac patients [59]. On the basis of growing evidence that demonstrates that CR's benefits may be affected by the interdependence of the body and mind, there is consensus about the need to assess and manage psychosocial risk factors during CR [63]. In the previous paragraph addressing psychological support in IHD, we reported some scientific evidence about the benefits of psychological treatment and relaxation therapy in the secondary prevention of IHD. Since depression may preclude participation in CR programmes, it is important to identify this mood disorder and help depressed patients to overcome this barrier by providing encouragement and enlisting the patient's family to help improve adherence [64]. The first step in planning an optimal CR programme for each patient is to assess the individual's clinical state and needs. The programme must include a supervised aerobic exercise training programme based upon the patient's clinical characteristics. In addition to formal exercise training, physical activity counselling should be offered to all patients. Other main components of a structured CR programme include nutritional counselling and smoking cessation intervention, both of which were addressed in the previous sections of this chapter. Overall, CR is recognized as one of the best-established models of care in modern healthcare systems for its effectiveness at reducing cardiovascular disease burden and improving lifestyles [65]. Unfortunately, despite the many proven clinical benefits of CR attendance, it is still globally underutilized [62]. The main reasons for this include referral problems, lack of awareness about the beneficial effects of CR, poor support for hesitant patients, and limited local resources. To increase CR attendance and broaden the number of patients who benefit from these programmes, alternative strategies for the delivery of CR are being developed. Smartphone-based homecare CR models have been found to be as effective as conventional CR at improving physiological and psychological health outcomes and increasing the use of CR after a myocardial infarction [66]. Overall, mobile technology can overcome some of the barriers to accessing CR and could be used to promote physical activity, self-management, and increased participation in CR programmes [67].

8.8 Closing Remarks

Psycho-education is a method of disease management that provides patients with the tools they need to take control of their health and healthcare. A complete psycho-educational intervention for IHD should include health education with nutrition and smoking cessation counselling, physical activity programmes, and emotional/psychosocial support. Cardiac rehabilitation is a secondary prevention intervention that focuses on the overall well-being of patients after a cardiac event. One of the core components of CR is the psychological support that is intended to both evaluate and manage psychosocial risk factors that are also cardiovascular risk factors.

Acknowledgement Conflicts of interest: None
Funding: None

References

1. Braunwald E (1980) Heart disease: a textbook of cardiovascular medicine. Saunders, Philadelphia
2. World Health Organization (2002) Joint WHO/FAO expert consultation on diet, nutrition and the prevention of chronic diseases. Report No. 916
3. Goldman CR (1988) Toward a definition of psychoeducation. Hosp Community Psychiatry 39: 666–668
4. McGillion M, Arthur H, Victor JC et al (2008) Effectiveness of psychoeducational interventions for improving symptoms, health-related quality of life, and psychological well being in patients with stable angina. Curr Cardiol Rev 4:1–11
5. Child A, Sanders J, Sigel P et al (2010) Meeting the psychological needs of cardiac patients: an integrated stepped-care approach within a cardiac rehabilitation setting. Br J Cardiol 17: 175–179
6. Perk J, De Backer G, Gohlke H et al (2012) European guidelines on cardiovascular disease prevention in clinical practice (version 2012). The fifth joint task force of the European society of cardiology and other societies on cardiovascular disease prevention in clinical practice (constituted by representatives of nine societies and by invited experts). Eur Heart J 33: 1635–1701

7. Artinian NT, Fletcher GF, Mozaffarian D et al (2010) Interventions to promote physical activity and dietary lifestyle changes for cardiovascular risk factor reduction in adults: a scientific statement from the American Heart Association. Circulation 122:406–441
8. Wadden TA, Vogt RA, Foster GD et al (1998) Exercise and the maintenance of weight loss: 1-year follow-up of a controlled clinical trial. J Consult Clin Psychol 66:429–433
9. Rozanski A (2014) Behavioral cardiology. Current advances and future directions. J Am Coll Cardiol 64:100–110
10. Smith SC Jr, Benjamin EJ, Bonow RO et al (2011) AHA/ACCF secondary prevention and risk reduction therapy for patients with coronary and other atherosclerotic vascular disease: 2011 update: a guideline from the American Heart Association and American College of Cardiology Foundation. Circulation 124:2458–2473
11. Woodruffe S, Neubeck L, Clark RA et al (2015) Australian cardiovascular health and rehabilitation association (ACRA) core components of cardiovascular disease secondary prevention and cardiac rehabilitation 2014. Heart Lung Circ. doi:10.1016/j.hlc.2014.12.008
12. Colivicchi F, Di Roma A, Uguccioni M et al (2010) Secondary cardiovascular prevention after acute coronary syndrome in clinical practice. G Ital Cardiol 11:3S–29S
13. Pavy B, Iliou MC, Vergès-Patois B et al (2012) French society of cardiology guidelines for cardiac rehabilitation in adults. Arch Cardiovasc Dis 105:309–328
14. Giannuzzi P, Mezzani A, Saner H, Working Group on Cardiac Rehabilitation and Exercise Physiology et al (2003) European society of cardiology. physical activity for primary and secondary prevention. Position paper of the working group on cardiac rehabilitation and exercise physiology of the European society of cardiology. Eur J Cardiovasc Prev Rehabil 10:319–327
15. Warren TY, Barry V, Hooker SP et al (2010) Sedentary behaviors increase risk of cardiovascular disease mortality in men. Med Sci Sports Exerc 42:879–885
16. Fletcher GF, Balady GJ, Amsterdam EA et al (2001) Exercise standards for testing and training: a statement for healthcare professionals from the American Heart Association. Circulation 104:1694–1740
17. Lippi G, Maffulli N (2009) Biological influence of physical exercise on hemostasis. Semin Thromb Hemost 35:269–276
18. Chen YW, Apostolakis S, Lip GY (2014) Exercise-induced changes in inflammatory processes: implications for thrombogenesis in cardiovascular disease. Ann Med 46:439–455
19. Billman GE (2009) Cardiac autonomic neural remodeling and susceptibility to sudden cardiac death: effect of endurance exercise training. Am J Physiol Heart Circ Physiol 297: H1171–H1193
20. Vanhees L, Geladas N, Hansen D et al (2012) Importance of characteristics and modalities of physical activity and exercise in the management of cardiovascular health in individuals with cardiovascular risk factors: recommendations from the EACPR. Part II. Eur J Prev Cardiol 19: 1005–1033
21. Heran BS, Chen JM, Ebrahim S et al (2011) Exercise-based cardiac rehabilitation for coronary heart disease. Cochrane Database Syst Rev 7:CD001800
22. Hambrecht R, Walther C, Mobius-Winkler S et al (2004) Percutaneous coronary angioplasty compared with exercise training in patients with stable coronary artery disease: a randomized trial. Circulation 109:1371–1378
23. Neves A, Alves AJ, Ribeiro F et al (2009) The effect of cardiac rehabilitation with relaxation therapy on psychological, hemodynamic, and hospital admission outcome variables. J Cardiopulm Rehabil Prev 29:304–309
24. van Dixhoorn J, White AA, Ernst E (2005) Relaxation therapy for rehabilitation and prevention in ischaemic heart disease: a systematic review and meta-analysis. Eur J Cardiovasc Prev Rehabil 12:193–202
25. Iqbal R, Anand S, Ounpuu S et al (2008) Dietary patterns and the risk of acute myocardial infarction in 52 countries: results of the INTERHEART study. Circulation 118:1929–1937

26. (1999) Dietary supplementation with n-3 polyunsaturated fatty acids and vitamin E after myocardial infarction: results of the GISSI Prevenzione trial. Gruppo Italiano per lo Studio della Sopravvivenza nell'Infarto miocardico. Lancet 354:447–455
27. Jakobsen MU, O'Reilly EJ, Heitmann BL et al (2009) Major types of dietary fat and risk of coronary heart disease: a pooled analysis of 11 cohort studies. Am J Clin Nutr 89:1425–1432
28. Nicklas TA, Qu H, Hughes SO et al (2011) Self-perceived lactose intolerance results in lower intakes of calcium and dairy foods and is associated with hypertension and diabetes in adults. Am J Clin Nutr 94:191–198
29. Qin LQ, Xu JY, Han SF et al (2015) Dairy consumption and risk of cardiovascular disease: an updated meta-analysis of prospective cohort studies. Asia Pac J Clin Nutr 24:90–100
30. Augustin LS, Kendall CW, Jenkins DJ et al (2015) Glycemic index, glycemic load and glycemic response: an international scientific consensus summit from the international carbohydrate quality consortium (ICQC). Nutr Metab Cardiovasc Dis 25:795–815
31. Weickert MO, Pfeiffer AF (2008) Metabolic effects of dietary fiber consumption and prevention of diabetes. J Nutr 138:439–442
32. Aaron KJ, Sanders PW (2013) Role of dietary salt and potassium intake in cardiovascular health and disease: a review of the evidence. Mayo Clin Proc 88:987–995
33. Dauchet L, Amouyel P, Hercberg S et al (2006) Fruit and vegetable consumption and risk of coronary heart disease: a meta-analysis of cohort studies. J Nutr 136:2588–2593
34. Mukamal KJ, Maclure M, Muller JE et al (2001) Prior alcohol consumption and mortality following acute myocardial infarction. JAMA 285:1965–1970
35. Di Castelnuovo A, Costanzo S, Bagnardi V et al (2006) Alcohol dosing and total mortality in men and women: an updated meta-analysis of 34 prospective studies. Arch Intern Med 166: 2437–2445
36. Sofi F, Abbate R, Gensini GF, Casini A (2010) Accruing evidence on benefits of adherence to the Mediterranean diet on health: an updated systematic review and meta-analysis. Am J Clin Nutr 92:1189–1196
37. Widmer RJ, Flammer AJ, Lerman LO et al (2015) The Mediterranean diet, its components, and cardiovascular disease. Am J Med 128:229–238
38. Critchley JA, Capewell S (2003) Mortality risk reduction associated with smoking cessation in patients with coronary heart disease: a systematic review. JAMA 290:86–97
39. Hiroyasu Iso H, Chigusa Date C, Akio Yamamoto A et al (2005) Smoking cessation and mortality from cardiovascular disease among Japanese men and women. The JACC study. Am J Epidemiol 161(2):170–179
40. 2008 PHS Guideline Update Panel, Liaisons, and Staff (2008) Treating tobacco use and dependence: 2008 update U.S. public health service clinical practice guideline executive summary. Respir Care 53(9):1217–1222
41. Nosen E, Woody SR (2013) Brief psycho-education affects circadian variability in nicotine craving during cessation. Drug Alcohol Depend 132(1–2):283–289
42. Prochaska JO, DiClemente CC (1982) Transtheoretical therapy: toward a more integrative model of change. Psychother Theory Res Pract 19:276–288
43. Cahill K, Lancaster T, Green N (2010) Stage-based interventions for smoking cessation. Cochrane Database Syst Rev 11:CD004492
44. Roncella A, Pristipino C, Cianfrocca C et al (2013) One-year results of the randomized, controlled, short-term psychotherapy in acute myocardial infarction (STEP-IN-AMI) trial. Int J Cardiol 170(2):132–139
45. Meneghetti A (2004) Ontopsychology handbook. Ontopsicologia Editrice, Rome
46. Roncella A, Giornetti A, Cianfrocca C et al (2009) Rationale and trial design of a randomized, controlled study on short-term psychotherapy after acute myocardial infarction: the STEP-IN-AMI trial (Short Term Psychotherapy in Acute Myocardial Infarction). J Cardiovasc Med (Hagerstown) 10(12):947–952
47. Williams RB (2010) Myocardial infarction and risk of suicide: another reason to develop and test ways to reduce distress in post myocardial-infarction patients. Circulation 122:2356–2358

48. Larsen KK, Agerbo E, Christensen B et al (2010) Myocardial infarction and risk of suicide: a population-based case- control study. Circulation 122:2388–2393
49. Bauer LK, Caro MA, Beach SR et al (2012) Effects of depression and anxiety improvement on adherence to medication and health behaviors in recently hospitalized cardiac patients. Am J Cardiol 109:1266–1271
50. Rozanski A, Blumenthal JA, Davidson KW et al (2005) The epidemiology, pathophysiology, and management of psychosocial risk factors in cardiac practice: the emerging field of behavioral cardiology. J Am Coll Cardiol 45(5):637–651
51. Peterson JC, Charlson ME, Hoffman Z et al (2012) A randomized controlled trial of positive-affect induction to promote physical activity after percutaneous coronary intervention. Arch Intern Med 172(4):329–336
52. Peterson JC, Charlson ME, Wells MT et al (2014) Depression, coronary artery disease, and physical activity: how much exercise is enough? Clin Ther 36(11):1518–1530
53. Milani RV, Lavie CJ (2007) Impact of cardiac rehabilitation on depression and its associated mortality. Am J Med 120:799–806
54. Blumenthal JA, Babyak MA, Carney RM et al (2004) Exercise, depression, and mortality after myocardial infarction in the ENRICHD trial. Med Sci Sports Exerc 36:746–755
55. Milani RV, Lavie CJ (2009) Reducing psychosocial stress: a novel mechanism of improving survival from exercise training. Am J Med 122:931–938
56. Hare DL, Toukhsati SR, Johansson P et al (2014) Depression and cardiovascular disease: a clinical review. Eur Heart J 35(21):1365–1372
57. Judith H, Lichtman LH, Bigger JT Jr et al (2008) Recommendations for screening, referral, and treatment: a science advisory from the American Heart Association Prevention Committee of the Council on cardiovascular nursing, council on clinical cardiology, council on epidemiology and prevention, and interdisciplinary council on quality of care and outcomes research: endorsed by the American Psychiatric Association. Circulation 118:1768–1775
58. Gulliksson M, Burell G, Vessby B et al (2011) Randomized controlled trial of cognitive behavioral therapy vs. standard treatment to prevent recurrent cardiovascular events in patients with coronary heart disease: Secondary Prevention in Uppsala Primary Health Care Project (SUPRIM). Arch Intern Med 171:134–140
59. Hellerstein HK, Ford AB (1957) Rehabilitation of the cardiac patient. JAMA 164:225–231
60. Balady GJ, Williams MA, Ades PA et al (2007) Core components of cardiac rehabilitation/secondary prevention programs: 2007 update: a scientific statement from the American Heart Association Exercise, Cardiac Rehabilitation, and Prevention Committee, the Council on Clinical Cardiology; the Councils on Cardiovascular Nursing, Epidemiology and Prevention, and Nutrition, Physical Activity, and Metabolism; and the American Association of Cardiovascular and Pulmonary Rehabilitation. Circulation 115:2675–2682
61. Dalal HM, Doherty P, Taylor RS (2015) Cardiac rehabilitation. BMJ 351:h5000. doi:10.1136/bmj.h5000
62. de Vries H, Kemps HMC, van Engen-Verheul MM et al (2015) Cardiac rehabilitation and survival in a large representative community cohort of Dutch patients. Eur Heart J 6: 1519–1528
63. Pogosova N, Saner H, Pedersen SS et al (2015) Psychosocial aspects in cardiac rehabilitation: from theory to practice. A position paper from the cardiac rehabilitation section of the European Association of Cardiovascular Prevention and Rehabilitation of the European Society of Cardiology. Eur J Prev Cardiol 22(10):1290–1306
64. Lichtman JH, Bigger JT Jr, Blumenthal JA et al (2008) Depression and coronary heart disease: recommendations for screening, referral, and treatment: a science advisory from the American Heart Association Prevention Committee of the Council on Cardiovascular Nursing, Council on Clinical Cardiology, Council on Epidemiology and Prevention, and Interdisciplinary Council on Quality of Care and Outcomes Research: endorsed by the American Psychiatric Association. Circulation 118(17):1768–1775

65. Arena R, Lavie CJ, Cahalin LP (2015) Transforming cardiac rehabilitation into broad-based healthy lifestyle programs to combat noncommunicable disease. Expert Rev Cardiovasc Ther 29:1–14
66. Varnfield M, Karunanithi M, Lee CK et al (2014) Smartphone-based home care model improved use of cardiac rehabilitation in postmyocardial infarction patients: results from a randomised controlled trial. Heart 100(22):1770–1779
67. Beatty AL, Fukuoka Y, Whooley MA (2013) Using mobile technology for cardiac rehabilitation: a review and framework for development and evaluation. J Am Heart Assoc 2(6):e000568

Psychiatric Pharmacotherapy in Coronary Artery Disease Patients

9

Roberto Latini and Silvio Garattini

The best thing about the future is that it comes one day at a time.

Abraham Lincoln

9.1 Introduction

A large quantity of evidence of different levels of strength has been gathered over the last four decades on the effects of antidepressant and antipsychotic drugs on the cardiovascular system [1–4]. In particular, attention has focused on the risk of sudden cardiac death and myocardial infarction (MI). While the causal relationship between several psychiatric drugs and sudden death via the induction of QT interval prolongation and potentially lethal ventricular arrhythmias like torsades de pointes (TdP) and the Brugada syndrome has been almost completely elucidated, the association with myocardial infarction is not so clear. This is mainly because most of the evidence comes from observational case–control and often retrospective studies, rather than from randomized controlled trials. It is impossible merely by means of observational studies to satisfactorily answer the following crucial questions:

1. Do antidepressants and antipsychotic agents simply identify patients with psychiatric disorders?
2. Which are the interactions between psychiatric disorders and psychiatric drugs on the risk of cardiovascular diseases and their outcomes?
3. Could effective psychiatric therapy not only improve mental symptoms but also decrease cardiovascular events?

R. Latini (✉) • S. Garattini
IRCCS Istituto di Ricerche Farmacologiche Mario Negri, Via Giuseppe La Masa 19, Milan, Italy
e-mail: roberto.latini@marionegri.it; silvio.garattini@marionegri.it

A. Roncella, C. Pristipino (eds.), *Psychotherapy for Ischemic Heart Disease*,
DOI 10.1007/978-3-319-33214-7_9

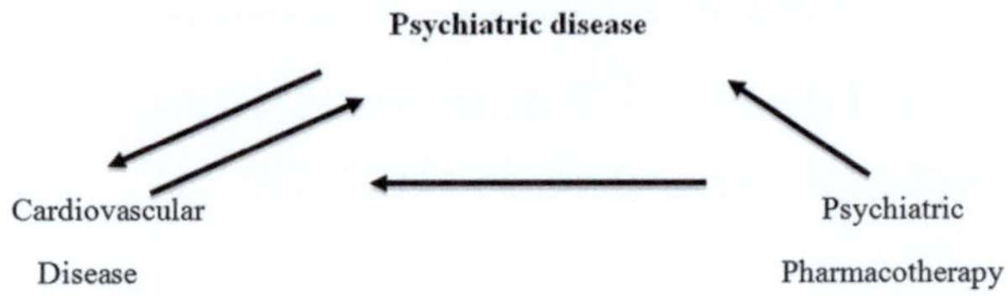

Fig. 9.1 The conundrum of psychiatric therapy

As a general reference, it should be kept in mind that over 45 % of patients in hospital after a myocardial infarction have depression.

The complexity of this conundrum is schematically depicted in Fig. 9.1.

In any case, based largely on concerns over QT prolongation and the development of life-threatening arrhythmias, a number of antipsychotic drugs have been temporarily or permanently withdrawn from the market or their use restricted, and strict rules for testing drugs for arrhythmogenic potential have been promoted.

The results of several studies suggest that psychiatric patients are exposed to an increased risk of cardiovascular events. Community-based studies have detected a two- to five-fold higher risk of ischemic heart disease in patients with mental illnesses than in the general population and a two- to three-fold greater risk of death from cardiovascular causes [4, 5]. These increased risks have been identified in different studies not only on depression or psychosis but also on epilepsy, although the evidence for epilepsy is much less compelling [6].

Since near consensus has been reached on these beliefs, psychiatric patients in need of antipsychotic or antidepressant drugs constitute a real therapeutic problem, which is rendered even more complex when they have cardiovascular comorbidities, coronary artery disease (CAD) in particular, given the associated high risk of sudden cardiac death.

The two main categories of mental disease, depression and psychosis, will be discussed separately in the present chapter.

9.2 Antidepressant Drugs

Heart disease is more prevalent in patients with depression, and its prognosis is worsened by this psychiatric comorbidity. An ideal treatment for depression would be one that simultaneously alleviates depression and decreases the risk of cardiovascular events. In general, antidepressants—particularly tricyclic drugs—are not recommended in patients with cardiovascular disease due to their reported adverse cardiac effects. However, newer selective serotonin reuptake inhibitors (SSRIs) might be associated with a lower risk of cardiovascular events, thereby lessening the increased risk associated with depression.

This statement is partly based on different cardiovascular effects of the two categories of antidepressants:

1. Tricyclic antidepressants increase heart rate, induce orthostatic hypotension, slow intraventricular conduction, and suppress ventricular premature complexes (arrhythmias).
2. SSRIs decrease heart rate to, albeit, only a slight degree; they also do not typically slow intracardiac conduction, do not affect blood pressure, and do not cause orthostatic hypotension.

In general, European guidelines on cardiovascular disease prevention suggest that efforts should be made to detect depression and that patients with clinically significant depressive disorders should be started on specific treatments [7]. Nonetheless, there is presently no clear evidence that adequate treatment of depression effectively reduces the associated increased risks of cardiovascular events.

It should be considered up front that, while there is no agreement on the association between certain antidepressive agents and the risk of myocardial infarction (MI), their association with lethal ventricular arrhythmias and consequent sudden death appears quite robust; and this is the main reason to avoid prescribing these agents in patients with preexisting ischemic heart disease.

9.2.1 Specific Studies

One cohort study prospectively examined whether a major depressive episode increased the risk of incident MI and evaluated the role of psychotropic medication use in this relationship [8]. A history of depression and psychotropic medication use were assessed in 1981, and self-reported MI was assessed in 1994. In this Baltimore-based study, 64 MIs were reported among 1551 respondents who had been free of heart disease in 1981. Comparing those with a history of dysphoria and those without, the odds ratio (OR) for an MI was 2.07 (95 % CI, 1.16–3.71), while the odds ratio associated with a history versus no history of a major depressive episode was 4.54 (95 % CI, 1.65–12.44), independent of coronary risk factors. Including drug treatment in the multivariate risk models, the association between psychotropic medication use and MI was no longer significant, thereby suggesting that the increased risk of MI might be attributable to the primary relationship between depression and ischemic heart disease.

Eighty-one outpatients with a diagnosis of major depressive disorder and documented ischemic heart disease were randomly assigned to either paroxetine, 20–30 mg/day, or nortriptyline targeted to a therapeutic plasma concentration of 50–150 ng/mL for 6 weeks [9]. Twenty-five (61 %) of 41 patients improved during treatment with paroxetine, versus 22 (55 %) of 40 on nortriptyline. Neither drug significantly affected blood pressure or conduction intervals. Paroxetine had no sustained effects on heart rate or rhythm or indices of heart rate variability. Conversely, patients treated with nortriptyline had a sustained 11 % increase in heart rate from a mean of 75 to 83 beats per minute ($p < 0.001$) and a reduction in heart rate variability, as measured by the standard deviation (SD) of all normal R–R intervals over a 24-h period, from 112 to 96 ($p < 0.01$). Adverse cardiac events occurred in one (2 %) of 41 patients treated with paroxetine versus seven (18 %) of 40 patients treated with nortriptyline ($p < 0.03$). Paroxetine and nortriptyline both proved to be effective as antidepressants in depressed patients with ischemic heart disease. However, nortriptyline treatment was associated with a significantly higher rate of serious adverse cardiac events relative to paroxetine.

In yet another case–control study, 933 men and women with ischemic heart disease were matched by age and sex to 5516 controls [10]. Odds ratios for ischemic heart disease were significantly elevated among patients who had, at some time, received a prescription for tricyclic antidepressants, even after adjusting for diabetes mellitus, hypertension, smoking, body mass index, and the use of SSRIs (OR = 1.56, 95 % CI 1.18–2.05). Patients who had ever taken dosulepin (dothiepin) had a significantly higher odds ratio for ischemic heart disease after adjusting for confounding factors and the use of other antidepressants (OR = 1.67, 95 % CI 1.17–2.36). There was no significant increase in the odds ratios for amitriptyline, lofepramine, or SSRIs on multivariate analysis.

The safety of SSRI antidepressants versus tricyclics has been assessed, since SSRIs appear to lack the adverse pro-arrhythmic effects of tricyclic antidepressants and are thought to inhibit platelet aggregation [11]. In a Danish, registry-based, case–control study, 8887 patients hospitalized for an MI for the first time between 1994 and 2002 were identified and matched by age and sex with 88,862 controls. In patients with a history of cardiovascular disease, nonsignificantly lower risks of MI were observed and differences by class of antidepressant remained uncertain. These associations were not apparent in people without a history of cardiovascular disease. The authors concluded that antidepressant use might be associated with a decreased risk of hospitalization for MI among persons with a history of cardiovascular disease; however, whether there were differences by class of antidepressant remained uncertain.

On the contrary, results of prospective, controlled clinical trials support the findings that SSRIs are beneficial in patients with ischemic heart disease. In one small placebo-controlled study, the SSRI sertraline reduced platelet/endothelial activation in depressed patients after an acute coronary syndrome [12]. These findings suggest that the ancillary effects of SSRIs may be an additional advantage in patients with depression and CAD.

Along the same line, in another placebo-controlled study on 127 patients with stable CAD, the SSRI escitalopram reduced the occurrence of mental stress-induced myocardial ischemia, while no difference was found for exercise-induced ischemia [13]. These results support and extend previous evidence on the beneficial effects of the modulation of central and peripheral serotoninergic function on ischemic heart disease symptoms. The findings may also help in elucidating the pathways that link depression/negative emotions and cardiovascular outcomes.

9.3 Antipsychotic Drugs

Since the early 1990s, a clear relationship has been established between some antipsychotics, prolongation of the QT interval on the ECG, and the development of an atypical polymorphic form of tachycardia known as *torsades de pointes* (TdP) and sudden cardiac death. Not all the antipsychotics exhibit the same risk: the newer atypical antipsychotics, olanzapine, risperidone, and quetiapine, display a much lower risk than the older antipsychotics, in particular phenothiazines, when given long term to sick patients.

Another issue is that of acute sedation of critically ill and agitated patients with intravenous haloperidol. In September 2007, the Food and Drug Administration (FDA) recommended continuous electrocardiographic monitoring for intravenous (IV) haloperidol to detect QT prolongation and TdP. It is well established that haloperidol may prolong the QT interval by blocking the repolarizing potassium IKr current. Although drugs that block the IKr channel can produce arrhythmia in healthy individuals, the risk is increased in patients with cardiac disease or an electrolyte imbalance (i.e., hypokalemia and hypomagnesemia), those concomitantly taking a pro-arrhythmic drug, and those on mechanical ventilation.

The FDA identified a total of 70 cases of IV haloperidol-associated QT prolongation and/or TdP [14]. There were 54 reports of TdP, with 42 of these events reportedly preceded by QT prolongation. When post-event QTc data were reported, QTc was prolonged by more than 450 msec in 96 % of cases. Three patients experienced sudden cardiac arrest. Sixty-eight patients (97 %) had additional risk factors for TdP/prolonged QT, most commonly taking some concomitant pro-arrhythmic agent. Patients experiencing TdP had received a cumulative dose of 5–645 mg, while patients with QT prolongation alone had received a cumulative dose of 2–1540 mg. While administration of IV haloperidol can be associated with QT prolongation/TdP, this complication most often takes place in the setting of concomitant risk factors. It is important to note that available data suggest that a total cumulative dose of IV haloperidol of <2 mg can be administered safely without ongoing electrocardiographic monitoring in patients without concomitant risk factors.

While regulatory agencies advise against the use of intravenous haloperidol, a review of the World Health Organization (WHO) global individual case safety report database (VigiBase) fails to reveal that the intravenous route is any more likely to be associated with adverse cardiac events. VigiBase data were analyzed for QT prolongation, TdP, and/or cardiac arrest involving intravenous haloperidol versus other routes of administration, as well as the antipsychotics olanzapine and quetiapine [15]. The absolute numbers of individual case safety reports of QT prolongation, TdP, and/or cardiac arrest were 365 cases for haloperidol, 489 for olanzapine, and 520 for quetiapine. Reporting rates for haloperidol did not increase over the last two decades. Thirty-two percent of the haloperidol cases involved oral, 16.4 % intramuscular, and 22.7 % intravenous administration. The difference in the reporting odds ratios for haloperidol and quetiapine was not statistically significant. Olanzapine was associated with a slightly lower reporting odds ratio. Even considering the limitation of pharmacovigilance studies, which rarely include a denominator, the recommendation against intravenous haloperidol warrants further study.

9.3.1 Specific Studies

Myocarditis and cardiomyopathy have most consistently been linked to treatment with clozapine [16]. A pharmacovigilance data mining study using the WHO database concluded that myocarditis and cardiomyopathy are significantly more often associated with clozapine than other antipsychotic medications (231 clozapine reports versus 89 for all the other antipsychotics combined). The clinical features of myocarditis are nonspecific. Although fever, tachycardia, chest pain, dyspnea, flu-like symptoms, eosinophilia, elevated cardiac enzyme levels, and ECG changes may all be present, no single finding is pathognomonic. The risk of developing cardiomyopathy has been estimated to be up to five times greater in patients treated with clozapine than that seen in the general population. It is possible for nonlethal, subclinical clozapine-induced myocarditis to progress to dilated cardiomyopathy.

All patients with a documented stroke and at least one prescription for any antipsychotic drug before the end of 2002 were registered in the WHO database. Ultimately, 6790 eligible patients were identified and included in final analysis [17]. Rate ratios were calculated for stroke comparing periods of time exposed to antipsychotics against unexposed periods. Use of any antipsychotic drug was associated with a risk ratio for stroke of 1.73 (95 % CI 1.60–1.87), including 1.69 (1.55–1.84) for typical antipsychotics and 2.32 (1.73–3.10) for atypical antipsychotics. In patients receiving any antipsychotic drug, the risk ratios were 3.50 (2.97–4.12) for those with dementia and 1.41 (1.29–1.55) for those without. All antipsychotics, therefore, seem to be associated with an increased risk of stroke, and this risk might be greater in patients receiving atypical versus typical antipsychotics. People with dementia also seem to be at a higher risk of an associated stroke than people without, so that the use of antipsychotics should, when possible, be avoided in such patients.

9.4 Age and Gender

Atypical antipsychotic agents have been associated with adverse cerebrovascular events, particularly in elderly dementia patients. However, limited evidence exists regarding the comparative cerebrovascular profiles of individual atypical agents, particularly in community settings.

A total of 2458 cerebrovascular events were identified in one study cohort: 1081 (21.38 %) in risperidone users, 816 (18.75 %) in olanzapine users, and 561 (21.05 %) in quetiapine users. After adjusting for propensity scores and other covariates, the Cox proportional hazards model revealed that the use of quetiapine [hazard ratio (HR) 0.88; 95 % CI 0.78, 0.99] but not risperidone (HR 1.05; 95 % CI

0.95, 1.16) was associated with a decreased risk of adverse cerebrovascular events relative to olanzapine, thereby suggesting that quetiapine might be somewhat safer, in terms of cerebrovascular event risk, than olanzapine in the elderly [18].

Prolongation of the QT interval is a common and serious adverse effect, associated with increased risk for ventricular arrhythmias, syncope, and sudden death. Women have a greater risk of QT prolongation than men. The occurrence of drug-induced QT prolongation presumably depends upon the specific regulation of channel expression by sex hormones. On the other hand, men seem to have a higher susceptibility to drug-related sudden cardiac death.

9.5 Clinical Guidelines/Recommendations

Patients with schizophrenia and bipolar disorders have a high prevalence of cardiovascular diseases and, at the same time, a lower chance of being prescribed appropriate cardiovascular drug therapy or treatments like percutaneous coronary angioplasty, stent implantation, or coronary artery bypass graft (CABG) surgery. This poor quality of care likely contributes to the excessive cardiovascular morbidity and mortality that is observed in patients with mental disorders, in particular the elderly. Therefore, it is advisable that each patient who is going to be started on an antipsychotic drug undergoes careful measurement of blood pressure and ECG for QTc measurement. As a general indication, a QTc >500 ms or an increase in QTc ≥60 ms above baseline is associated with a significantly increased risk of TdP, ventricular fibrillation, and sudden cardiac death. These concerns should be kept in mind considering also the well-known unwanted metabolic effects of antipsychotics—like abnormalities in lipid and glucose metabolism—which further increase the cardiovascular risks of the treated patient [19].

Guidelines to evaluating QT interval prolongation and the pro-arrhythmic potential of antiarrhythmic drugs were published in 2005. With few exceptions, all new drugs must undergo a "thorough" QT (TQT) study. However, the majority of presently used drugs were developed and released before TQT studies were mandatory. Additionally, even a well-performed TQT study cannot rule out pro-arrhythmic effects when the drug is used on a large scale in clinical situations where patients often receive multiple medications and have comorbid substance abuse or even preexisting heart diseases. Most importantly, several antipsychotics and antidepressants on the market are known to induce QT prolongation. On this basis, psychiatrists and other physicians need to be able to assess and handle the potential for drug-induced QT prolongation. In the TQT studies, drug-induced QT interval prolongation is used as a surrogate risk marker, and the regulatory threshold level of concern is an increase of roughly 5 ms above baseline, while a QT duration above 500 ms or an increase of ≥60 ms above baseline is commonly used as a threshold value in clinical practice. The exact criteria used for the evaluation in the TQT study depend on the indication for the tested drug. Several common cardiovascular conditions—including ischemic heart disease, arterial hypertension, heart failure, and bradyarrhythmias, but also a broad range of less common conditions like cardiomyopathies and primary arrhythmias—predispose patients to the development of drug-induced arrhythmias. Interactions with other concomitantly used drugs, including potassium- and magnesium-wasting diuretics, CYP3A4 inhibitors, and other QT-prolonging drugs (e.g., antibiotics and antifungals), can also increase the likelihood of serious arrhythmia.

To improve patient safety, clinical guidelines integrating these many potentially interacting factors are warranted, and collaboration between psychiatrists and cardiologists is needed. Such guidelines must be clinically manageable and proven to reduce the risk of drug-induced arrhythmias when administered to patients with a psychiatric disorder.

Notwithstanding the negative cardiovascular impact of several antidepressant and antipsychotic drugs, many studies have shown that the prevalence of depression is higher in patients with cardiovascular disease than in the general population, with figures ranging from 17 to 47 %. For example, depression is associated with more than a twofold increase in mortality among patients who survive an acute myocardial infarction [20]. Since depression has been demonstrated to increase morbidity and mortality in cardiovascular disease, and to worsen already-impaired quality of life, these patients cannot be deprived of pharmacologic and psychotherapeutic care. For these reasons, patients with CAD or heart failure must be evaluated and treated for depression, when indicated. Randomized trials have shown that therapy, mostly with newer antidepressants, is well tolerated and safe in cardiac patients and can improve quality of life; however, the size of the trials reported to date does not allow for us to conclude that antidepressant therapy improves survival and/or morbidity [21, 22].

9.6 Conclusions

A number of antipsychotic and antidepressant drugs are known to increase the risk of ventricular arrhythmias and sudden cardiac death. This effect is manifested through the prolongation of the QT interval and/or the induction of TdP arrhythmias. Offending drugs include (1) typical antipsychotics like chlorpromazine, pimozide, thioridazine, perphenazine, trifluoperazine, haloperidol, and droperidol; (2) atypical antipsychotics like clozapine, quetiapine, risperidone, sultopride, ziprasidone, and loxapine; (3) tricyclic antidepressants like amitriptyline, amoxapine, clomipramine, desipramine, citalopram, doxepin, imipramine, nortriptyline, and trimipramine; and (4) other antidepressants like fluoxetine, sertraline, and venlafaxine. Antipsychotics can increase cardiac risk even at low doses, whereas antidepressants do this generally only at high doses or in the setting of drug combinations, especially in patients with preexisting cardiovascular disease. This being said, not all antipsychotics appear to exhibit the same level of risk, though considerable debate continues over this [23].

These observations call for the need for careful clinical histories, as well as for ECGs at baseline and after drug administration, in particular in psychiatric patients at increased cardiovascular risk, including those with a predisposition to QT prolongation. High-risk antipsychotics and antidepressants should be avoided in patients with known congenital LQTS or BS, as well as in the setting of an acute systemic disease, including acute cardiac infarction patients and those with renal dysfunction.

9.7 Perspectives

Most of the evidence on the adverse effects of psychiatric drugs in patients with CAD comes from case–control studies or from data registries; and most of the data were collected retrospectively. Given the limited potential to control for confounders in such studies, prospective, long-term, adequately sized, placebo-controlled, or otherwise comparative studies are warranted. A prerequisite for the success of such studies will be close collaborations between psychiatrists and cardiologists.

Large-scale, multicenter trials are still needed to assess whether antidepressants or antipsychotics can, on one hand, decrease the risk of cardiovascular disease in psychiatric patients and, on the other, improve clinical outcomes in patients with ischemic heart disease or heart failure. For this reason, at present no evidence-based therapeutic guidelines can be made available to either the cardiologist or psychiatrist.

References

1. Krantz DS, Whittaker KS, Francis JL et al (2009) Psychotropic medication use and risk of adverse cardiovascular events in women with suspected coronary artery disease: outcomes from the women's ischemia syndrome evaluation (WISE) study. Heart 95(23):1901–1906
2. Honkola J, Hookana E, Malinen S et al (2012) Psychotropic medications and the risk of sudden cardiac death during an acute coronary event. Eur Heart J 33(6):745–751
3. Fanoe S, Kristensen D, Fink-Jensen A et al (2014) Risk of arrhythmia induced by psychotropic medications: a proposal for clinical management. Eur Heart J 35(20):1306–1315
4. Hennekens CH, Hennekens AR, Hollar D, Casey DE (2005) Schizophrenia and increased risks of cardiovascular disease. Am Heart J 150(6):1115-1121
5. Lin ST, Chen CC, Tsang HY et al (2014) Association between antipsychotic use and risk of acute myocardial infarction: a nationwide case-crossover study. Circulation 130(3):235–243
6. Olesen JB, Abildstrøm SZ, Erdal J et al (2011) Effects of epilepsy and selected antiepileptic drugs on risk of myocardial infarction, stroke, and death in patients with or without previous stroke: a nationwide cohort study. Pharmacoepidemiol Drug Saf 20:964–971
7. Perk J, De Backer G, Gohlke H, European Association for Cardiovascular Prevention and Rehabilitation (EACPR), ESC Committee for Practice Guidelines (CPG) et al (2012) European guidelines on cardiovascular disease prevention in clinical practice (version 2012). The fifth joint task force of the European society of cardiology and other societies on cardiovascular disease prevention in clinical practice (constituted by representatives of nine societies and by invited experts). Eur Heart J 33(13):1635–1701
8. Pratt LA, Ford DE, Crum RM et al (1996) Depression, psychotropic medication, and risk of myocardial infarction. Prospective data from the Baltimore ECA follow-up. Circulation 94(12):3123–3129

9. Roose SP, Laghrissi-Thode F et al (1998) Comparison of paroxetine and nortriptyline in depressed patients with ischemic heart disease. JAMA 279(4):287–291
10. Hippisley-Cox J, Pringle M, Hammersley V et al (2001) Antidepressants as risk factor for ischaemic heart disease: case-control study in primary care. BMJ 323(7314):666–669
11. Monster TB, Johnsen SP, Olsen ML et al (2004) Antidepressants and risk of first-time hospitalization for myocardial infarction: a population-based case-control study. Am J Med 117(10): 732–737
12. Serebruany VL, Glassman AH, Malinin AI, Sertraline AntiDepressant Heart Attack Randomized Trial Study Group et al (2003) Platelet/endothelial biomarkers in depressed patients treated with the selective serotonin reuptake inhibitor sertraline after acute coronary events: the sertraline antidepressant heart attack randomized trial (SADHART) platelet substudy. Circulation 108(8):939–944
13. Jiang W, Velazquez EJ, Kuchibhatla M et al (2013) Effect of escitalopram on mental stress-induced myocardial ischemia: results of the REMIT trial. JAMA 309(20):2139–2149
14. Meyer-Massetti C, Cheng CM, Sharpe BA et al (2010) The FDA extended warning for intravenous haloperidol and torsades de pointes: how should institutions respond? J Hosp Med 5(4): E8–E16
15. Meyer-Massetti C, Vaerini S, Rätz Bravo AE et al (2011) Comparative safety of antipsychotics in the WHO pharmacovigilance database: the haloperidol case. Int J Clin Pharm 33(5): 806–814
16. Fitzsimons J, Berk M, Lambert T et al (2005) A review of clozapine safety. Expert Opin Drug Saf 4(4):731–744
17. Douglas IJ, Smeeth L (2008) Exposure to antipsychotics and risk of stroke: self controlled case series study. BMJ 337:a1227
18. Chatterjee S, Chen H, Johnson ML, Aparasu RR (2012) Comparative risk of cerebrovascular adverse events in community-dwelling older adults using risperidone, olanzapine and quetiapine: a multiple propensity score-adjusted retrospective cohort study. Drugs Aging 29(10): 807–817
19. De Hert M, Detraux J, van Winkel R et al (2011) Metabolic and cardiovascular adverse effects associated with antipsychotic drugs. Nat Rev Endocrinol 8(2):114–126
20. Celano CM, Huffamn JC (2011) Depression and cardiac disease. A review. Cardiol Rev 19(3): 130–142
21. Kim JM, Bae KY, Stewart R et al (2015) Escitalopram treatment for depressive disorder following acute coronary syndrome: a 24-week double-blind, placebo-controlled trial. J Clin Psychiatry 76(1):62–68
22. Blumenthal JA, Sherwood A, Babyak MA et al (2012) Exercise and pharmacological treatment of depressive symptoms in patients with coronary heart disease: results from the UPBEAT (Understanding the prognostic benefits of exercise and antidepressant therapy) study. J Am Coll Cardiol 60(12):1053–1063
23. Leucht S, Cipriani A, Spineli L et al (2013) Comparative efficacy and tolerability of 15 antipsychotic drugs in schizophrenia: a multiple-treatments meta-analysis. Lancet 382:951–962

Evidence-Based Psychotherapy in Ischemic Heart Disease: Umbrella Review and Updated Meta-Analysis

10

Giuseppe Biondi-Zoccai, Marianna Mazza, Leonardo Roever, Jan van Dixhoorn, Giacomo Frati, and Antonio Abbate

A good head and a good heart are always a formidable combination.

Nelson Mandela

10.1 Introduction

The management of ischemic heart disease has seen momentous improvements over the last few decades [1]. However, the booming elderly population and refinements in complex management strategies have often transformed a major mortality burden into a similarly impactful morbidity burden, primarily manifested as heart failure [2]. For instance, the chances of a patient with an anterior

G. Biondi-Zoccai, MD, MStat (✉) • G. Frati, MD, MSc
Department of Medico-Surgical Sciences and Biotechnologies, Sapienza University of Rome, Corso della Repubblica 79, 04100 Latina, Italy

Department of AngioCardioNeurology, IRCCS Neuromed, Pozzilli, Italy
e-mail: giuseppe.biondizoccai@uniroma1.it; giacomo.frati@uniroma1.it

M. Mazza, MD, PhD
Institute of Psychiatry, Catholic University, Rome, Italy
e-mail: mariannamazza@hotmail.com

L. Roever, MHS
Department of Clinical Research, Federal University of Uberlândia, Uberlândia, Brazil
e-mail: leonardoroever@hotmail.com

J. van Dixhoorn, MD, PhD
Centre for Breathing Therapy, Amersfoort, The Netherlands
e-mail: j.dixhoorn@versatel.nl

A. Abbate, MD, PhD
Division of Cardiology, VCU Pauley Heart Center, Virginia Commonwealth University, Richmond, VA, USA
e-mail: antonio.abbate@vcuhealth.org

A. Roncella, C. Pristipino (eds.), *Psychotherapy for Ischemic Heart Disease*,
DOI 10.1007/978-3-319-33214-7_10

myocardial infarction (MI) surviving to hospital discharge have improved dramatically; however, such successes have exponentially increased the number of patients with recent or prior myocardial infarction with or at substantial risk for heart failure.

Beyond lifestyle changes, drug therapy, surgery, and the use of implantable or non-implantable medical devices, psychological interventions in general and psychotherapy in particular hold the promise of providing complementary or even synergistic benefits to patients with or at risk for ischemic heart disease [3–6]. Indeed, psychotherapy—which is used in the present work to identify any type of psychological intervention not intended to have a direct cardiovascular effect—may provide direct beneficial effects for the neurogenic and psychogenic determinants of atherothrombosis and myocardial ischemia in particular, as well as cardiovascular function in general [3–5, 7] (see Chaps. 1 and 3). Even if this is not our perspective, psychotherapy could be highly beneficial even if it could simply improve adherence to evidence-based treatments and limit the untoward psychological effects of cardiovascular disease on patients and relatives. There is, however, a dire need for clarity on this topic, as this type of intervention is obviously at risk of suboptimal standardization or confounding due to placebo and small study effects [8]. Indeed, while it is reasonable to expect that psychotherapy may have beneficial impacts on anxiety and depression dimensions, with ensuing clinically relevant improvements in quality of life, it remains unclear whether it can also improve cardiovascular outcomes such as death, myocardial infarction, and the like.

Systematic reviews have the capacity to summarize the evidence base on a specific clinical topic while enabling the explicit selection, abstraction, and appraisal of the single sources of evidence. When combined with pairwise or network meta-analysis, these reviews can provide more precise and accurate effect estimates while appraising consistency and the impact of select moderators [9]. Umbrella reviews represent another, most recent development in the field of evidence synthesis [10]. They basically consist of overviews of systematic reviews and can provide a comprehensive evidence platform to appraise the risk-benefit profile of a clinical intervention while enabling careful quantitative analysis and synthesis with pairwise and network meta-analysis. Both systematic reviews with meta-analyses and umbrella reviews can be combined pragmatically to timely and accurately summarize the evidence base for a specific clinical topic [11]. We thus conducted an umbrella review and updated meta-analysis on the impact of psychotherapy in patients with ischemic heart disease.

10.2 Methods of Umbrella Review and Updated Meta-Analysis

10.2.1 Design

This work was designed a priori and conducted according to established methods [12]. Specifically, we aimed to conduct a detailed umbrella review of systematic reviews and meta-analyses, compounded by an updated meta-analysis of randomized clinical trials (RCTs), focusing on the risk-benefit balance of psychotherapy for ischemic heart disease.

10.2.2 Search

We searched for systematic reviews focusing on the role of psychotherapy in the prevention of major adverse cardiovascular events in ischemic heart disease indexed in PubMed on April 18, 2015, according to the following established search strategy: ((coronary AND (artery OR revascularization)) OR (ischemic OR ischaemic) AND (heart) AND (psychodynamic OR interpersonal OR psychoanal* OR psycho-anal* OR (brief AND dynamic) OR cognitive OR behavioral OR behavioural) AND (psychotherapy)) AND systematic[sb]. Notably, the "systematic[sb]" term automatically calls an extensive search string developed by Shojania et al. [13].

We then searched for randomized clinical trials focusing on the role of psychotherapy in the prevention of major adverse cardiovascular events in ischemic heart disease and published after the time frame of inclusion of the most recent systematic review identified by the above search. Specifically, PubMed was searched on April 18, 2015, according to the following established search strategy [14]: (coronary AND (artery OR revascularization)) OR (ischemic OR ischaemic) AND (heart) AND (psychodynamic OR interpersonal OR psychoanal* OR psycho-anal* OR (brief AND dynamic) OR cognitive OR behavioral OR behavioural) AND (psychotherapy) AND (randomized controlled trial[pt] OR controlled clinical trial[pt] OR randomized controlled trials[mh] OR random allocation[mh] OR double-blind method[mh] OR single-blind method[mh] OR clinical trial[pt] OR clinical trials[mh] OR (clinical trial[tw] OR ((singl*[tw] OR doubl*[tw] OR trebl*[tw] OR tripl*[tw]) AND (mask*[tw] OR blind[tw])) OR (latin square[tw]) OR placebos[mh] OR placebo*[tw] OR random*[tw] OR research design[mh:noexp] OR follow-up studies[mh] OR prospective studies[mh] OR cross-over studies [mh] OR control*[tw] OR prospectiv*[tw] OR volunteer*[tw]) NOT (animal [mh] NOT human[mh]) NOT (comment[pt] OR editorial[pt] OR meta-analysis [pt] OR practice-guideline[pt] OR review[pt])). No language restrictions were enforced. Searches were conducted by two experienced reviewers with divergences solved after consensus.

10.2.3 Abstraction

We abstracted key details on studies, patients, treatments, and outcomes from the included trials. In particular, we defined major adverse cardiovascular events as the composite of death, myocardial infarction, and revascularization. Individual components of major adverse cardiovascular events were also extracted. Data abstraction was conducted by two experienced reviewers with divergences again resolved after consensus.

10.2.4 Appraisal

The validity of systematic reviews was appraised with the *A Measurement Tool to Assess Systematic Reviews* (AMSTAR) tool, focusing on a priori design, duplicate study selection and data extraction, the comprehensiveness of the literature search performed, status of publication, list of studies (included and excluded), characteristics of the included studies, scientific quality of the included studies reported and used appropriately, appropriate methods for combining the study findings, assessment of likelihood of publication bias, and conflicts of interest [15].

The validity of randomized trials was appraised with the *Cochrane Risk of Bias* tool, which explicitly distinguishes between the following domains: adequacy of sequence generation; adequacy of allocation concealment; adequacy of blinding of participants, personnel, and outcome assessors (with assessments made for each main outcome or class of outcomes); adequacy of incomplete outcome data (with assessments made for each main outcome or class of outcomes); adequacy of outcome reporting; and risk of other sources of bias [16].

Data appraisal was again conducted by two experienced reviewers with divergences resolved after consensus.

10.2.5 Analysis

Continuous variables are reported as mean values and categorical variables as counts. Risk estimates for dichotomous variables were computed with a random effect method to obtain odds ratios (OR) with 95 % confidence intervals and corresponding p values for effect. Statistical heterogeneity was appraised by computing I^2 and performing the Breslow-Day test. Small study effects were appraised visually with a funnel plot and the Egger test. Statistical significance was set at the two-tailed 0.05 level for effect and the two-tailed 0.10 level for heterogeneity and small study effects. Computations were performed using the statistical software program Stata 13 (StataCorp, College Station, TX, USA).

10.3 Results

10.3.1 Umbrella Review of Systematic Reviews

Our search yielded a total of 11 systematic reviews, of which three were included, with a fourth review retrieved by snowballing (Tables 10.1 and 10.2) [3–6]. Specifically, Linden and colleagues reported on 23 randomized clinical trials including a total of 1259 patients who received a mixture of psychological therapies like cognitive/behavioral therapy, counseling, education, psychotherapy, relaxation therapy, stress management training (STM), and type A behavior modification [3]. Outcomes of interest were anxiety, blood lipids, blood pressure, depression, heart rate, major adverse cardiac events, and psychological distress. The key findings were that psychotherapy was associated with significant improvements in heart rate, blood lipids, major adverse cardiac events, and psychological distress. However, the risks of placebo effect and selective reporting were not appraised in detail and cannot be discarded in this work. Moreover, the inclusion of studies that were conducted before modern treatments for ischemic heart disease which had been introduced limits the current external validity of the review.

Dusseldorp et al. [4] reported on 37 studies (both randomized and nonrandomized) and 8998 patients, including, as interventions of interest, counseling, education, exercise training, relaxation therapy, and stress management training. They reported on the following outcomes: angina, anxiety, blood lipids, blood pressure, diet, depression, exercise, major adverse cardiac events, psychological distress, smoking, and weight. Notably, they found that patients in the intervention groups had significant improvements in angina, blood lipids, blood pressure, depression, major adverse cardiac events, smoking, and weight. However, the risks of selection bias, placebo effects, and selective reporting were not appraised and cannot be discarded, and the inclusion of studies conducted before modern treatments for ischemic heart disease which had been introduced again limits the current external validity of this review.

Van Dixhoorn and colleagues included a total of 27 studies (both randomized clinical trials and observational studies) incorporating 2269 patients [5]. The interventions of interest were cognitive/behavioral therapy, relaxation therapy, and stress management training. The outcomes of interest were angina, anxiety, arrhythmia, blood lipids, blood pressure, exercise tolerance, heart rate, heart rate variability, ischemia, major adverse cardiac events, and return to work. In this meta-analysis, psychotherapy was associated with significant improvements in angina, anxiety, arrhythmia, depression, exercise tolerance, heart rate, ischemia, blood lipids, major adverse cardiac events, and return to work. However, the risks of placebo effects and selective reporting were not appraised in detail and cannot be discarded. Moreover, as with the previous analyses, the inclusion of studies conducted before modern treatments for ischemic heart disease which had been introduced limits the current external validity of the review.

Finally, Whalley et al. included 24 randomized clinical trials involving a total of 9087 patients, focusing on cognitive/behavioral therapy, counseling, education,

Table 10.1 Salient features of previously published systematic reviews on psychotherapy for ischemic heart disease

Review	Patients	Studies	Follow-up (years)	Time frame	Included studies	Types of intervention	Outcomes of interest	Key findings	Additional details/ commence
Linden (1996)	1259	23	2	1968–1996	RCTs only	• Cognitive/ behavioral therapy • Counseling • Education • Psychotherapy • Relaxation therapy/SMT • Type A behavior modification	• Anxiety • Blood pressure • Depression • Heart rate • Lipids • MACE • Psychological distress	Psychotherapy was associated with improvements in: • Heart rate • Lipids • MACE • Psychological distress	• The risks of placebo effect and selective reporting were not appraised in detail and cannot be appraised • The inclusion of studies conducted before modern treatment for ischemic heart disease which had been introduced limits the current external validity of the review
Dusseldorp (1999)	8998	37	5	1974–1997	Both non-RCTs and RCTs	• Counseling • Education • Exercise training • Relaxation therapy/SMT	• Angina • Anxiety • Blood pressure • Diet • Depression • Lipids • Exercise	Psychotherapy was associated with improvements in: • Angina • Blood pressure	• The risks of selected bias, placebo effect, and selective reporting were not appraised and cannot be discarded

							• MACE • Psychological distress • Smoking • Weight	• Depression • Lipids • MACE • Smoking • Weight	• The inclusion of studies conducted before modern treatment for ischemic heart disease which had been introduced limits the current external validity of the review
Van Dixhoorn (2005)	2269	27	2	1970–2005	Both non-RCTs and RCTs	• Cognitive/ behavioral therapy • Relaxation therapy/SMT	• Angina • Anxiety • Arrhythmia • Blood pressure • Depression • Exercise tolerance • Heart rate • Ischemia • Lipids • MACE • Return to work	Psychotherapy was associated with improvements in • Angina • Anxiety • Arrhythmia • Exercise tolerance • Heart rate • Heart rate variability • Ischemia • Lipids • MACE • Return to work	• The risk of selection bias, placebo effect and selective reporting were not appraised in detail and cannot be discarded • The inclusion of studies conducted before modern treatment for ischemic heart disease had been introduced limits the current external validity of the review
Whalley (2011)	9087	24	2	1987–2008	RCTs only	• Cognitive/ behavioral therapy • Counseling • Education	• Anxiety • Depression • MACE • Quality of life • Stress	Psychotherapy was associated with improvements in	• The risk of a placebo effect was not appraised in detail and cannot be discarded

(continued)

Table 10.1 (continued)

Review	Patients	Studies	Follow-up (years)	Time frame	Included studies	Types of intervention	Outcomes of interest	Key findings	Additional details/ commence
						• Psychotherapy • Relaxation therapy/SMT • Type A behavior modification	• Type A behavior	• Anxiety • Depression	• Evidence of small study effects was apparent for selected outcome (e.g. death) • The inclusion of studies conducted before modern treatment for ischemic heart disease had been introduced limits the current external validity of the review

MACE major adverse cardiovascular events (i.e., the composite of death, myocardial infarction, stroke, and revascularization), *RCT* randomized clinical trial, *STM* stress management training

Table 10.2 Validity of published systematic reviews on psychotherapy for ischemic heart disease, according to assessing the methodological quality of systematic reviews (AMSTAR tool)

Review	Was "a priori" design provided?	Was there duplicate study selection and data extraction?	Was a comprehensive literature search performed?	Was the status of publication used as an inclusion criterion?	Was a list of studies provided?	Were the characteristics of the included studies provided?	Was the scientific quality of the included studies assessed and documented?	Was the scientific quality of the included studies used appropriately in formulating conclusion?	Were the methods used to combine the findings of studies appropriate?	Was the likelihood of publication bias assessed?	Was the conflict of interest stated?	Overall score
Linden (1996)	No	No	No	Yes	Yes	Yes	No	No	Yes	No	No	3/11
Dusseldorp (1999)	No	No	No	Yes	Yes	Yes	Yes	Yes	Yes	No	No	5/11
Van Dixhoorn (2005)	No	Yes	Yes	No	Yes	Yes	Yes	Yes	Yes	Yes	No	9/11
Whalley (2011)	Yes	Yes	Yes	Yes	Yes	Yes	Yes	Yes	Yes	Yes	Yes	11/11

psychotherapy, relaxation therapy, stress management training, and type A behavior modification [6]. They focused on the following outcomes: anxiety, depression, major adverse cardiac events, quality of life, stress, and type A behavior. Meta-analysis suggested that psychotherapy was associated with significant improvements in anxiety and depression. Nonetheless, the risk of placebo effect was not appraised in detail and cannot be discarded; evidence of small study effects was apparent for selected outcomes (e.g., death); and the inclusion of studies conducted before modern treatments for ischemic heart disease which had been introduced again limits the current external validity of the review.

10.3.2 Systematic Review and Meta-Analysis of Randomized Clinical Trials

The search for randomized clinical trials identified 82 potential citations, with five randomized trials (851 patients) not included in the most recent and comprehensive systematic review by Whalley et al. (Table 10.3) [17–21]. Thus, a total of 24 randomized trials were ultimately included, for a comprehensive set of 9275 subjects providing data on major adverse cardiac events [17–39]. Patient diagnoses included stable ischemic heart disease, recent coronary revascularization, and acute coronary syndromes. The interventions of interest were group or individual cognitive-behavioral therapy, disease adjustment, education, relaxation, stress management therapy, and type A behavior modification. Most studies enrolled a majority of male patients, with the notable exceptions of Burell et al. [23], Claesson et al. [25], Koertge et al. [31], and Orth-Gomér et al. [20]. Trial quality was highly variable, especially in the earliest ones that were also conducted during a therapeutic era devoid of many contemporary treatments for ischemic heart disease, like drug-eluting coronary stents, platelet P2Y12 receptor antagonists, and statins (Table 10.4).

Meta-analysis revealed psychotherapy to be associated with a significant reduction in the risk of death over the course of follow-up [odds ratio = 0.743 (95 % confidence interval 0.588–0.940), p for effect = 0.013, p for heterogeneity = 0.253, $I^2 = 16.8$ %] (Table 10.5, Figs. 10.1 and 10.2). However, this analysis was substantially undermined by statistically significant evidence of small study effects ($p = 0.007$) (Fig. 10.3). Conversely, no significant effect of psychotherapy was identified focusing on myocardial infarction [odds ratio = 0.804 (0.630–1.027), p for effect = 0.080, p for heterogeneity = 0.173, $I^2 = 26–2$ %, p for small study effects = 0.245] (Figs. 10.4, 10.5, and 10.6) or revascularization [odds ratio = 0.877 (0.693–1.109), p for effect = 0.274, p for heterogeneity = 0.200, $I^2 = 23.5$ %, p for small study effects = 0.448] (Figs. 10.7, 10.8, and 10.9). Psychotherapy was associated with significant benefits for major adverse cardiac events [odds ratio = 0.715 (0.540–0.946), p for effect = 0.019] (Figs. 10.10 and 10.11). However, this analysis was also limited by the evidence of significant heterogeneity (p for heterogeneity = 0.014, $I^2 = 54.9$ %) and evidence of small study effects ($p = 0.094$) (Fig. 10.12).

Table 10.3 Key features of recent randomized trials on psychotherapy for ischemic heart disease

Study	Design	Setting	Patients	Follow-up (years)	Diagnosis	Intervention(s)	Age (years)	Females (%)	Diabetics
Albus (2009)	RCT	Multi-center	77	7	Stable CAD	Group cognitive-behavioral therapy for 12 months	54	12	NA
Appels (EX-IT, 2005)	RCT	Multi-center	727	1.5	PCI	Group cognitive-behavioral therapy, education, relaxation, and type A behavior modification for 28 contact hours	53	23	NA
Berkman (ENRICHD, 2000)	RCT	Multicenter	2481	NA	AMI	Group and individual cognitive-behavioral therapy, education, relaxation, and type A behavior modification for 18 contact hours	61	34	NA
Burell (1996)	RCT	Multicenter	261	3	CABG	Group cognitive-behavioral therapy, education, relaxation, and type A behavior modification for 75 contact hours	58	86	NA
Burgess (1987)	RCT	Single-center	180	0.25	AMI	Individual cognitive-behavioral therapy, education, relaxation, and type A behavior modification for 3 months	51	15	NA
Claesson (2005)	RCT	Single-center	198	1	Stable or unstable CAD	Group cognitive-behavioral therapy, education, relaxation, and type A behavior modification for 40 contact hours	61	100	NA

(continued)

Table 10.3 (continued)

Study	Design	Setting	Patients	Follow-up (years)	Diagnosis	Intervention(s)	Age (years)	Females (%)	Diabetics
Cowan (2001)	RCT	Single-center	133	NA	Out of hospital cardiac arrest	Individual cognitive-behavioral therapy, education, relaxation, and type A behavior modification for 16.5 contact hours	NA	27	NA
Friedman (RCCP 1982)	RCT	Single center	862	NA	AMI	Cognitive-behavioral therapy, relaxation, and type A behavior modification for 57 contact hours	53	8	NA
Gulliksson (SUPRIM 2011)	RCT	Single center	362	7.8	Stable or unstable CAD	Cognitive-behavioral therapy for 40 contact hours spanning 1 year	62	23	15 %
Hofman Bang (1999)	RCT	Single center	93	NA	PCI	Group and individual cognitive-behavioral therapy, education, relaxation, and type A behavior modification for 1 month	53	16	NA
Ibrahim (1974)	RCT	Single center	118	NA	AMI	Group cognitive-behavioral therapy, education, relaxation, and type A behavior modification for 74 contact hours	52	10	NA
Jones (1996)	RCT	Multicenter	2328	NA	AMI	Group cognitive-behavioral therapy, education, and relaxation for 14 contact hours	NA	27	NA

Koertge (2009)	RCT	Single center	247	NA	AMI, PCI or CABG	Group cognitive-behavioral therapy, education, relaxation, and type A behavior modification for 40 contact hours	62	100	NA
Mayou (2002)	RCT	Single center	114	NA	AMI	Behavior change, disease adjustment, and education therapy for 2.4 contact hours	58	22	NA
McLaughlin (2005)	RCT	Single center	100	NA	ACS	Cognitive-behavioral therapy, counseling, relaxation training, and education for 3 contact hours	60	33	NA
Michalsen (2005)	RCT	Single center	105	NA	Stable or unstable CAD	Cognitive-behavioral therapy, relaxation, and type A behavior modification for 96 contact hours	59	23	NA
Neves (2009)	RCT	Single center	81	2	Stable or unstable CAD	Group relaxation therapy for 3 months	60	15	NA
Oldenburg (1995)	RCT	Single center	46	1	AMI	Counseling, relaxation training, and education for 12 months	56	11	NA
Orth-Gomér (SWITCHD 2009)	RCT	Multicenter	237	7	AMI, PCI or CABG	Group cognitive-behavioral therapy for 12 months	62	100	12 %
Rahe (1979)	RCT	Single center	44	NA	AMI	Group cognitive-behavioral therapy and relaxation for 3 months	53	11	NA

(continued)

Table 10.3 (continued)

Study	Design	Setting	Patients	Follow-up (years)	Diagnosis	Intervention(s)	Age (years)	Females (%)	Diabetics
Sebregts (2005)	RCT	Single center	204	NA	AMI or CABG	Group cognitive-behavioral therapy, education, relaxation, and type A behavior modification for 20 contact hours	55	14	NA
STEP-IN-AMI (2013)	RCT	Single center	101	1	AMI (1 week after complete revascularization)	Group and individual psychotherapy lasting up to 6 months	55	11	16 %
Stem (1983)	RCT	Single center	64	NA	AMI	Education, relaxation therapy, and type A behavior modification for 14 contact hours	53	15	NA
Van Dixhoorn (1999)	RCT	Single center	156	NA	AMI	Relaxation therapy for 6 contact hours	56	6	NA

AMI acute myocardial infarction, *CABG* coronary artery bypass grafting, *CAD* coronary artery disease, *NA* not available or applicable, *PCI* percutaneous coronary intervention, *RCT* randomized clinical trial

Table 10.4 Assessment of the validity of recent randomized trials on psychotherapy for ischemic heart disease, according to the Cochrane Collaboration Risk of Bias tool

Study	Sequence generation	Allocation concealment	Blinding of participants, personnel, and outcome assessors	Incomplete outcome data	Selective outcome reporting	Other sources of bias
Albus (2009)	Computer generated	Independent research nurse	Not reported	All patients apparently analyzed	No	No
Appels (EXIT, 2005)	Computer generated	Independent research nurse	Blinding of outcome assessors	Analysis according to intention to treat	Yes	No
Berkman (ENRICHD, 2000)	Unclear	Unclear	Unclear	Unclear	Unclear	No
Burell (1996)	Unclear	Centralized phone service	Unclear	Unclear	No	No
Burgess (1987)	Unclear	Sealed envelopes	Unclear	Analysis according to intention to treat	No	No
Claesson (2005)	Unclear	Unclear	Unclear	Unclear	No	No
Cowan (2001)	Unclear	Centralized phone service	Blinding of outcome assessors	Analysis according to intention to treat	No	No
Friedman (RCCP, 1982)	Random numbers	Unclear	Unclear	Unclear	No	No
Gulliksson (SUPRIM, 2011)	Computer generated	Sealed envelopes	National civil registry record linkage	All patients apparently analyzed	No	No
Hofman Bang (1999)	Unclear	Unclear	Unclear	Unclear	No	No
Ibrahim (1974)	Alternate allocation	Unclear	Unclear	Unclear	No	No
Jones (1996)	Unclear	Centralized phone service	Blinding of outcome assessors	Unclear	No	No

(continued)

Table 10.4 (continued)

Study	Sequence generation	Allocation concealment	Blinding of participants, personnel, and outcome assessors	Incomplete outcome data	Selective outcome reporting	Other sources of bias
Koertge (2009)	Random numbers	Sealed envelopes	Blinding of outcome assessors	Analysis according to intention to treat	No	No
Mayou (2002)	Random numbers	Sealed envelopes	Unclear	Analysis according to intention to treat	Unclear	No
McLaughlin (2005)	Coin flip	Unclear	Interactive phone service	Analysis according to intention to treat	No	No
Michalsen (2005)	Computer generated	Unclear	Unclear	Analysis according to per protocol	No	No
Neves (2009)	Unclear	Unclear	Not reported	All patients apparently analyzed	No	No
Oldenburg (1995)	Alternative allocation	High risk	Unclear	Unclear	No	No
Orth-Gomér (SWITCHD, 2009)	Random numbers	Independent research person	Not reported	All patients apparently analyzed	No	No
Rahe (1979)	Unclear	Unclear	Unclear	High risk	No	No
Sebregts (2005)	Unclear	Sealed envelopes	Blinding of outcome assessors	Seven patients randomized but excluded from the study	No	No
STEP-IN-AMI (2013)	Unclear	Sealed envelopes	Blinding of outcome assessors	Analysis according to intention to treat	No	No
Stern (1983)	Unclear	Unclear	Not reported	All patients apparently analyzed	No	No
Van Dixhoorn (1999)	Unclear	Unclear	Not reported	All patients apparently analyzed	No	No

Table 10.5 Meta-analysis of psychotherapy for ischemic heart disease

Outcome	Odds ratio			*P* for heterogeneity	Inconsistency (I^2) (%)	*P* for small study effects
	Point estimate	95 % confidence interval	*P* for effect			
Death	0.743	0.588–0.940	0.013	0.253	16.8	0.007
Myocardial infarction	0.804	0.630–1.027	0.080	0.173	26.2	0.245
Revascularization	0.877	0.693–1.109	0.274	0.200	23.5	0.448
Death, myocardial infarction, or revascularization	0.715	0.540–0.946	0.019	0.014	54.9	0.094

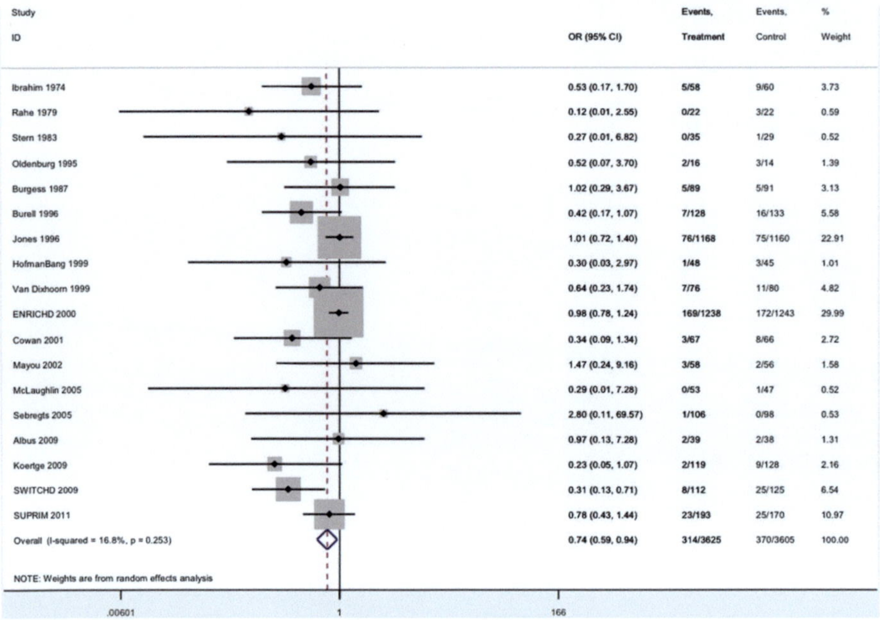

Fig. 10.1 Forest plot for the risk of death (*CI* confidence interval, *OR* odds ratio; treatment: psychotherapy)

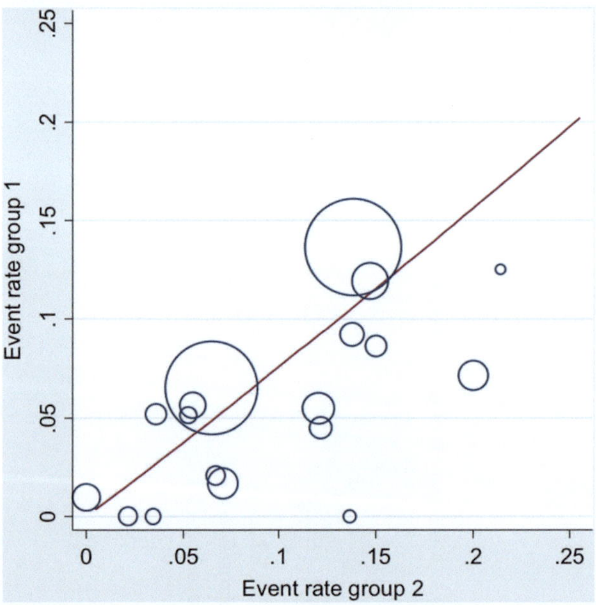

Fig. 10.2 L'Abbe plot for the risk of death (group 1, psychotherapy; group 2, control group; *line*, pooled odds ratio line)

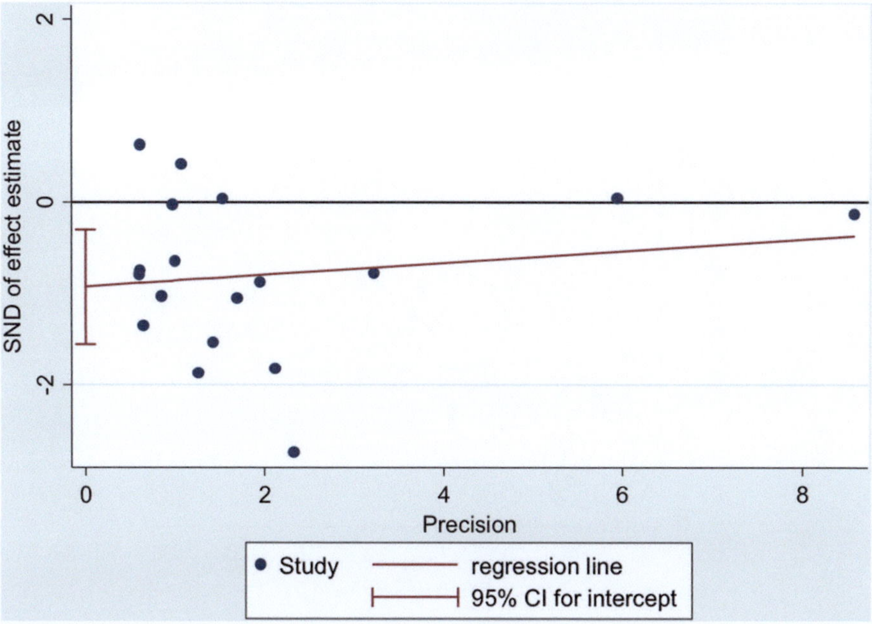

Fig. 10.3 Funnel plot for the risk of death (*CI* confidence interval, *SND* standardized normal deviate)

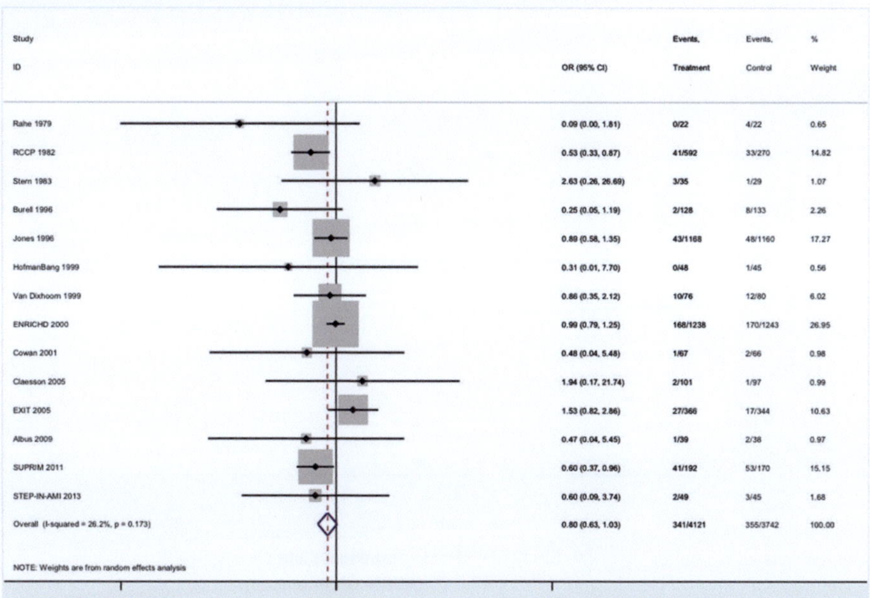

Fig. 10.4 Forest plot for the risk of myocardial infarction (*CI* confidence interval, *OR* odds ratio; treatment: psychotherapy)

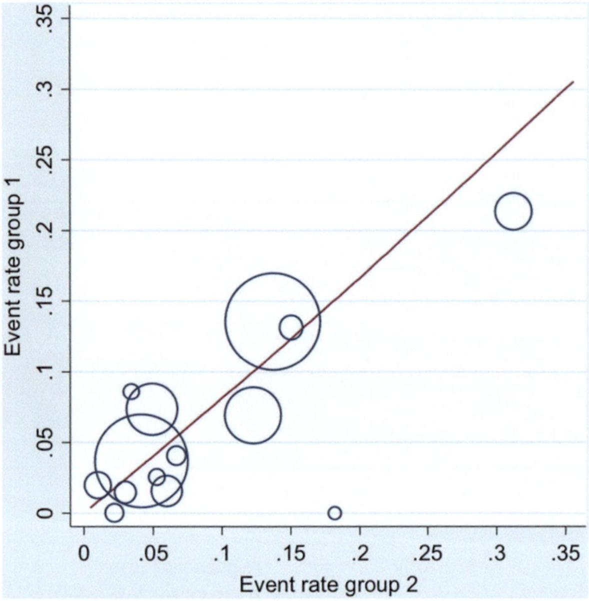

Fig. 10.5 L'Abbe plot for the risk of myocardial infarction (group 1, psychotherapy; group 2, control group; *line*, pooled odds ratio line)

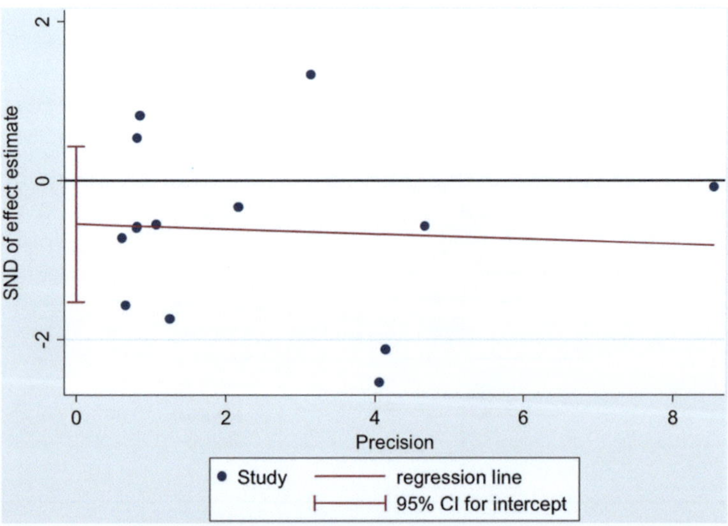

Fig. 10.6 Funnel plot for the risk of myocardial infarction (*CI* confidence interval, *SND* standardized normal deviate)

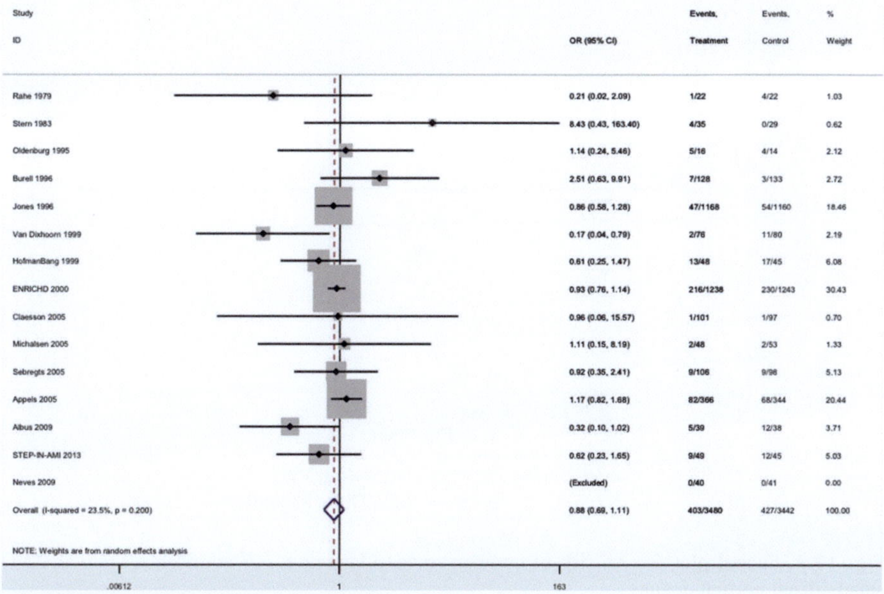

Fig. 10.7 Forest plot for the risk of coronary revascularization (*CI* confidence interval, *OR* odds ratio; treatment: psychotherapy)

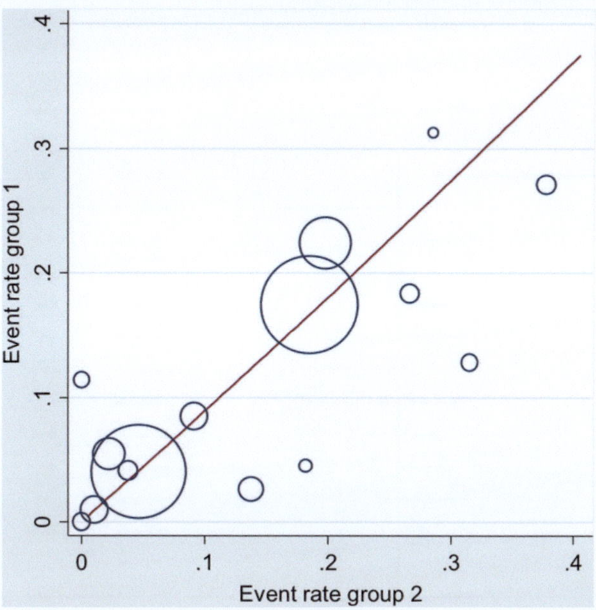

Fig. 10.8 L'Abbe plot for the risk of coronary revascularization (group 1, psychotherapy; group 2, control group; *line*, pooled odds ratio line)

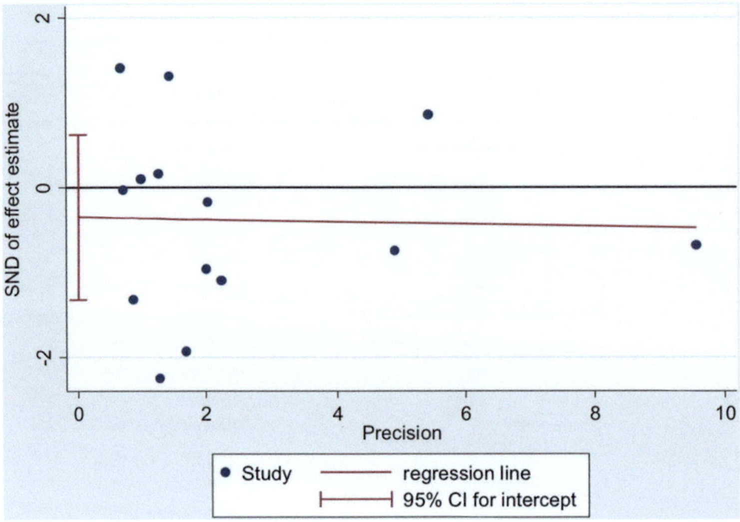

Fig. 10.9 Funnel plot for the risk of coronary revascularization (*CI* confidence interval, *SND* standardized normal deviate)

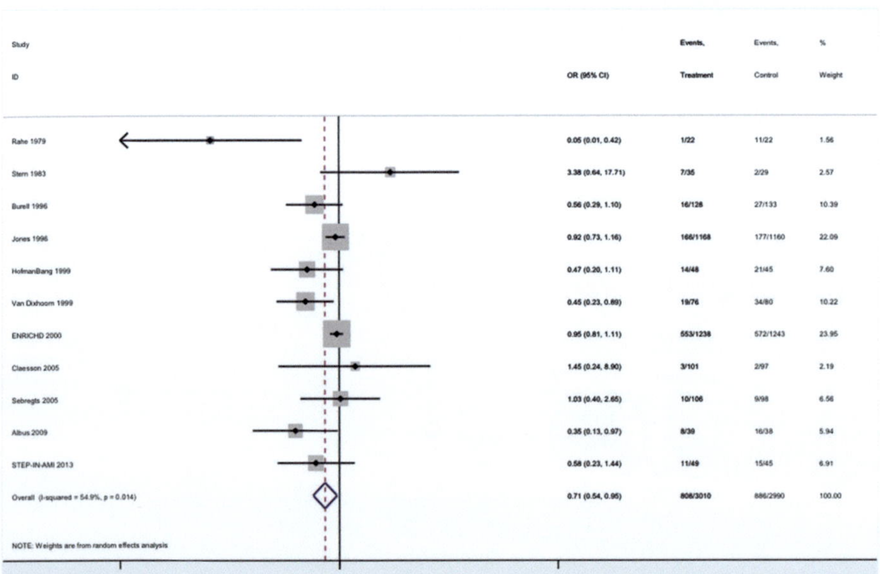

Fig. 10.10 Forest plot for the risk of major adverse cardiac events (*CI* confidence interval, *OR* odds ratio; treatment: psychotherapy)

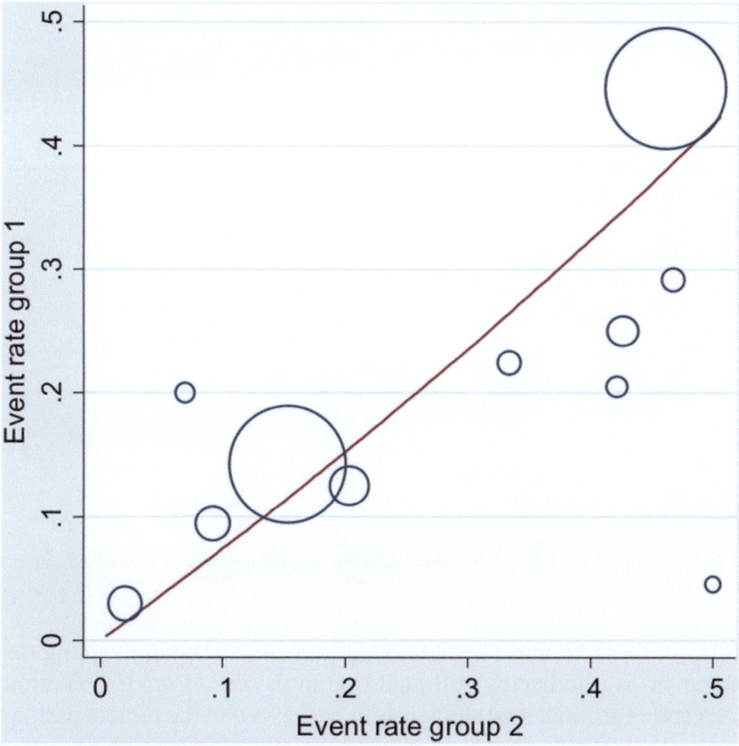

Fig. 10.11 L'Abbe plot for the risk of major adverse cardiac events (group 1, psychotherapy; group 2, control group; *line*, pooled odds ratio line)

10.4 Discussion

The present comprehensive umbrella review and updated meta-analysis provide an accurate, precise, and updated estimate of the risk-benefit balance of psychotherapy and ancillary psychological interventions in patients with ischemic heart disease. Specifically, we found four published systematic reviews on this topic and in particular a high-quality Cochrane review [3–6]. These analyses highlighted a substantial potential of psychotherapy to improve anxiety and depression, whereas the impact of this treatment modality on other clinical outcomes, including major adverse cardiac events, was not as clear-cut. Moreover, our updated meta-analysis of randomized clinical trials, including more than 9000 patients and including only studies providing details on hard cardiovascular events, suggested that psychotherapy could be associated with improved mortality and morbidity in patients with ischemic heart disease.

However, the apparent presence of small study effects and/or heterogeneity in the risks of death and major adverse cardiac events casts a shadow of doubt on the

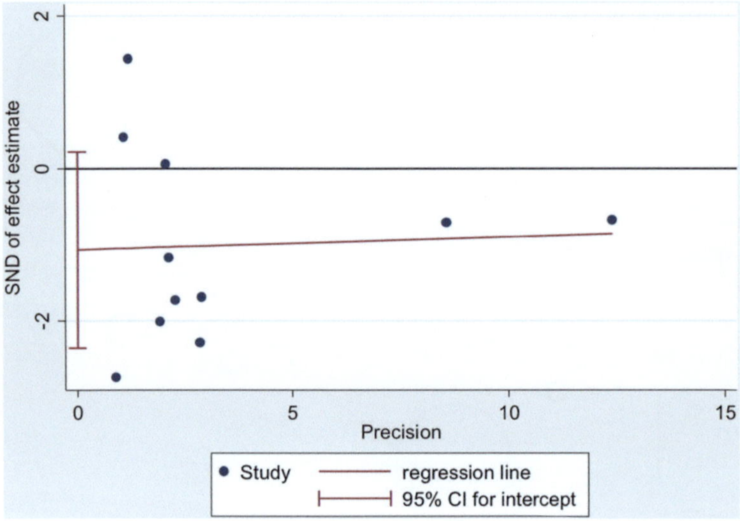

Fig. 10.12 Funnel plot for the risk of major adverse cardiac events (*CI* confidence interval, *SND* standardized normal deviate)

true validity of these findings. In addition, it is unclear whether the purported beneficial effects of psychotherapy still hold true in the era of modern cardiovascular care, as several of the included studies were performed in the remote past, when the use of dual antiplatelet therapy, beta-blockers, angiotensin-converting enzyme inhibitors, and statins was erratic or absent altogether. Thus, while it is conceivable that the benefits of psychotherapy for ischemic heart disease are substantial, further large multicenter trials are required to definitively clarify whether such potential benefits outweigh the corresponding risks and costs.

The potentially favorable results of psychotherapy for ischemic heart disease should not come as a surprise. Indeed, there is no question that ischemic heart disease has a strong psychological component [40–42] (see the already-cited Chap. 1), and psychotherapy is intended to minimize psychological stress and facilitate normal psychological processes [39, 43, 44]. In addition, the duration of follow-up appears particularly important in this setting, as psychotherapy could lead to beneficial lifestyle changes midterm, which could translate into momentous benefits long term for hard clinical endpoints. At present, a multitude of psychological interventions are used to treat cardiac patients (group therapy, individual cognitive-behavioral therapy, short-term dynamic psychotherapy, psychoeducation, counseling), reflecting uncertainty about the exact mechanisms by which negative emotions affect cardiac outcomes [6]. Many trials are relatively small and present short-term follow-up only [45], notwithstanding the major difficulty of conducting large and pragmatic trials focusing on psychotherapy. Moreover, the details of intervention and methodology are often poorly reported. The question of how psychotherapy and ancillary psychological interventions might improve outcomes in patients with ischemic heart disease remains unanswered.

Yet, the potential exists for modern technologies to act synergistically with psychotherapy. Accordingly, we could foresee a comprehensive post-discharge care plan in the future which involves, beyond drug, device or surgical therapy, cardiopulmonary rehabilitation plus formal psychological interventions. This could be even more impactful in the current era dominated by the successes of modern cardiovascular care for acute coronary syndromes, which often translates into a veritable epidemic of chronic ischemic heart disease and heart failure. Notably, there is no free lunch and the care with which psychotherapy is provided to these patients remains paramount. Indeed, administering psychological support through non-dedicated personnel may even have detrimental effects or, at best, prove inconsequential [27]. Accordingly, the online/telemedicine provision of psychotherapy is not foreseeable, as direct and constant contact between the practitioner and patient is crucial to ensuring that nonverbal communication contributes to the success of psychotherapy sessions (see Chap. 17).

10.5 Conclusions

Despite our ambitions, the current work has several shortcomings, including those typical of both systematic and umbrella reviews [46–50]. In addition, since any meta-analysis or overview of reviews clearly reflects the quality and breadth of the primary research evaluated, this umbrella review and updated meta-analysis cannot redress the limitations of the original trials included, some of which were at risk of significant bias (e.g., those allocating patients according to an alternate assignment scheme).

Nonetheless, though psychotherapy and ancillary psychological interventions might improve the prognosis of patients with ischemic heart disease, several unsettled issues remain, particularly the real impact of psychotherapy and psychological interventions in the current era of modern, multifaceted cardiovascular care. Further large trials are therefore still needed to definitely gauge the risk-benefit profile of this type of intervention in the setting of ischemic heart disease.

Acknowledgments Conflicts of interest: None
Funding: None

References

1. Wilson JF (2014) In the clinic. Stable ischemic heart disease. Ann Intern Med 160:ITC1-1-16
2. Gerber Y, Weston SA, Redfield MM et al (2015) A contemporary appraisal of the heart failure epidemic in Olmsted County, Minnesota, 2000 to 2010. JAMA Intern Med 175:996–1004
3. Linden W, Stossel C, Maurice J (1996) Psychosocial interventions for patients with coronary artery disease: a meta-analysis. Arch Intern Med 156:745–752

4. Dusseldorp E, van Elderen T, Maes S, Meulman J, Kraaij V (1999) A meta-analysis of psychoeducational programs for coronary heart disease patients. Health Psychol 18:506–519
5. van Dixhoorn J, White A (2005) Relaxation therapy for rehabilitation and prevention in ischaemic heart disease: a systematic review and meta-analysis. Eur J Cardiovasc Prev Rehabil 12:193–202
6. Whalley B, Rees K, Davies P et al (2011) Psychological interventions for coronary heart disease. Cochrane Database Syst Rev 8:CD002902
7. Pereira VH, Cerqueira JJ, Palha JA, Sousa N (2013) Stressed brain, diseased heart: a review on the pathophysiologic mechanisms of neurocardiology. Int J Cardiol 166:30–37
8. Pinto VL, Brunini TM, Ferraz MR, Okinga A, Mendes-Ribeiro AC (2008) Depression and cardiovascular disease: role of nitric oxide. Cardiovasc Hematol Agents Med Chem 6:142–149
9. Biondi-Zoccai G, Peruzzi M, Giordano A, Frati G (2014) Commentary: transcatheter renal sympathetic denervation for resistant arterial hypertension: when sham brings shame? J Endovasc Ther 21:197–201
10. Biondi-Zoccai G (ed) (2014) Network meta-analysis: evidence synthesis with mixed treatment comparison. Nova, Hauppauge, NY
11. Whittemore R, Chao A, Jang M, Minges KE, Park C (2014) Methods for knowledge synthesis: an overview. Heart Lung 43:453–461
12. Griebeler ML, Morey-Vargas OL, Brito JP et al (2014) Pharmacologic interventions for painful diabetic neuropathy: an umbrella systematic review and comparative effectiveness network meta-analysis. Ann Intern Med 161:639–649
13. Moher D, Liberati A, Tetzlaff J, Altman DG, PRISMA Group (2009) Preferred reporting items for systematic reviews and meta-analyses: the PRISMA statement. BMJ 339:b2535
14. Shojania KG, Bero LA (2001) Taking advantage of the explosion of systematic reviews: an efficient MEDLINE search strategy. Eff Clin Pract 4:157–162
15. Biondi-Zoccai GG, Agostoni P, Abbate A, Testa L, Burzotta F (2005) A simple hint to improve Robinson and Dickersin's highly sensitive PubMed search strategy for controlled clinical trials. Int J Epidemiol 34:224–225
16. Shea BJ, Grimshaw JM, Wells GA et al (2007) Development of AMSTAR: a measurement tool to assess the methodological quality of systematic reviews. BMC Med Res Methodol 7:10
17. Albus C, Theissen P, Hellmich M et al (2009) Long-term effects of a multimodal behavioral intervention on myocardial perfusion—a randomized controlled trial. Int J Behav Med 16: 219–226
18. Gulliksson M, Burell G, Vessby B, Lundin L, Toss H, Svärdsudd K (2011) Randomized controlled trial of cognitive behavioral therapy vs. standard treatment to prevent recurrent cardiovascular events in patients with coronary heart disease: Secondary Prevention in Uppsala Primary Health Care project (SUPRIM). Arch Intern Med 171:134–140
19. Neves A, Alves AJ, Ribeiro F, Gomes JL, Oliveira J (2009) The effect of cardiac rehabilitation with relaxation therapy on psychological, hemodynamic, and hospital admission outcome variables. J Cardiopulm Rehabil Prev 29:304–309
20. Orth-Gomér K, Schneiderman N, Wang HX et al (2009) Stress reduction prolongs life in women with coronary disease: the Stockholm Women's Intervention Trial for Coronary Heart Disease (SWITCHD). Circ Cardiovasc Qual Outcomes 2:25–32
21. Roncella A, Pristipino C, Cianfrocca C et al (2013) One-year results of the randomized, controlled, short-term psychotherapy in acute myocardial infarction (STEP-IN-AMI) trial. Int J Cardiol 170:132–139
22. Appels A, Bär F, van der Pol G et al (2005) Effects of treating exhaustion in angioplasty patients on new coronary events: results of the randomized Exhaustion Intervention Trial (EXIT). Psychosom Med 67:217–223
23. Burell G (1995) Behaviour modification after coronary artery bypass graft surgery: effects on cardiac morbidity and mortality. J Rehabil Sci 8:39–40
24. Burgess AW, Lerner DJ, D'Agostino RB, Vokonas PS (1987) A randomized control trial of cardiac rehabilitation. Soc Sci Med 24:359–370

25. Claesson M, Birgander LS, Lindahl B et al (2005) Women's hearts—stress management for women with ischemic heart disease: explanatory analyses of a randomized controlled trial. J Cardiopulm Rehabil 25:93–102
26. Cowan MJ, Pike KC, Kogan BH (2001) Psychosocial nursing therapy following sudden cardiac arrest: impact on two-year survival. Nurse Res 50:68–76
27. Berkman LF, Blumenthal J, Burg M, Enhancing Recovery in Coronary Heart Disease Patients Investigators (ENRICHD) et al (2003) Effects of treating depression and low perceived social support on clinical events after myocardial infarction: the enhancing recovery in coronary heart disease patients (ENRICHD) randomized trial. JAMA 289:3106–3116
28. Hofman-Bang C, Lisspers J, Nordlander R et al (1999) Two-year results of a controlled study of residential rehabilitation for patients treated with percutaneous transluminal coronary angioplasty—a randomized study of a multifactorial programme. Eur Heart J 20:1465–1474
29. Ibrahim MA, Feldman JG, Sultz HA et al (1974) Management after myocardial infarction: a controlled trial of the effect of group psychotherapy. Int J Psychiatry Med 5:253–268
30. Jones DA, West RR (1996) Psychological rehabilitation after myocardial infarction: multicentre randomised controlled trial. BMJ 313:1517–1521
31. Koertge J, Janszky I, Sundin O et al (2008) Effects of a stress management program on vital exhaustion and depression in women with coronary heart disease: a randomized controlled intervention study. J Intern Med 263:281–293
32. Mayou RA, Thompson DR, Clements A et al (2002) Guideline-based early rehabilitation after myocardial infarction. A pragmatic randomised controlled trial. J Psychosom Res 52:89–95
33. McLaughlin TJ, Aupont O, Bambauer KZ et al (2005) Improving psychologic adjustment to chronic illness in cardiac patients. The role of depression and anxiety. J Gen Intern Med 20: 1084–1090
34. Michalsen A, Grossman P, Lehmann N et al (2005) Psychological and quality-of-life outcomes from a comprehensive stress reduction and lifestyle program in patients with coronary artery disease: results of a randomized trial. Psychother Psychosom 74:344–352
35. Oldenburg B, Perkins RJ, Andrews G (1985) Controlled trial of psychological intervention in myocardial infarction. J Consult Clin Psychol 53:852–859
36. Rahe RH, Ward HW, Hayes V (1979) Brief group therapy in myocardial infarction rehabilitation: three- to four-year follow-up of a controlled trial. Psychosom Med 41:229–242
37. Sebregts EH, Falger PR, Appels A et al (2005) Psychological effects of a short behavior modification program in patients with acute myocardial infarction or coronary artery bypass grafting. A randomized controlled trial. J Psychosom Res 58:417–424
38. Stern MJ, Gorman PA, Kaslow L (1983) The group counseling v exercise therapy study. A controlled intervention with subjects following myocardial infarction. Arch Intern Med 143: 1719–1725
39. van Dixhoorn JJ, Duivenvoorden HJ (1999) Effect of relaxation therapy on cardiac events after myocardial infarction: a 5-year follow-up study. J Cardiopulm Rehabil 19:178–185
40. Rosengren A, Hawken S, Ounpuu S et al (2004) Association of psychosocial risk factors with risk of acute myocardial infarction in 11 119 cases and 13 648 controls from 52 countries (the INTERHEART study): case–control study. Lancet 364:953–962
41. Gidron Y, Gilutz H, Berger R, Huleihel M (2002) Molecular and cellular interface between behavior and acute coronary syndromes. Cardiovasc Res 56:15–21
42. Pignalberi C, Patti G, Chimenti C, Maseri A (1998) Role of different determinants of psychological distress in acute coronary syndromes. J Am Coll Cardiol 32:613–619
43. Lehrer PM, Woolfolk RL (1993) Principles and practice of stress management. Guilford Press, New York
44. Cozolino L (2010) The neuroscience of psychotherapy: healing the social brain. W.W. Norton, New York
45. Kisely SR, Campbell LA, Yelland MJ, Paydar A (2012) Psychological interventions for symptomatic management of non-specific chest pain in patients with normal coronary anatomy. Cochrane Database Syst Rev 6:CD004101

46. Biondi-Zoccai G, Lotrionte M, Landoni G, Modena MG (2011) The rough guide to systematic reviews and meta-analyses. HSR Proc Intensive Care Cardiovasc Anesth 3:161–173
47. Biondi-Zoccai GG, Lotrionte M, Abbate A et al (2006) Compliance with QUOROM and quality of reporting of overlapping meta-analyses on the role of acetylcysteine in the prevention of contrast associated nephropathy: case study. BMJ 332:202–209
48. Biondi-Zoccai G, Abbate A, Peruzzi M, Frati G (2014) Commentary: observations, trials, and meta-analyses: the life cycle of evidence-based endovascular therapy. J Endovasc Ther 21: 693–696
49. Biondi-Zoccai G, Landoni G, Modena MG (2011) A journey into clinical evidence: from case reports to mixed treatment comparisons. HSR Proc Intensive Care Cardiovasc Anesth 3:93–96
50. Armijo-Olivo S, Ospina M, da Costa BR et al (2014) Poor reliability between Cochrane reviewers and blinded external reviewers when applying the Cochrane risk of bias tool in physical therapy trials. PLoS One 9:e96920

Cognitive and Behavioral Psychotherapy in Coronary Artery Disease

11

Marinella Sommaruga

Healing is best accomplished when art and science are conjoined, when body and spirit are probed together.
Bernard Lown (Bernard Lown, The Lost Art of Healing)

11.1 Introduction

Coronary artery disease (CAD) is the most common form of heart disease. Although the management of physical problems in patients with CAD is important, the psychosocial effects of this disease are very important also. Patients often have to cope with radical changes in their health status and, for this reason, may experience a wide range of negative emotional reactions, like anger, anxiety, fear, and depression. Many fail to return to their previous work, leisure, or level of sexual activity, even if they are physically fit enough to engage in these activities. Moreover, over the last 30 years, psychosocial risk factors—including negative emotions, stress and negative mental mind-sets (including depressive symptoms, anxiety, pessimism, anger, and hostility), and inadequate psychosocial and living conditions (like low socioeconomic status and social isolation)—have also been found to be associated with CAD [1, 2].

As a consequence, many position papers [1–3] and psychological guidelines [4] underline the need for the effective management of these psychosocial risk factors, which includes screening for them and implementing different psychological intervention programs like counseling, motivational interviews, health psychoeducation, and psychotherapy.

M. Sommaruga, PsyD (✉)
Clinical Psychology and Social Support Unit, Salvatore Maugeri Foundation, Care and Research Institute of Milan, Via Camaldoli 64, 20138 Milan, Italy
e-mail: marinella.sommaruga@fsm.it

A. Roncella, C. Pristipino (eds.), *Psychotherapy for Ischemic Heart Disease*,
DOI 10.1007/978-3-319-33214-7_11

A large number of "multidisciplinary" studies [5, 6] have been conducted to determine the effectiveness of psychosocial interventions for the primary and secondary prevention of CAD, but often the effects of psychosocial components cannot be formally extracted from these studies. Some studies have identified positive effects on quality of life, health behaviors, and somatic risk profile, while others have documented protective effects against cardiovascular morbidity and mortality. Some studies showed small-to-moderate improvements in depression and anxiety, a small reduction in cardiac mortality risk, and a reduction in all-cause mortality risk for men, but not women. Men appear to profit more from such interventions than women; this being said, there are fewer studies on women than men.

Linden et al. [6] found that programs that were initiated at least 2 months after a cardiac event yielded greater effects on the rate of future events than those initiated immediately afterward. Meanwhile, Welton et al. [7] conducted systematic literature searches to update an earlier Cochrane review. They classified the components of interventions into six types: usual care, educational, behavioral, cognitive, relaxation, and support. Most interventions were a combination of these components. There was evidence that psychological interventions were effective at reducing total cholesterol and standardized mean anxiety scores, that interventions with behavioral components were effective at reducing the odds of all-cause mortality and nonfatal myocardial infarction, and that interventions with behavioral and/or cognitive components reduced standardized mean depression scores.

Many of the evidence-based techniques that have been developed as management strategies to promote healthy behaviors and enhance psychosocial well-being were derived from cognitive-behavioral therapy (CBT). These have included interventions either involving or targeting health counseling, smoking cessation and weight management, self-monitoring, stress management, etc. An integrative model of psychotherapy and medical practices proposed by the GICR–IACPR (Italian Association for Cardiovascular Prevention, Rehabilitation and Epidemiology)—demonstrating the steps of a psychological intervention for CAD patients, particularly within a cardiac rehabilitation setting in Italy—is described in Chap. 22.

11.2 Cognitive and Behavioral Psychotherapy

CBT encompasses a range of therapies derived from cognitive-behavioral models of disorders, whereby the patient works collaboratively with a therapist using a shared formulation to achieve specific treatment goals. Such goals may include recognizing the impact of behavioral and/or thinking patterns on feeling states and encouraging alternative cognitive and/or behavioral coping skills to reduce the severity of target symptoms and problems.

The core premise of this treatment approach, which was pioneered by Beck [8] and Ellis [9], holds that maladaptive cognitions contribute to the maintenance of emotional distress and behavioral problems.

The basis of cognitive therapy is *cognitive restructuring*, which involves the identification of schemas and automatic thoughts, and the restructuring of these thoughts into more realistic and adaptive cognitions [10].

In addition to cognitive restructuring, *behavioral activation*, which involves the assignment and scheduling of weekly activities, helps patients to resume activities they have discontinued and engage in new activities.

Problem-solving techniques are also used to help patients make choices when they are faced with difficult situations or everyday decisions that have become overwhelming.

Positive self-statements can be taught to help boost patient's self-esteem.

Distraction and refocusing are used to assist patients when they have difficulty concentrating or if they are experiencing an overload of emotion.

Relaxation therapy [11] is a well-established psychological therapy for alleviating psychological distress in patients with chronic illness. Among the various relaxation techniques available, progressive muscle relaxation (PMR) follows procedures that were standardized and validated by Bernstein and Borkovic, based upon a classic muscle relaxation program developed by Jacobson. Other basic relaxation techniques include imagery exercises.

Although relaxation therapy has been shown to be effective for CAD patients, only a few randomized controlled trials or meta-analyses of small studies have been conducted to assess the role of relaxation training on health outcomes in heart disease patients with psychological problems.

Mindfulness-based cognitive therapy (MBCT) was developed as a manualized group skills training program that would address vulnerability between episodes of recurrent major depression [12, 13]. MBCT integrates aspects of CBT for depression into the mindfulness-based stress reduction (MBSR) program developed by Kabat-Zinn [14]. MBCT includes simple breathing, meditation, and yoga stretches to help participants become more aware of the present moment, including getting in touch with moment-to-moment changes in their mind and body. MBCT also includes basic education about depression and several exercises drawn from cognitive therapy. These more structured exercises make MBCT different from mindfulness meditation, but the approach is embedded within and seeks to remain true to the insight meditation tradition that has been taught for two and a half thousand years. MBCT helps individuals to develop the capacity to allow distressing moods, thoughts, and sensations to come and go, without having to battle against them. It also helps them to stay in touch with the present moment.

Metacognitive Therapy (MCT) is a recent development for understanding the causes of mental health problems and treating them [15]. Metacognition is the component of cognition that controls mental processes and thinking. Most people have some direct conscious experience of metacognition. MCT helps patients to develop new ways of controlling their attention, relating to negative thoughts and beliefs, and modifying metacognitive beliefs that give rise to unhelpful thinking patterns.

Acceptance and Commitment Therapy (ACT) is a "third-wave" behavioral and cognitive therapy [16, 17] that uses acceptance and mindfulness strategies, together with commitment and behavior change strategies, to increase psychological flexibility. Psychological flexibility means contacting the present moment fully as a conscious human being and, based upon what the situation affords, changing or persisting in certain behaviors in the service of chosen values.

Applications of "acceptance-based" interventions have proven efficacious for chronic physical conditions [18].

All of these ACT-based interventions have brief treatment durations and are often administered within a group setting. The length of treatment varies (e.g., from 3-h workshops to 3-week retreats). While traditional CBT attempts to dispute, change, and restructure the content of negative thoughts, ACT attempts to change the relationship between the person and his own thoughts and feelings. ACT appears to be particularly promising for increasing adherence to low-risk lifestyles among cardiac patients (e.g., low fat diet, smoking cessation, medication adherence).

One important ACT process that is useful for explaining behavior change is the connection with key personal values, defined as long-term desired qualities of living [16]. When an individual loses contact with his life values, he may sacrifice long-term behavioral goals and values (e.g., adopting a healthy lifestyle) to satisfy salient short-term goals (e.g., reducing present discomfort). Short- and long-term distress tolerance is necessary to adopt healthy (but strenuous) lifestyle changes.

Thus, *modern CBT* contains a range of specific models and approaches to treat disorders and combines a variety of cognitive, behavioral, and emotion-focused techniques. Although these strategies greatly emphasize cognitive factors, physiological, emotional, and behavioral components are also recognized for the role that they play in the maintenance of the disorder [19].

CBT is a well-documented, evidence-based treatment for anxiety disorders. In CBT, patients are taught to restructure anxiety-provoking thoughts that lead to panic attacks, are taught relaxation techniques to counteract stress and anxiety, and are given exposure therapy to desensitize themselves to stressful stimuli [20]. A Cochrane review [21] concluded that therapy based on CBT principles was effective at reducing anxiety symptoms for the short-term treatment of General Anxiety Disorder (GAD).

CBT is also often used successfully for the treatment of depressive disorders. Meta-analyses and extensive literature reviews have found that using CBT is comparable to using medication alone, in terms of reducing depressive symptoms. Other studies have yielded similar findings, even among patients experiencing recurrent or more severe levels of depression [22–24].

CBT is recommended by the National Institute of Clinical Excellence (NICE) for anxiety disorders and depression and has other effective uses across many mental health problems [25]. In light of evidence that some individuals respond well to "low-intensity" interventions, NICE also advocates a stepped-care approach to the delivery of psychological therapies for mild to moderate depression and certain anxiety disorders. Treatment for anxiety and depression typically lasts 12–14 sessions, during which the therapist works with the client to examine and modify negative thoughts, biases, and behaviors that underlie symptoms. Homework is a part of treatment and often consists of recording thoughts, changing patterns of behavior, activity scheduling, and conducting "behavioral experiments" to test distorted beliefs. In a recent review of meta-analyses [19] examining CBT for a range of problems, Hayes et al. showed that, in general, the evidence base of CBT was very strong for treating anxiety disorders, depression, and several other mental health problems.

11.3 Cognitive and Behavioral Psychotherapy for CAD

Depression and anxiety are the most common psychological problems observed in CAD patients, and CBT should be instituted at the beginning of care to improve mental health care among CAD populations [26].

11.3.1 Depression and Depressive Symptoms

Treatment options for depression and depressive symptoms include psychological counseling (including CBT), antidepressant drugs [primarily selective serotonin reuptake inhibitors (SSRIs)], and physical activity [5, 27]. However, while psychological and antidepressant pharmacologic treatment can reduce depressive symptoms, their impact reducing the incidence of myocardial infarction, both cardiac and all-cause mortality, and the need for cardiac surgery is less clear [5, 28–30]. As explained in Chap. 9, "*antidepressant and antipsychotic drugs improve quality of life but not necessarily survival of patients with ischemic heart disease, and for almost any antidepressant and antipsychotic drug adverse impact on the cardiovascular system has been reported.*"

Several controlled studies have investigated the effectiveness of psychotherapeutic interventions treating significant depressive syndromes in CAD patients. Positive yet moderate effects on depressive symptoms were identified in most of these studies, which evaluated various techniques like CBT [31–34], interpersonal therapy [35], and "collaborative treatment" [36].

This conclusion was also drawn by the authors of a recent Cochrane review [29]. The authors, in fact, concluded that both psychological interventions and pharmaceuticals (SSRIs) might exert small yet clinically meaningful effects on depression outcomes in CAD patients. They were unable to identify any significant beneficial effects in terms of reducing either mortality rates or the incidence of cardiac events. Overall, however, the evidence is sparse due to the low number of high-quality trials per outcome and the heterogeneity of examined populations and interventions. Despite the fact that depression is considered to be an independent etiological and prognostic risk factor for CAD, and that there are a number of well-accepted evidence-based treatments for depression, there have been few trials that have investigated the impact of treating depression in CAD patients.

In the *Enhancing Recovery in Coronary Heart Disease* (ENRICHD) trial, 2481 recent myocardial infarction patients with depression and/or low social support randomly received either CBT (and SSRI antidepressants, if indicated) or usual care. Significant but modest improvements in depression and social support were found among the CBT-treated patients. There was no benefit in terms of cardiac outcomes or mortality after 29 months of follow-up, however, and cardiac outcomes appeared to be worse among women [31]. Nonetheless, methodological issues have since been raised, indicating that these results do not prove the ineffectiveness of CBT.

This finding, in fact, has been attributed to the unexpectedly vigorous treatment of the supposed usual care control group with antidepressant therapy, cardiac rehabilitation, and psychological support as part of routine medical care, thereby reducing group differences [37]. Another possible reason that the CBT intervention failed to affect survival could be the large number of patients with mild, transient depression who were enrolled in the study, which may have diluted results. Finally, the results were also weakened by enhanced survival rates from improved secondary prevention management in this medically well-managed study group.

A randomized controlled study on the effects of exercise and stress management training on markers of cardiovascular risk in patients with CAD [38] demonstrated a reduction of depression and psychological distress, together with improvements in some markers of cardiovascular risk in intervention patients.

In a recent systematic review, Dickens et al. [39] tried to identify the characteristics of psychological interventions that improve depression and depressive symptoms among people with CAD. Results demonstrated that psychological interventions improved depression, although the effect was small. Problem solving, general education, skills training, cognitive-behavioral therapy, and relaxation had small effects on CAD patients who were recruited irrespective of their depression status. Among high-quality trials of depressed CAD patients, only CBT generated significant albeit small effects.

11.3.2 Anxiety

Recently, Tully et al. [40] found that GAD was second to depression as the most common mental health problem among cardiac patients seeking psychological support.

Despite CBT being a frontline anxiety disorder treatment option in non-CAD populations [41], limited work has been performed in heart disease patients [42]. Indeed, behavioral exposure and symptom induction, such as through hyperventilation exercises, form a key component of the CBT model for panic disorder [43]. However, both the safety and tolerability of symptom induction still need to be demonstrated in CAD patients, considering that a panic attack in the midst of a panic challenge test might lead to reversible myocardial perfusion defects in patients with positive cardiac stress tests [44]. Also, elsewhere it was noted that worry induction in GAD treatment may theoretically lead to changes in heart rate and systolic blood pressure, the safety of which should also be demonstrated [45].

Nevertheless, the challenges of GAD treatments in CAD patients were well described in the first GAD prognostic study reported by Frasure-Smith and Lesperance [46]. In addition, CBT is useful and effective for teaching anger management skills when treating individuals with Type A personality and can also assist in weaning patients off benzodiazepines, helping to ensure greater self-reliance and mastery over anxiety symptoms [20].

11.3.3 Stress Management and Behavioral Medicine

Benson was the first to systematically study the physiologic changes that occur with the practice of meditation and mind/body therapies. He coined this physiologic state that counteracts the "stress response" as the "relaxation response" [47]. He also integrated relaxation training and CBT into clinical group programs, with goals ranging from reducing cardiac risk factors to helping patients with infertility, HIV, and cancer. These programs have been shown to reduce the amount of money spent on unnecessary medical procedures and work-ups, improve compliance with treatment, and reduce the risk factors of stress and an unhealthy lifestyle [48].

The Recurrent Coronary Prevention Project for reducing Type A behavior [49] was one of the first behavioral medicine trials that has attempted to incorporate stress reduction, relaxation training/CBT, and lifestyle modification for heart disease.

In Ornish's Lifestyle Heart Trial [50, 51], those participants who maintained lifestyle changes achieved a regression of coronary artery stenosis at 1-, 4-, and 5-year follow-up. Meanwhile, Edelman et al. [52] demonstrated that, after 10 months of a personalized health plan consisting of mindfulness meditation, relaxation training, stress management, and health education and coaching, patients in the active treatment group had lowered their risk of cardiac events, lost more weight, and exercised more frequently than those in a usual care group.

On January 28, 2011, following the release of results from the *Secondary Prevention in Uppsala Primary Health Care project* (SUPRIM) study [53], in which CBT produced a 41 % reduction in fatal and nonfatal first recurrent cardiovascular events, the European Society of Cardiology believed stress management programs should be made more widely available across Europe for patients with CAD. In the SUPRIM study, investigators had randomly assigned 362 men and women, who had been discharged from hospital after an ischemic heart disease event, to either usual care and CBT ($n = 192$) or usual care with no additional therapy ($n = 170$). Usual care included medications to lower blood pressure and cholesterol and to prevent blood clots. The CBT program, which was delivered in 22-h sessions, focused on reducing daily stress, time urgency, and hostility. The program included five specific goals of education, self-monitoring, skills training, cognitive restructuring, and spiritual development. After a mean follow-up of

94 months, the group undergoing CBT had a lower rate of fatal and nonfatal first recurrent cardiac events, fewer recurrent acute myocardial infarctions, and a non-significant lowering in all-cause mortality.

Orth-Gomér et al. [54] enrolled 30 consecutive patients, 11 women and 19 men, hospitalized for an acute coronary syndrome, in a cognitive, behavioral intervention stress management program that consisted of ten 2-h sessions. The investigators identified no gender differences in the preplanned programs, but discussion styles varied between women and men. Women were more open and more personal, and discussed family issues more frequently than job issues, even though all of the women were employed outside their homes. Conversely, men largely talked about concrete, practical issues—mostly about their jobs—and not directly about their feelings. The daily stresses of life decreased significantly for both men and women, but more so for women. Depressive thoughts were low at baseline, and there was no change over time. In contrast, anxiety scores were high at baseline and decreased significantly, but again more so among women than men.

Recently, Murphy et al. [55] developed a "*Beating Heart Problems*" cognitive-behavioral therapy and motivational interviewing (MI) program to help patients to develop behavioral and cognitive self-management skills. The "Beating Heart Problems" program is a face-to-face CBT and MI group program comprised of 8 weekly sessions lasting 1.5 h each. Its modules address physical activity, diet, medication adherence, smoking cessation, depression, anxiety, anger, and social support. Within each module, patients undertake exercises that enable them to review situations in their lives to identify, challenge, and change the unhelpful thoughts and faulty beliefs (cognitions) associated with risk factors and negative emotions. The CBT and MI "tools" are used to assist participants with behavior changes and mood management. In particular, patients are supported in their construction of action plans for implementing practical health behaviors, including goal setting, and in their identification of motivators for change, resources, barriers, rewards, and relapse-prevention strategies. Patients underwent risk factor screening 6 weeks after hospital discharge (before randomization) and again 4 and 12 months later. Versus the control group, treatment group patients tended toward greater reduction in their 2-year risk of a recurrent cardiac event at both 4- and 12-month follow-up. Significant benefits related to dietary fat intake and functional capacity were also evident.

When treating the psychosocial aspects of cardiovascular disease, women benefit from different interventions than men do. Most recently, the beneficial effect of psychotherapy on the incidence of cardiac events was proven for women with CAD.

Orth-Gomér et al. [56] implemented a stress reduction program for women and investigated its efficacy enhancing survival in women with CAD. They randomized 237 women (mean age 62 years) who had been hospitalized in Stockholm for acute myocardial infarction or revascularization to either a group-based cognitive-behavioral intervention or usual care. Women who had experienced an acute coronary event received either 20 group-based sessions (4–8 women per group) for 1 year or usual care only. Over a mean of 7 years after entering the study, women in usual care had a mortality rate of 20 %, whereas those in the psychosocial intervention had a mortality rate of just 7 %. No woman was lost to follow-up. After multivariate control for clinical prognostic factors in the *Stockholm Women's Intervention Trial for Coronary Heart Disease* (SWITCHD), a group-based psychosocial intervention program for women with CAD was shown to improve survival. The results of this study suggest that even women with severe CAD can benefit from psychosocial interventions specifically targeted to reduce stress and enhance their social support skills.

Blom et al. [57] investigated the effects of a 1-year stress management program on daily stress behaviors and social support among 247 female patients ≤75 years old with CAD. Women in the intervention group (who received 20 group sessions of stress management therapy, each session lasting 2 h) experienced a more pronounced reduction in self-rated daily stress behaviors over time than usual healthcare controls.

Over the last few years, there has been a growth of interest in mindfulness-based psychotherapeutic approaches across a range of medical problems. Tacon et al. [58] reported significant reductions in anxiety and negative affect and improvements in emotional control and coping among women with heart disease participating in a pilot group receiving MBSR.

Another study, a randomized controlled trial, examined the effects of an MBSR program in patients with CAD [59]. The authors observed a significant reduction in symptoms of anxiety and depression, perceived stress, blood pressure, and body mass index in patients in the MBSR group after completion of the intervention. At 3-month follow-up, those therapeutic gains were maintained.

Using interpretive phenomenological analysis (IPA) of participant experiences, Griffiths et al. [60] assessed the first-reported MBCT group adapted for cardiac rehabilitation. Five men and one woman (the number in accordance with IPA sample sizes) joined the MBCT group consisting of an 8-week program adapted for a cardiac population (2 h per week). Adaptations to the program included tailoring information handouts toward emotions experienced by cardiac patients (e.g., health-related worry and rumination), modification of the walking and supine meditation exercises, and the removal of yoga. In place of yoga, stretching and breathing exercises were included and further adapted to involve sitting rather than standing stretches. Qualitative analysis identified the development of awareness, commitment, within-group experiences relating to the material, and acceptance as central experiential themes.

Only one study has been reported on ACT, conducted by Goodwin and colleagues [61]. It evaluated an acceptance-based program for cardiac patients and provided initial evidence documenting effective increases in heart-healthy behaviors. Sixteen patients participated in four sessions, each lasting 90 min and focused on developing mindfulness and distress tolerance skills, and strengthening commitment to health-related behavior changes. Participants in this study were highly satisfied with the intervention. In particular, results showed large improvements in diet and moderate increases in physical activity from pre- to posttreatment. However, given the absence of a control group and the small sample size of this initial investigation, large-scale randomized clinical trials are needed to test the efficacy of ACT-based interventions in cardiac patients. This was the first evaluation of an ACT program aimed at increasing heart-healthy behaviors among cardiac patients.

Finally, it is important to underline the results of a meta-analysis published by Biondi-Zoccai et al. (see Chap. 10). They concluded that psychotherapy and ancillary psychological interventions may indeed improve the prognosis of patients with ischemic heart disease, but also that several unsettled issues remain. In particular is the question of what the real impact psychotherapy and psychological interventions have in the current era of modern, multifaceted cardiovascular care.

11.4 Current Studies

Analysis of the literature also shows that promising new studies are currently in progress.

Enhancing Standard Cardiac Rehabilitation with Stress Management Training in Patients with Heart Disease (ENHANCED) is a randomized clinical trial evaluating the effects of stress management training on changes in biomarkers of cardiac risk and quality of life among patients enrolled in traditional exercise-based cardiac rehabilitation [62]. The patients are being evaluated and randomized to cardiac rehabilitation enhanced by stress management training (including sessions devoted to relaxation training, cognitive restructuring, communication skills, and problem solving) or to standard exercise-based cardiac rehabilitation (12 weeks of treatment).

Another multicenter psychotherapy trial (SPIRR-CAD) has as its aim trying to answer the question of whether a stepwise psychotherapy intervention, combining individual and group psychotherapy based on psychodynamic principles, and incorporating cognitive–behavioral elements, can improve symptoms of depression in patients with CAD better than usual treatment [63]. In addition, Albus et al. will investigate whether successful treatment translates into reduced physiological and behavioral coronary risk factors, physiological risk markers, and improved quality of life. Furthermore, they will investigate whether the intervention is associated with reduced healthcare costs, and whether personality, gender, and genetic polymorphisms predict treatment outcomes.

Finally, the ACT on HEART study [64] is the first randomized clinical trial designed to evaluate the efficacy of a brief group-administered ACT-based program promoting health behavior change and psychological well-being among cardiac patients. Results will address the effectiveness of a brief treatment created to simultaneously impact multiple cardiovascular risk factors. Conducted within the context of clinical practice, this trial will potentially, empirically clarify whether psychological support improves quality of life and reduces mortality and morbidity rates among cardiac patients.

11.5 Conclusions

CBT appears to be effective at reducing psychological symptoms in CAD patients, but further studies are required, especially directed toward subgroups of patients with different needs. Furthermore, some studies have demonstrated that gender-specific treatments can be effective to meet the unique needs of females, addressing issues like emotional processing, being listened to, and attention to family role issues (see also Chap. 6), though these results also require confirmation. Finally, current studies, based on the second and third waves of cognitive and behavioral therapies, might even reveal new directions.

Based upon this evidence, it is clearly warranted that cardiologists and mental health professionals, in the future, collaborate more and integrate treatment for anxiety, depression, stress, and anger/hostility into the everyday practice of cardiology.

References

1. Pogosova N, Saner H, Pedersen SSF, on behalf of the Cardiac Rehabilitation Section of the European Association of Cardiovascular Prevention and Rehabilitation of the European Society of Cardiology et al (2015) Psychosocial aspects in cardiac rehabilitation From theory to practice. A position paper from the Cardiac Rehabilitation Section of the European Association of Cardiovascular Prevention and Rehabilitation of the European Society of Cardiology. Eur J Prev Cardiol 22(10):1290–1306
2. Rozanski A (2014) Behavioral cardiology current advances and future directions. J Am Coll Cardiol 64(1):100–110
3. Ladwig KH, Lederbogen F, Albus C et al (2014) Position paper on the importance of psychosocial factors in cardiology update 2013. Ger Med Sci 7:12 (Doc09)
4. Task Force per le Attività di Psicologia in Cardiologia Riabilitativa e Preventiva, Gruppo Italiano di Cardiologia Riabilitativa e Preventiva (2003) Guidelines for psychology activities in cardiologic rehabilitation and prevention. Monaldi Arch Chest Dis 60(3):184–234
5. Whalley B, Thompson DR, Taylor RS (2014) Psychological interventions for coronary heart disease: Cochrane systematic review and meta-analysis. Int J Behav Med 21(1):109–121
6. Linden W, Phillips MJ, Leclerc J (2007) Psychological treatment of cardiac patients: a meta-analysis. Eur Heart J 28(24):2972–2984
7. Welton NJ, Caldwell DM, Adamopoulos E, Vedhara K (2009) Mixed treatment comparison meta-analysis of complex interventions psychological interventions in coronary heart disease. Am J Epidemiol 169(9):1158–1165
8. Beck AT (1970) Cognitive therapy nature and relation to behavior therapy. Behav Ther 1: 1184–1200
9. Ellis A (1962) Reason and emotion in psychotherapy. Lyle Stuart, New York
10. Young JE, Weinberger AD, Beck ET (2001) Clinical handbook of psychological disorders: a step-by-step treatment manual, 3rd edn. Guilford, New York, pp 264–308
11. van Dixhoorn J, White A (2005) Relaxation therapy for rehabilitation and prevention in ischaemic heart disease: a systematic review and meta-analysis. Eur J Cardiovasc Prev Rehabil 12(3):193–202
12. Segal ZV, Williams JMG, Teasdale JD (2002) Mindfulness- based cognitive therapy for depression: a new approach to preventing relapse. Guilford, New York
13. Williams JMG, Teasdale JD, Segal ZV, Kabat-Zinn J (2007) The mindful way through depression: freeing yourself from chronic unhappiness. Guilford, New York

14. Kabat-Zinn J (1990) Full catastrophe living: how to cope with stress, pain and illness using mindfulness meditation. Bantam Dell, A Division of Random House, New York
15. Fisher P, Wells A (2009) Metacognitive therapy. Routledge Taylor and Francis Group, New York
16. Hayes SC, Luoma JB, Bond FW et al (2006) Acceptance and commitment therapy model, processes and outcomes. Behav Res Ther 44(1):1–25
17. Powers MB, Zum Vorde Sive Vording MB, Emmelkamp PM (2009) Acceptance and commitment therapy: a meta-analytic review. Psychother Psychosom 78(2):73–80
18. Prevedini AB, Presti G, Rabitti E et al (2011) Acceptance and commitment therapy (ACT): the foundation of the therapeutic model and an overview of its contribution to the treatment of patients with chronic physical diseases. G Ital Med Lav Ergon 33(1):A53–A63
19. Hofmann SG, Asnaani A, Vonk IJ et al (2012) The efficacy of CBT: a review of meta-analyses. Cognit Ther Res 36(5):427–440
20. Janeway D (2009) An integrated approach to the diagnosis and treatment of anxiety within the practice of cardiology. Cardiol Rev 17(1):36–43
21. Hunot V, Churchill R, Silva de Lima M, Teixeira V (2007) Psychological therapies for generalised anxiety disorder. Cochrane Database Syst Rev 24(1):CD001848
22. Bekke-Hansen S, Trockel M, Burg MM, Taylor CB (2012) Depressive symptom dimensions and cardiac prognosis following myocardial infarction: results from the ENRICHD clinical trial. Psychol Med 42(1):51–60. doi:10.1017/S0033291711001000
23. Robinson LA, Berman JS, Neimeyer RA (1990) Psychotherapy for the treatment of depression a comprehensive review of controlled outcome research. Psychol Bull 10:830–849
24. De Rubeis RJ, Hollon SD, Amsterdam JD et al (2005) Cognitive therapy vs. medication in the treatment of moderate to severe depression. Arch Gen Psychiatry 62(4):409–416
25. Clark DM (2011) Implementing NICE guidelines for the psychological treatment of depression and anxiety disorders: the IAPT experience. Int Rev Psychiatry 23(4):318–327
26. Tully PJ, Selkow T, Bengel J, Rafanelli C (2014) A dynamic view of comorbid depression and generalized anxiety disorder symptom change in chronic heart failure: the discrete effects of CBT, exercise rehabilitation, and psychotropic medication. Disabil Rehabil 37(7):585–592
27. Elderon L, Whooley MA (2013) Depression and cardiovascular disease. Prog Cardiovasc Dis 55:511–523
28. Rutledge T, Redwine LS, Linke SE et al (2013) A meta-analysis of mental health treatments and cardiac rehabilitation for improving clinical outcomes and depression among patients with coronary heart disease. Psychosom Med 75:335–349
29. Baumeister H, Hutter N, Bengel J (2011) Psychological and pharmacological interventions for depression in patients with coronary artery disease. Cochrane Database Syst Rev 9:CD008012
30. Mazza M, Lotrionte M, Biondi-Zoccai G et al (2010) Selective serotonin reuptake inhibitors provide significant lower re-hospitalization rates in patients recovering from acute coronary syndromes evidence from a meta analysis. J Psychopharmacol 24:1785–1792
31. Berkman LF, Blumenthal J, Burg et al (2003) Enhancing recovery in coronary heart disease patients investigators (ENRICHD). Effects of treating depression and low perceived social support on clinical events after myocardial infarction the enhancing recovery in coronary heart disease patients (ENRICHD) randomized trial. JAMA 289(23):3106–3116
32. Barth J, Paul J, Härter M, Bengel J (2005) Inpatient psychotherapeutic treatment for cardiac patients with depression in Germany–short term results. Psychosoc Med 2:Doc04
33. Freedland KE, Skala JA, Carney RM et al (2009) Treatment of depression after coronary artery bypass surgery a randomized controlled trial. Arch Gen Psychiatry 66(4):387–396
34. Davidson KW, Rieckmann N, Clemow L et al (2010) Enhanced depression care for patients with acute coronary syndrome and persistent depressive symptoms coronary psychosocial evaluation studies randomized controlled trial. Arch Intern Med 170(7):600–608
35. Lespérance F, Frasure-Smith N, Koszycki D, CREATE Investigators et al (2007) Effects of citalopram and interpersonal psychotherapy on depression in patients with coronary artery

disease the Canadian Cardiac Randomized Evaluation of Antidepressant and Psychotherapy Efficacy (CREATE) trial. JAMA 297(4):367–379
36. Rollman BL, Belnap BH, LeMenager MS et al (2009) Telephone-delivered collaborative care for treating post-CABG depression: a randomized controlled trial. JAMA 302(19):2095–2103
37. Rozanski A, Blumenthal JA, Davidson KW et al (2005) The epidemiology, pathophysiology, and management of psychosocial risk factors in cardiac practice: the emerging field of behavioural cardiology. J Am Coll Cardiol 45(5):637–651
38. Blumenthal JA, Sherwood A, Babyak MA et al (2005) Effects of exercise and stress management training on markers of cardiovascular risk in patients with ischaemic heart disease: a randomized controlled trial. J Am Med Assoc 293(13):1626–1634
39. Dickens C, Cherrington A, Adeyemi I et al (2013) Characteristics of psychological interventions that improve depression in people with coronary heart disease: a systematic review and meta-regression. Psychosom Med 75(2):211–221
40. Tully PJ, Cosh SM, Baumeister H (2014) The anxious heart in whose mind? A systematic review and meta-regression of factors associated with anxiety disorder diagnosis, treatment and morbidity risk in coronary heart disease. J Psychosom Res 77(6):439–448
41. Lessard MJ, Marchand A, Pelland ME et al (2012) Comparing two brief psychological interventions to usual care in panic disorder patients presenting to the emergency department with chest pain. Behav Cogn Psychother 40:129–147
42. Sardinha A, Araújo CGS, Soares-Filho GLF, Nardi AE (2011) Anxiety, panic disorder and coronary artery disease issues concerning physical exercise and CBT. Expert Rev Cardiovasc Ther 9:165–175
43. Wells A (1997) Panic disorder. In: Wells A (ed) Cognitive therapy of anxiety disorders a practice manual and conceptual guide. Wiley, Sussex, pp 98–132
44. Fleet RP, Lesperance F, Arsenault A et al (2005) Myocardial perfusion study of panic attacks in patients with coronary artery disease. Am J Cardiol 96:1064–1068
45. Shemesh E, Annunziato RA, Weatherley BD et al (2011) A randomized controlled trial of the safety and promise of cognitive–behavioral therapy using imaginal exposure in patients with post-traumatic stress disorder resulting from cardiovascular illness. J Clin Psychiatry 72: 168–174
46. Frasure-Smith N, Lespérance F (2008) Depression and anxiety as predictors of 2-year cardiac events in patients with stable coronary artery disease. Arch Gen Psychiatry 65:62–71
47. Benson H (1984) Beyond the relaxation response. Berkley Books, New York
48. Hellman CJ, Budd M, Borysenko J et al (1990) A study of the effectiveness of two group behavioral medicine interventions for patients with psychosomatic complaints. Behav Med 16: 165–173
49. Friedman M, Thoreson CE, Gill JJ et al (1986) Alteration of Type-A behavior and its effect on cardiac recurrences in post-myocardial infarction patients: summary results of the recurrent coronary prevention project. Am Heart J 132:653–665
50. Ornish D, Brown SE, Scherwitz LW et al (1990) Can lifestyle changes reverse coronary heart disease? Lancet 336(8708):129–133
51. Ornish D, Brown SE, Billings JH et al (1993) Can lifestyle changes reverse coronary atherosclerosis? Four year results of the lifestyle heart trial abstract. Circulation 8:83–85
52. Edelman D, Oddone E, Liebowitz RS et al (2006) A multidimensional integrative medicine intervention to improve cardiovascular risk. J Gen Intern Med 21:728–734
53. Gulliksson M, Burell G, Vessby B et al (2011) Randomized controlled trial of CBT vs. standard treatment to prevent recurrent cardiovascular events in patients with coronary heart disease. Secondary Prevention in Uppsala Primary Health Care project (SUPRIM). Arch Intern Med 171(2):134–140
54. Orth-Gomér K (2012) Behavioral interventions for coronary heart disease patients. Biopsychosoc Med 6(1):5
55. Murphy BM, Worcester MU, Higgins RO et al (2013) Reduction in 2-year recurrent risk score and improved behavioral outcomes after participation in the "Beating Heart Problems" self-

management program: results of a randomized controlled trial. J Cardiopulm Rehabil Prev 33(4):220–228

56. Orth-Gomér K, Schneiderman N, Wang HX et al (2009) Stress reduction prolongs life in women with coronary disease: the Stockholm Women's Intervention Trial for Coronary Heart Disease (SWITCHD). Circ Cardiovasc Qual Outcomes 2(1):25–32
57. Blom M, Georgiades A, Janszky I et al (2009) Daily stress and social support among women with CAD: results from a 1-year randomized controlled stress management intervention study. Int J Behav Med 16(3):227–235
58. Tacon AM, McComb J, Caldera Y, Randolph P (2003) Mindfulness meditation, anxiety reduction, and heart disease: a pilot study. Fam Community Health 26:25–33
59. Parswani MJ, Sharma MP, Iyengar S (2013) Mindfulness-based stress reduction program in coronary heart disease: a randomized control trial. Int J Yoga 6(2):111–117
60. Griffiths K, Camic PM, Hutton JM (2009) Participant experiences of a mindfulness-based cognitive therapy group for cardiac rehabilitation. J Health Psychol 14(5):675–681
61. Goodwin CL, Forman EM, Herbert JD et al (2012) A pilot study examining the initial effectiveness of a brief acceptance-based behavior therapy for modifying diet and physical activity among cardiac patients. Behav Modif 36(2):199–217
62. Blumenthal JA, Wang JT, Babyak M et al (2010) Enhancing standard cardiac rehabilitation with stress management training: background, methods, and design for the enhanced study. J Cardiopulm Rehabil Prev 30(2):77–84
63. Albus C, Beutel ME, Deter HC et al (2011) A stepwise psychotherapy intervention for reducing risk in coronary artery disease (SPIRR-CAD)-rationale and design of a multicenter, randomized trial in depressed patients with CAD. J Psychosom Res 71(4):215–222
64. Spatola CA, Manzoni GM, Castelnuovo G et al (2014) The ACT on HEART study: rationale and design of a randomized controlled clinical trial comparing a brief intervention based on acceptance and commitment therapy to usual secondary prevention care of coronary heart disease. Health Qual Life Outcomes 12:22

Mind–Body Practices for the Prevention and Treatment of Cardiovascular Disease 12

Andrew B. Newberg and Stephen Olex

> *. . . this very old perspective—that the mind and body are actually different sides of the same coin—. . .goes all the way back to the origins of medicine.*
>
> Dr. Jon Kabat-Zinn (Kabat-Zinn J, and Moyers B (2002) Meditation. In: Moyers B (ed) Healing and the Mind. Broadway Books, New York, p 115–144)

12.1 Introduction

Mind–body practices have existed for hundreds or, in many cases, thousands of years and in the current era appear to be growing in popularity. This continued relevance is likely related not only to religious and spiritual connections but also to the effectiveness of the practices. Traditionally, improved health is not the goal of many mind–body practices. However, in recent decades there has been increased interest in these practices in the scientific community because the effects that they produce appear to be physiologically beneficial. This interest has been especially strong with regard to cardiovascular disease. In this chapter, the potential mechanisms of benefit of mind–body practices on the cardiovascular system will

Excerpts of the authors' previous work *Meditation: Should a Cardiologist Care?* are reprinted here in the *Potential Mechanisms of Cardiovascular Benefit for Mind-Body Practices* and *Meditation* sections with the permission of Elsevier (Olex et al., Int J Cardiol 168(3):1805–1810, 2013).

A.B. Newberg, MD
Integrative Medicine/Nuclear Medicine, Brind-Marcus Center of Integrative Medicine, Thomas Jefferson University Hospital, Villanova, PA 19085, USA
e-mail: andrew.newberg@jefferson.edu

S. Olex, MD (✉)
Integrative Cardiology, Brind-Marcus Center of Integrative Medicine, Thomas Jefferson University Hospital, Villanova, PA 19085, USA
e-mail: stephen.olex@jefferson.edu

A. Roncella, C. Pristipino (eds.), *Psychotherapy for Ischemic Heart Disease*,
DOI 10.1007/978-3-319-33214-7_12

be explored, and the data supporting the use of certain mind–body practices in the prevention and treatment of cardiovascular disease will be examined.

12.2 Potential Mechanisms of Cardiovascular Benefit

For ease of discussion, the potential mechanisms of benefit are separated here. Nonetheless, substantial overlap exists in this section and throughout the chapter, largely because it is an extraordinarily complex singular entity—the mind–body process—that is being described from different vantage points (Table 12.1).

12.2.1 Effects on the Autonomic Nervous System and the Hypothalamic–Pituitary–Adrenal (HPA) Axis

Since mind–body practices can exert beneficial effects on the autonomic nervous system [1–3] and decrease the stress response, they have the potential to decrease the deleterious cardiovascular effects of autonomic imbalance and stress hormone production. For a review of stress response mechanisms involved in ischemic heart disease, please refer to Chap. 3.

12.2.2 Effects on Traditional Cardiovascular Risk Factors

Whether through autonomic meditated mechanisms, through direct effects of movement on the body, or through additional mechanisms, mind–body practices have the potential to improve traditional cardiovascular risk factors, including hypertension, elevated blood glucose, and dyslipidemia.

12.2.3 Anti-inflammatory Reflex

Inflammation appears to play a central role in atherosclerotic plaque progression, vulnerability, and thrombogenicity [4, 5] and has been implicated in the

Table 12.1 Potential mechanisms of cardiovascular benefits from mind–body practices

Reduced sympathetic/increased parasympathetic tone
Reduced blood pressure
Improved traditional cardiovascular risk factor profile
Decreased arrhythmias
Decreased deleterious effects of chronic psychological distress
Decreased deleterious effects of acute and chronic stress
Reduced cortisol
Decreased inflammation
Increased telomere length
Increase in healthy lifestyle choices
Improved relationships/increased social connection

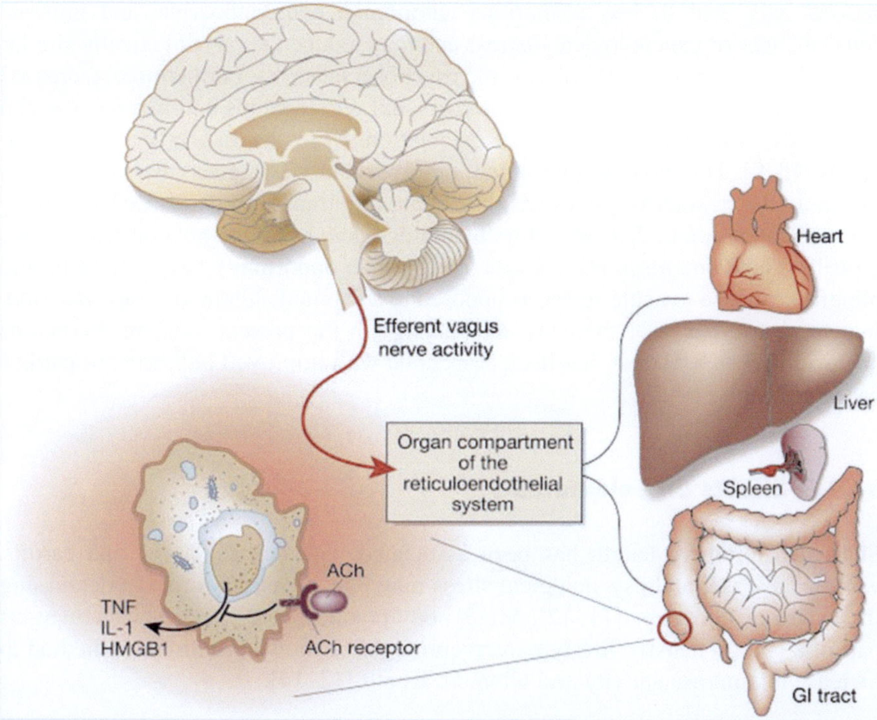

Fig. 12.1 Efferent limb of the anti-inflammatory reflex. Efferent vagal activity leads to acetylcholine (ACh) release in organs of the reticuloendothelial system, resulting in inhibition of pro-inflammatory cytokine release by tissue macrophages (Reproduced with permission from Tracey, 2002)

pathophysiology of heart failure [6]. Data suggest that the vagus nerve represents the efferent and afferent limbs of a cholinergic anti-inflammatory reflex that serves to decrease the detrimental effects of excessive pro-inflammatory stimulation [7] (Fig. 12.1). Mind–body practices that favorably affect autonomic tone have the potential to benefit the cardiovascular system via this reflex [1]. For a review of inflammation/immunity mechanisms involved in ischemic heart disease, please refer to the already cited Chap. 3.

12.2.4 Effects on the Mind–Heart Connection

Mind–body practices, by affecting the mind, have the potential to benefit the cardiovascular system through the mind–heart connection. Beyond simple relaxation techniques, mind–body practices like yoga and mindfulness can become a way of life for many individuals, influencing many if not all aspects of a person's life and affecting how he or she interacts with the world. As such, they have the potential for numerous downstream health benefits. Improved mental health in general may lead to less deleterious autonomic, neuroendocrine, and immune consequences of psychological distress and may reduce the physiologically similar detrimental effects of acute and chronic psychosocial stress. Furthermore, increased well-being may lead to improved interpersonal relationships and increased social connections, factors having known associations with the risk of cardiovascular disease [8, 9]. The moment-to-moment mind and body awareness that is cultivated in certain mind–body practices has the potential to transform one's life by increasing one's attention to diverse factors including what, how, and how much one eats, as well as how one responds to stress, allowing an opportunity for a conscious and mindful response to acute stress, as opposed to a habitual, automatic stress reaction. Increased awareness of thoughts and feelings in the present moment, known as *dispositional mindfulness*, has been associated with improved indicators of cardiovascular health [10].

12.2.5 Effects on Telomeres

Shortened telomere length has been associated with cellular aging and cardiovascular disease, and psychological stress may play a causative role in decreasing the length of telomeres [11, 12]. Mind–body practices and stress management, as part of a comprehensive lifestyle intervention, have shown promise as a method to increase telomerase activity and telomere length [12–14].

12.3 Mind–Body Practices and Cardiovascular Implications

12.3.1 Meditation

Meditation refers to a family of practices that may share many similarities but can have differences in underlying methods and goals. Meditative practices may involve focused attention, during which the practitioner directs his or her awareness on breathing, an object, or a word or phrase known as a *mantra*. Mindfulness meditation involves cultivating awareness of present moment experience, whether positive, negative, or neutral, so as to counteract the tendency of the human mind to be lost in thought and unaware of what is occurring in any moment. Religious and spiritual associations are not requisite for practice. It also should be recognized that the basis of many, if not all practices, is the training of the brain and body, a process that appears to have profound effects on both structure and function.

Much of the scientific research on meditation focuses on either mindfulness meditation or Transcendental meditation® (TM®). *Mindfulness* has been defined by Dr. Jon Kabat-Zinn as "the awareness that emerges through paying attention on purpose, in the present moment, and non-judgmentally to the unfolding of experience moment by moment" [15]. *Mindfulness-Based Stress Reduction* (MBSR) is an 8-week course developed by Kabat-Zinn at the University of Massachusetts Medical School in 1979 [16]. The course involves weekly meetings and the daily home practice of mindfulness meditation practices, including a body scan meditation, gentle yoga, and sitting meditation, as well as informal exercises designed to cultivate awareness in daily life. *Transcendental meditation*® (TM®) is a widely practiced and extensively researched mantra-based meditation program in which a word or phrase is mentally repeated as an object of focus.

Hypertension

Evidence suggests that meditation can acutely lower blood pressure to a modest degree during practice [17]. It is possible that those with baseline elevated systemic vascular resistance and/or autonomic imbalance may experience a more dramatic acute effect. An ambulatory blood pressure recording of a hypertensive woman who practiced TM® revealed a marked decrease in pressure during her meditation practice [18] (Fig. 12.2).

The regular practice of meditation does appear to reduce baseline blood pressure. The effect of regular practice of TM® on baseline blood pressure has received considerable attention in recent decades. Trials of TM® in those with normal blood pressure and those with hypertension have demonstrated significant reductions in both systolic and diastolic pressure [19–23]. However, several studies on TM® have been criticized for their poor quality and possible researcher bias [24, 25]. Data compiled from three studies on TM® that are considered more robust methodologically have demonstrated clinically significant reductions in both systolic (6 mmHg reduction) and diastolic (3.4 mmHg reduction) pressure [26]. The data on MBSR for hypertension are limited and the results have been mixed, with more data needed and upcoming [27–32].

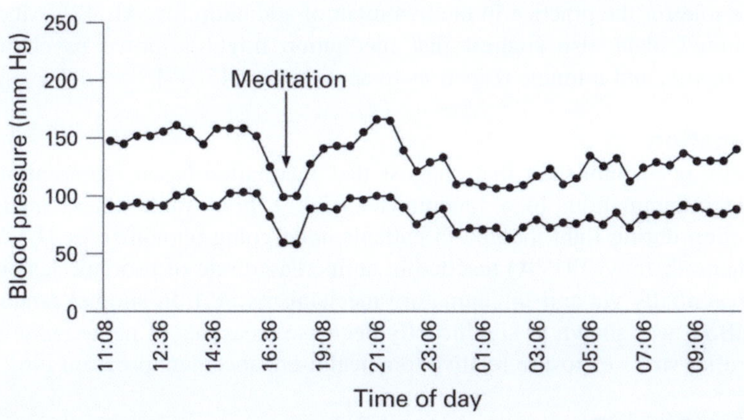

Fig. 12.2 Ambulatory blood pressure monitoring of a hypertensive woman who experienced a striking decrease in daytime blood pressure to values lower than those recorded during sleep. Upon review, the decrease corresponded to the woman's meditation practice (Reproduced with permission from Dear et al. 2008)

Autonomic Nervous System and the Hypothalmic–Pituitary–Adrenal (HPA) Axis

Described as a wakeful hypometabolic state [2], meditation practices can acutely exert a significant influence on autonomic tone via parasympathetic activation [33]. The regular practice of meditation may affect baseline autonomic balance favorably [34], though this has not been well studied. Decreased cortisol levels in those who meditate have been noted [19, 34]. Heart rate variability, a measure of the variation in instantaneous heart rate over time, allows a view into the functioning of the autonomic nervous system and autonomic balance. In general, autonomic imbalance with sympathetic dominance is related to decreased heart rate variability, while healthy autonomic balance is associated with increased heart rate variability. A more in-depth discussion of the effects of meditation on heart rate variability is outside the scope of this chapter and has been presented elsewhere [1]. Meditation practices can acutely influence and increase heart rate variability [35] and may, through slower breathing rates, exert beneficial effects on the baroreflex and chemoreflex [36–38]. It is quite possible that regular meditation may increase baseline heart rate variability and have a long-term beneficial effect on autonomic reflexes; however, to date, this potential has not been well studied in the literature.

Mind–Heart Connection

Subjectively reported benefits of meditation include relaxation and stress relief, increased concentration and attention, increased self-control, positive mood, emotional stability, increased resiliency to stress and negative events, and overall enhanced psycho-emotional balance [39]. There is objective evidence of meditation and mindfulness-induced effects in both the short and the long term on functional and structural brain plasticity [39, 40]. Clinically, there are promising data on the effects of meditation for depression, anxiety, pain, and stress/distress, and there is a possible role for the practice in the treatment of addiction [39, 41, 42]. Albeit still very limited, data also suggest that meditation might improve psychological, hemodynamic, and immune responses to acute stress [43, 44].

Inflammation

Data have been published that suggest that meditation-based interventions can decrease inflammation. In a randomized trial, a brief mindfulness meditation intervention during light therapy in patients undergoing phototherapy (UVB) and photochemotherapy (PUVA) resulted in an increased rate of psoriatic lesion resolution potentially via anti-inflammatory mechanisms [45]. In another randomized trial, MBSR was shown to significantly decrease measures of neurogenic inflammation after stress exposure relative to a health-enhancement program [46].

Coronary Artery Disease and Heart Failure

Data on the effects of meditation on clinical endpoints in established cardiovascular disease are limited but promising. One small randomized controlled study examined the effects of MBSR on patients with coronary artery disease and detected reductions in BMI, blood pressure, and perceived stress, as well as in levels of anxiety and depression [47]. Another small study examined the effects of TM® in African Americans (≥55 years) who had an ejection fraction less than 40 % [48] and found that the meditation group experienced significant improvements in the primary endpoint of 6-min walk test score. The *Support Education and Research in Chronic Heart Failure* (SEARCH) Study demonstrated significantly improved symptoms of heart failure at one year in patients who had undertaken a mindfulness meditation program, relative to controls [49].

12.3.2 Yoga

Yoga is an ancient mind–body discipline, originating in India, in which meditation, breath control, and specific postures are traditionally utilized for spiritual growth [50]. Yoga holds great intuitive appeal for the prevention and treatment of cardiovascular disease as the discipline appears to exert beneficial autonomic effects [3] and may increase baseline heart rate variability [51], in addition to providing physical activity, mental health benefits, and stress reduction [52]. Since yoga has been demonstrated to be accessible to those with lower physical tolerance, the practice also has the potential to benefit patients with limited functional capacity who might not be able to do aerobic exercises [53].

Traditional Cardiovascular Risk Factors

Though there are limitations in the data, an accumulating body of evidence suggests that yoga benefits cardiovascular disease risk factors. Among the more robust evidence is a large 2014 review and meta-analysis [53] in which statistically significant decreases were noted, relative to controls, in body mass index, systolic blood pressure (−5.21 mmHg), diastolic blood pressure (−4.98 mmHg), low-density lipoprotein cholesterol, body weight, total cholesterol, triglycerides, and heart rate, along with a significant increase in high-density lipoprotein cholesterol. No effect was apparent for fasting glucose or hemoglobin A1c. Of note, there were no statistically significant differences between yoga and exercise. Meanwhile, another review published the same year did identify beneficial effects on HgBA1c and insulin resistance [54]. Although these data are very promising, randomized controlled trials of yoga are limited by their small size, short duration, and low to moderate methodological quality [50, 53].

Mind–Heart Connection

Yoga has the potential to benefit the cardiovascular system via the mind–heart connection. It has been noted to have positive psychological effects on depression and anxiety and has the potential to improve the acute stress response to psychosocial stress, though the latter has not been well studied [52].

Inflammation

There is accumulating evidence supporting the anti-inflammatory effects of yoga. In one study, more experienced yoga practitioners had lower levels of Il-6 in response to the stressor lipopolysaccharide, while novices were more likely to have detectable levels of C-reactive protein [55]. Another study of patients with left ventricular systolic dysfunction and NYHA class I–III heart failure identified statistically significant reductions in IL-6 and high sensitivity C-reactive protein [56].

Arrhythmias

In an important uncontrolled trial that assessed the effect of yoga on paroxysmal atrial fibrillation (AF), yoga significantly decreased symptomatic AF episodes, symptomatic non-AF episodes, asymptomatic AF episodes, depression, and anxiety and improved other measures of quality of life. Preliminary data also suggest that yoga might decrease defibrillator shocks [57, 58].

Coronary Artery Disease and Heart Failure

The data are limited but encouraging regarding the effects of yoga on established cardiovascular disease. These data suggest that yoga improves risk factors, as well as anxiety, depression, and stress when utilized within the context of a postoperative cardiac rehabilitation program in patients who have undergone coronary bypass [59]. A 2014 review of four randomized trials investigated the effects of yoga on patients with coronary artery disease and heart failure [60]. One trial identified increased exercise tolerance with yoga, while another detected decreased angina frequency in the yoga group, findings that were based on very low quality evidence. The review authors gave a weak recommendation for yoga for coronary artery disease, while calling for additional research [60]. Meanwhile, in the two heart failure trials, a total of 59 patients with chronic heart failure underwent Hatha yoga interventions. In both of these trials, exercise time and maximum oxygen consumption improved in the yoga group as did the patients' quality of life, but, again, the studies were of low methodological quality. And once again a weak recommendation was given for yoga in heart failure patients, with the need for further research emphasized [60]. In a subsequent randomized trial in stable heart failure patients, yoga was found to enhance left ventricular function while reducing levels of the N-terminal pro-hormone brain natriuretic peptide (NT-proBNP) [61].

12.3.3 Tai Chi

Tai Chi is a mind–body practice and martial art that originated in China. It consists of three components: movement, meditation, and breathing. The practice is considered to be a low-impact exercise of low to moderate intensity that can be performed by older adults and those with chronic disease [62, 63]. As Tai Chi appears to have beneficial effects on the mind and body through physical activity, stress relief, and improving autonomic balance [63, 64], there has been understandable interest in its use for the prevention and treatment of cardiovascular disease.

Hypertension

Evidence exists to suggest that Tai Chi can benefit hypertension, though additional data are needed. In a 2008 pooled analysis of 26 studies published in English or Chinese, Tai Chi was noted to exert a beneficial effect on blood pressure, with systolic decreases of 7–32 mmHg and diastolic decreases of 2.4–18 mmHg in those with hypertension and systolic decreases of 4–18 mmHg and diastolic decreases of 2.3–7.5 mmHg in non-cardiovascular or healthy populations [65]. The authors of a 2014 Cochrane review who analyzed the effects of Tai Chi on blood pressure and lipids noted that some studies demonstrated beneficial effects on cardiovascular risk factors, but also that firm conclusions regarding the positive effects of Tai Chi could not be made secondary to the heterogeneity and quality of the trials [63]. More high-quality trials with longer term follow-up were called for.

Mind–Heart Connection

It appears that Tai Chi has positive effects on the mind component of the mind–heart connection. Positive effects have been documented for depression, anxiety, and stress, albeit with data that have significant limitations [66]. Data also suggest that Tai Chi improves stress reactivity [67].

Inflammation and Cortisol

Very limited data suggest that Tai Chi may decrease markers of inflammation and that its practice might decrease cortisol production [68, 69].

Coronary Artery Disease and Heart Failure

Few trials have looked at the effects of Tai Chi on those with established coronary artery disease. In one study of 126 patients with acute myocardial infarction, Tai Chi was found to reduce both systolic and diastolic blood pressure and to be safe after an acute myocardial infarction [62, 70]. In another study, the postoperative initiation of a 12-month Tai Chi program after coronary artery bypass graft surgery (CABG) was associated with a significant increase in cardio-respiratory function [71].

A handful of trials have examined the effects of Tai Chi on patients with congestive heart failure. In a recent meta-analysis of four randomized trials, Tai Chi significantly improved quality of life, but did not reduce brain natriuretic peptide (BNP) or blood pressure. It also failed to increase 6-min walking distance or peak oxygen uptake [72]. In a more recent small study of patients with heart failure with preserved ejection fraction, Tai Chi improved the 6-min walk distance and depression more than aerobic exercise, but there was no inter-group difference in peak oxygen uptake [73].

12.3.4 Stress Reduction/Comprehensive Lifestyle Programs

Comprehensive lifestyle programs exert significant beneficial effects in patients with established disease and have been noted to be cost-efficient [74]. In a well-known study published in 1983 in JAMA, Dr. Dean Ornish demonstrated increases in the duration of exercise, total work performed, and maximal ejection fraction with exercise, as well as a reduction in angina frequency in 23 patients with ischemic heart disease after 24 days of an intervention that consisted of intensive dietary changes as well as stress management techniques, including stretching/relaxation exercises and meditation [75]. Ornish subsequently noted regression of coronary artery disease with intensive lifestyle changes (documented by coronary angiogram) [76], a finding that has since been replicated [77]. A large meta-analysis published in 1996 investigated the effects of adding psychosocial interventions—including stress management training, relaxation therapy, and psychotherapy—to usual care within a standard rehabilitation regimen in patients with coronary artery disease and identified reductions in morbidity, mortality, and psychological distress [78]. Chronic diseases like cardiovascular disease are very likely ideally approached from an integrated multi-intervention approach that incorporates traditional medical therapy, dietary changes, exercise, and mind–body practices and/or stress management techniques.

12.4 Conclusions

More high-quality studies are needed of mind–body practices in cardiovascular disease, whether alone or as part of a comprehensive integrated lifestyle intervention. Ideally, these studies would be randomized with intermediate or longer term follow-up and would look not only at changes in physiologic parameters and laboratory data, but also at relevant and crucial endpoints in cardiovascular disease including arrhythmias, nonfatal and fatal myocardial infarctions, hospitalizations, and cardiac mortality in addition to quality of life parameters. It is probable that the significant beneficial effects of mind–body practices identified for such diverse factors as blood pressure, autonomic function, arrhythmia, inflammation, response to stress, mood, interpersonal relationships, lifestyle, and telomere length will result in reduced cardiovascular morbidity and mortality.

Given that our goals as clinicians are to help patients live better and longer, there appears to be sufficient evidence regarding mind–body practices to recommend them based upon the former, and growing evidence suggesting the potential for the latter [1]. As cardiovascular data evolve, mind–body practices can be confidently considered for the promotion of overall mind and body health. Many, if not all, mind–body practices are accessible even to those with limited functional capacity. Consequently, they have the potential to significantly benefit the lives of many patients.

References

1. Olex S, Newberg A, Figueredo VM (2013) Meditation: should a cardiologist care? Int J Cardiol 168(3):1805–1810
2. Jevning R, Wallace RK, Beidebach M (1992) The physiology of meditation: a review. A wakeful hypometabolic integrated response. Neurosci Biobehav Rev 16(3):415–424
3. Khattab K, Khattab AA, Ortak J et al (2007) Iyengar yoga increases cardiac parasympathetic nervous modulation among healthy yoga practitioners. Evid Based Complement Alternat Med 4(4):511–517
4. Libby P (2002) Inflammation in atherosclerosis. Nature 420(6917):868–874
5. Mizuno Y, Jacob RF, Mason PR (2011) Inflammation and the development of atherosclerosis. J Atheroscler Thromb 18(5):351–358
6. Emani S, Binkley PF (2010) Mind-body medicine in chronic heart failure: a translational science challenge. Circ Heart Fail 3(6):715–725
7. Tracey KJ (2002) The inflammatory reflex. Nature 420(6917):853–859
8. Udell JA, Steg PG, Scirica BM et al (2012) Living alone and cardiovascular risk in outpatients at risk of or with atherothrombosis. Arch Intern Med 172(14):1086–1095
9. Albus C (2010) Psychological and social factors in coronary heart disease. Ann Med 42(7): 487–494
10. Loucks EB, Britton WB, Howe CJ et al (2014) Positive associations of dispositional mindfulness with cardiovascular health: the new England family study. Int J Behav Med 22(4): 540–550
11. Kiecolt-Glaser JK, Glaser R (2010) Psychological stress, telomeres, and telomerase. Brain Behav Immun 24(4):529–530
12. Lavretsky H, Siddarth P, Nazarian N et al (2013) A pilot study of yogic meditation for family dementia caregivers with depressive symptoms: effects on mental health, cognition, and telomerase activity. Int J Geriatr Psychiatry 28(1):57–65
13. Ornish D, Lin J, Chan JM et al (2013) Effect of comprehensive lifestyle changes on telomerase activity and telomere length in men with biopsy-proven low-risk prostate cancer: 5-year follow-up of a descriptive pilot study. Lancet Oncol 14(11):1112–1120
14. Jacobs TL, Epel ES, Lin J et al (2011) Intensive meditation training, immune cell telomerase activity, and psychological mediators. Psychoneuroendocrinology 36(5):664–681
15. Kabat-Zinn J (2003) Mindfulness-based interventions in context: past, present and future. Clin Psychol Sci Pract 10:144–156
16. Kabat-Zinn J (2013) Full catastrophe living—using the wisdom of your body and mind to face stress, pain, and illness. Bantam Books, New York
17. Barnes VA, Treiber FA, Turner JR et al (1999) Acute effects of transcendental meditation on hemodynamic functioning in middle-aged adults. Psychosom Med 61(4):525–531
18. Dear JW, Gough K, Webb DJ (2008) Transcendental meditation and hypertension. Postgrad Med J 84(994):417
19. Murphy M, Donovan S (eds) (1999) The physical and psychological effects of meditation: a review of contemporary research with a comprehensive bibliography, 1931–1996, 2nd edn. Institute of Noetic Sciences, Sausalito
20. Bagga OP, Gandhi A (1983) A comparative study of the effect of transcendental meditation (T.M.) and Shavasana practice on cardiovascular system. Indian Heart J 35(1):39–45
21. Alexander CN, Langer EJ, Newman RI et al (1989) Transcendental meditation, mindfulness, and longevity: an experimental study with the elderly. J Pers Soc Psychol 57(6):950–964
22. Wenneberg SR, Schneider RH, Walton KG et al (1997) A controlled study of the effects of the transcendental meditation program on cardiovascular reactivity and ambulatory blood pressure. Int J Neurosci 89(1–2):15–28
23. Castillo-Richmond A, Schneider RH, Alexander CN et al (2000) Effects of stress reduction on carotid atherosclerosis in hypertensive African Americans. Stroke 31(3):568–573

24. Parati G, Steptoe A (2004) Stress reduction and blood pressure control in hypertension: a role for transcendental meditation? J Hypertens 22(11):2057–2060
25. Canter PH, Ernst E (2004) Insufficient evidence to conclude whether or not transcendental meditation decreases blood pressure: results of a systematic review of randomized clinical trials. J Hypertens 22(11):2049–2054
26. Anderson JW, Liu C, Kryscio RJ (2008) Blood pressure response to transcendental meditation: a meta-analysis. Am J Hypertens 21(3):310–316
27. NIH RePORTER (2015) National Institute of Health, Bethesda. http://projectreporter.nih.gov/project_info_description.cfm?aid=8703899&icde=23100189&ddparam=&ddvalue=&ddsub=&cr=1&csb=default&cs=ASC. Accessed 9 July 2015
28. Carlson LE, Speca M, Faris P et al (2007) One year pre-post intervention follow-up of psychological, immune, endocrine and blood pressure outcomes of mindfulness-based stress reduction (MBSR) in breast and prostate cancer outpatients. Brain Behav Immun 21(8): 1038–1049
29. Rosenzweig S, Reibel DK, Greeson JM et al (2007) Mindfulness-based stress reduction is associated with improved glycemic control in type 2 diabetes mellitus: a pilot study. Altern Ther Health Med 13(5):36–38
30. Palta P, Page G, Piferi RL et al (2012) Evaluation of a mindfulness-based intervention program to decrease blood pressure in low-income African-American older adults. J Urban Health 89(2):308–316
31. Hughes JW, Fresco DM, Myerscough R et al (2013) Randomized controlled trial of mindfulness-based stress reduction for prehypertension. Psychosom Med 75(8):721–728
32. Blom K, Baker B, How M et al (2014) Hypertension analysis of stress reduction using mindfulness meditation and yoga: results from the HARMONY randomized controlled trial. Am J Hypertens 27(1):122–129
33. Young JD, Taylor E (1998) Meditation as a voluntary hypometabolic state of biological estivation. News Physiol Sci 13:149–153
34. Sudsuang R, Chentanez V, Veluvan K (1991) Effect of Buddhist meditation on serum cortisol and total protein levels, blood pressure, pulse rate, lung volume and reaction time. Physiol Behav 50(3):543–548
35. Phongsuphap S, Pongsupap Y, Chandanamattha P et al (2008) Changes in heart rate variability during concentration meditation. Int J Cardiol 130(3):481–484
36. Lehrer PM, Gevirtz R (2014) Heart rate variability biofeedback: how and why does it work? Front Psychol 5:756
37. Sharma M, Frishman WH, Gandhi K (2011) RESPeRATE: non-pharmacological treatment of hypertension. Cardiol Rev 19(2):47–51
38. Cernes R, Zimlichman R (2015) RESPeRATE: the role of paced breathing in hypertension treatment. J Am Soc Hypertens 9(1):38–47
39. Rubia K (2009) The neurobiology of meditation and its clinical effectiveness in psychiatric disorders. Biol Psychol 82(1):1–11
40. Marchand WR (2014) Neural mechanisms of mindfulness and meditation: evidence from neuroimaging studies. World J Radiol 6(7):471–479
41. Goyal M, Singh S, Sibinga EM et al (2014) Meditation programs for psychological stress and well-being: a systematic review and meta-analysis. JAMA Intern Med 174(3):357–368
42. Khanna S, Greeson JM (2013) A narrative review of yoga and mindfulness as complementary therapies for addiction. Complement Ther Med 21(3):244–252
43. Barnes VA, Treiber FA, Davis H (2001) Impact of transcendental meditation on cardiovascular function at rest and during acute stress in adolescents with high normal blood pressure. J Psychosom Res 51(4):597–605
44. Pace TW, Negi LT, Adame DD et al (2009) Effect of compassion meditation on neuroendocrine, innate immune and behavioral responses to psychosocial stress. Psychoneuroendocrinology 34(1):87–98

45. Kabat-Zinn J, Wheeler E, Light T et al (1998) Influence of a mindfulness meditation-based stress reduction intervention on rates of skin clearing in patients with moderate to severe psoriasis undergoing phototherapy (UVB) and photochemotherapy (PUVA). Psychosom Med 60(5): 625–632
46. Rosenkranz MA, Davidson RJ, Maccoon DG et al (2013) A comparison of mindfulness-based stress reduction and an active control in modulation of neurogenic inflammation. Brain Behav Immun 27(1):174–184
47. Parswani MJ, Sharma MP, Iyengar S (2013) Mindfulness-based stress reduction program in coronary heart disease: a randomized control trial. Int J Yoga 6(2):111–117
48. Jayadevappa R, Johnson JC, Bloom BS et al (2007) Effectiveness of transcendental meditation on functional capacity and quality of life of African Americans with congestive heart failure: a randomized control study. Ethn Dis 17(1):72–77
49. Sullivan MJ, Wood L, Terry J et al (2009) The support, education, and research in chronic heart failure study (SEARCH): a mindfulness-based psychoeducational intervention improves depression and clinical symptoms in patients with chronic heart failure. Am Heart J 157(1): 84–90
50. Hartley L, Dyakova M, Holmes J et al (2014) Yoga for the primary prevention of cardiovascular disease. Cochrane Database Syst Rev 5:Cd010072
51. Muralikrishnan K, Balakrishnan B, Balasubramanian K et al (2012) Measurement of the effect of Isha Yoga on cardiac autonomic nervous system using short-term heart rate variability. J Ayurveda Integr Med 3(2):91–96
52. Skowronek IB, Mounsey A, Handler L (2014) Clinical inquiry: can yoga reduce symptoms of anxiety and depression? J Fam Pract 63(7):398–407
53. Chu P, Gotink RA, Yeh GY et al (2014) The effectiveness of yoga in modifying risk factors for cardiovascular disease and metabolic syndrome: a systematic review and meta-analysis of randomized controlled trials. Eur J Prev Cardiol. pii:2047487314562741 [Epub ahead of print]
54. Cramer H, Lauche R, Haller H et al (2014) Effects of yoga on cardiovascular disease risk factors: a systematic review and meta-analysis. Int J Cardiol 173(2):170–183
55. Kiecolt-Glaser JK, Christian L, Preston H et al (2010) Stress, inflammation, and yoga practice. Psychosom Med 72(2):113–121
56. Pullen PR, Nagamia SH, Mehta PK et al (2008) Effects of yoga on inflammation and exercise capacity in patients with chronic heart failure. J Card Fail 14(5):407–413
57. Toise SC, Sears SF, Schoenfeld MH et al (2014) Psychosocial and cardiac outcomes of yoga for ICD patients: a randomized clinical control trial. Pacing Clin Electrophysiol 37(1):48–62
58. Dabhade AM, Pawar BH, Ghunage MS et al (2012) Effect of pranayama (breathing exercise) on arrhythmias in the human heart. Explore (NY) 8(1):12–15
59. Raghuram N, Parachuri VN, Swarnagowri MV et al (2014) Yoga based cardiac rehabilitation after coronary artery bypass surgery: one-year results on LVEF, lipid profile and psychological states—a randomized controlled study. Indian Heart J 66(5):490–502
60. Cramer H, Lauche R, Haller H et al (2014) A systematic review of yoga for heart disease. Eur J Prev Cardiol 22(3):284–295
61. Krishna BH, Pal P, Pal G et al (2014) A randomized controlled trial to study the effect of yoga therapy on cardiac function and N terminal pro BNP in heart failure. Integr Med Insights 9:1–6
62. Lan C, Chen SY, Wong MK et al (2013) Tai chi chuan exercise for patients with cardiovascular disease. Evid Based Complement Alternat Med 983208
63. Hartley L, Flowers N, Lee MS et al (2014) Tai chi for primary prevention of cardiovascular disease. Cochrane Database Syst Rev 4:Cd010366
64. Motivala SJ, Sollers J, Thayer J et al (2006) Tai Chi Chih acutely decreases sympathetic nervous system activity in older adults. J Gerontol A Biol Sci Med Sci 61(11):1177–1180
65. Yeh GY, Wang C, Wayne PM et al (2008) The effect of tai chi exercise on blood pressure: a systematic review. Prev Cardiol 11(2):82–89
66. Wang F, Lee EK, Wu T et al (2014) The effects of tai chi on depression, anxiety, and psychological well-being: a systematic review and meta-analysis. Int J Behav Med 21(4):605–617

67. Nedeljkovic M, Ausfeld-Hafter B, Streitberger K et al (2012) Taiji practice attenuates psychobiological stress reactivity—a randomized controlled trial in healthy subjects. Psychoneuroendocrinology 37(8):1171–1180
68. Irwin MR, Olmstead R (2012) Mitigating cellular inflammation in older adults: a randomized controlled trial of Tai Chi Chih. Am J Geriatr Psychiatry 20(9):764–772
69. Campo RA, Light KC, O'Connor K et al (2015) Blood pressure, salivary cortisol, and inflammatory cytokine outcomes in senior female cancer survivors enrolled in a tai chi chih randomized controlled trial. J Cancer Surviv 9(1):115–125
70. Channer KS, Barrow D, Barrow R et al (1996) Changes in haemodynamic parameters following Tai Chi Chuan and aerobic exercise in patients recovering from acute myocardial infarction. Postgrad Med J 72(848):349–351
71. Lan C, Chen SY, Lai JS et al (1999) The effect of Tai Chi on cardiorespiratory function in patients with coronary artery bypass surgery. Med Sci Sports Exerc 31(5):634–638
72. Pan L, Yan J, Guo Y et al (2013) Effects of Tai Chi training on exercise capacity and quality of life in patients with chronic heart failure: a meta-analysis. Eur J Heart Fail 15(3):316–323
73. Yeh GY, Wood MJ, Wayne PM et al (2013) Tai chi in patients with heart failure with preserved ejection fraction. Congest Heart Fail 19(2):77–84
74. Zeng W, Stason WB, Fournier S et al (2013) Benefits and costs of intensive lifestyle modification programs for symptomatic coronary disease in medicare beneficiaries. Am Heart J 165(5):785–792
75. Ornish D, Scherwitz LW, Doody RS et al (1983) Effects of stress management training and dietary changes in treating ischemic heart disease. JAMA 249(1):54–59
76. Ornish D, Scherwitz LW, Billings JH et al (1998) Intensive lifestyle changes for reversal of coronary heart disease. JAMA 280(23):2001–2007
77. Gupta SK, Sawhney RC, Rai L et al (2011) Regression of coronary atherosclerosis through healthy lifestyle in coronary artery disease patients—Mount Abu Open Heart Trial. Indian Heart J 63(5):461–469
78. Linden W, Stossel C, Maurice J (1996) Psychosocial interventions for patients with coronary artery disease: a meta-analysis. Arch Intern Med 156(7):745–752

Short-Term Psychotherapy in Patients with Acute Myocardial Infarction

13

Adriana Roncella

> *...anguish, love, jealous, worry, and similar mental states are accompanied by emaciation, wasting away, and other bodily changes predisposing to disease and consumption in men. A mental disturbance provoking pain, excessive joy, hope or anxiety extends to the heart, where it affects its temper, and rate, impairing general nutrition and vigor.*
> William Harvey [William Harvey (1628) "Anatomical studies on the motion of the heart and blood" (English translation by Chauncey D. Leake). 1928, third edition, second printing 1949, Charles C. Thomas, Publisher, Springfield, Illinois]

13.1 Introduction

Since the middle of the last century, a vast quantity of scientific studies on psychosocial risk factors and cardiac diseases have been conducted worldwide. Among this research have been numerous clinical trials on a variety of psychotherapeutic methods, and, among these approaches, the ones most often examined have been behavioral, cognitive, and interpersonal therapy. These approaches have been proven effective at improving psychological symptoms. However, it remains uncertain whether their efficacy extends to patients' medical and, more specifically, cardiac outcomes. Taken together, these studies show that some psychological interventions (like "stress management") might improve the prognosis of patients with coronary artery disease (CAD). However, the great heterogeneity that has existed within the studies' subject samples necessitates further confirmation in each specific subgroup of cardiac disease patients, like those with an acute myocardial

A. Roncella, MD (✉)
Department of Cardiovascular Disease, San Filippo Neri Hospital, Via G. Martinotti 20, 00135 Rome, Italy
e-mail: adrianaroncella@hotmail.it

A. Roncella, C. Pristipino (eds.), *Psychotherapy for Ischemic Heart Disease*,
DOI 10.1007/978-3-319-33214-7_13

infarction (AMI), in whom the pathophysiology underlying the clinical manifestations of disease is variable. In addition, these studies spanned many years, during which considerable progress has been made in the pharmacological and interventional treatment of ischemic heart disease, overall associated with significant improvements in outcomes. This is especially true of AMIs, wherein the latest treatments might outweigh the benefits of supplementary psychological treatment. Moreover, any formal, published assessments of humanistic-existential psychotherapy approaches remain missing.

After carefully evaluating all the previous scientific research, we designed and orchestrated a randomized clinical trial to assess the value of short-term psychotherapy in patients with an AMI who had been treated with either an urgent or emergent percutaneous coronary intervention, within the Department of Cardiovascular Disease at San Filippo Neri Hospital in Rome [1].

We utilized for the first time, a humanistic-existential psychotherapy derived from the ontopsychological method.

The chapter then details and explains the specific psychotherapy approach used.

13.2 The STEP-IN-AMI Trial

This controlled randomized study, published in 2013 in the International Journal of Cardiology [2], for the first time documented the benefits of an original humanistic-existential form of short-term psychotherapy, improving both medical and cardiological prognosis and cardiac and psychological symptoms of patients with AMI. This benefit was observed at 1 year after the index event and was above and beyond the benefits generated utilizing the more advanced medical, interventional, and rehabilitation interventions available at that time.

The protocol was approved by the ethics committee of San Filippo Neri Hospital in Rome in 2004 [1], and enrollment of patients was completed in 2011. Briefly, 101 patients age $\leq$70 years, and enrolled within 1 week of complete revascularization with urgent/emergent angioplasty for an AMI, were randomized to receive either standard cardiac care (SCC) plus short-term humanistic-existential psychotherapy (STP) or SCC (controls) alone.

The primary composite endpoint was the 1-year incidence of new cardiac events, which included re-infarction, death, stroke, revascularization, life-threatening ventricular arrhythmias, and the recurrence of either typical and clinically significant angina or other clinically significant new comorbid conditions. Secondary endpoints were rates for individual components of the primary outcome, the incidence of rehospitalizations for cardiac problems, New York Heart Association (NYHA) class, and psychometric test scores at follow-up.

Ninety-four patients were then analyzed at 1 year. At 1-year follow-up, STP patients had experienced a lower incidence of the primary endpoint, relative to controls (21/49, 42.9 % vs. 35/45, 77.8 % patients; $p = 0.0006$, respectively; NNT = 3). This benefit was attributable to the lower incidence of recurrent angina and of new comorbid conditions in the STP group (14/49, 28.6 % vs. 22/45, 48.9 %

patients, $p = 0.04$, NNT = 5; and 5/49, 10.2 % vs. 25/45, 55.6 %, $p = 0.0001$, NNT = 3, respectively). Patients administered STP also had statistically fewer rehospitalizations, a better NYHA class, higher quality of life, and lower depression scores.

Five-year follow-up is under way to assess longer term outcomes, and the evaluation of the results will be completed in 2016. If larger studies remain necessary to confirm the generalizability of these results, this study is one of the most strikingly positive studies in the field of psychotherapy (see Chap. 10). Moreover, it introduces an innovative psychotherapeutic approach into the field of Cardiac Psychology.

13.3 The Psychotherapeutic Approach

On the basis of acquired experience, synthetic but complete and very practical insights into the psychotherapy approach, which was adopted in the STEP-IN-AMI trial, are presented in this chapter, as a means to assist other psychologists and physicians who would like to expand their knowledge and practice of Cardiac Psychology.

As written above we utilized, for the first time, a humanistic-existential psychotherapy derived from the ontopsychological method [3] and specifically adapted by the psychotherapist herself to the context of research in the field of cardiac psychology. We developed a standardized, basic model of STP that could be easily reproduced and delivered within the Italian national healthcare system.

Psychotherapy was performed by a single skilled and licensed psychotherapist, with the help of clinical staff, both psychologists and nurses. The administration of psychoactive drugs was not part of the protocol, but, in patients already being treated pharmaceutically, psychiatric drugs were not discontinued. All patients were invited to participate in a cardiac rehabilitation program; those who refused the program received educational training and lifestyle change recommendations.

The *ontopsychological method* is a complex and original synthesis in part derived from psychoanalysis, analytical psychology, and the humanistic-existential approach as was initially elaborated by Abraham Maslow [4]. With the ontopsychological approach, the human being is considered a complex system that consists of the union of psyche and body, where anything happening in the body may influence the psyche and vice versa, as demonstrated by several studies in the field of psychoneuroendocrinoimmunology [5–7]. With this view, a psychotherapeutic intervention must improve not only psychological symptoms, quality of life, and cardiac prognosis (the main endpoints considered in previous psychological interventions in patients with ischemic heart disease) but also global health to be considered effective in cardiac patients.

For an overview of the method, the original published International Journal of Cardiology report is displayed here [2]. "*Psychotherapy was delivered initially in individual and then group sessions over a 6-month period after the incident AMI. Individual meetings focused on personal history, as emotionally lived by the patient, and on understanding basic expressions of the unconscious dimension, through the interpretation of body and oneiric language. The number of individual meetings was tailored to the specific needs and problems of each patient, ranging from 3 to 11 meetings over a 3-month period.*

The shortest cycle, which was 3 single sessions, involved a 31-year old man, who exhibited great resistance to the analysis; whereas the longest cycle of 11 sessions occurred with a 56-year old man with clinically-relevant depression and two suicide attempts. Over the duration of this brief course of treatment, the psychotherapist helps the patient to gain insights and elaborate on conflicts that need to be resolved, as well as on dysfunctional behaviors and interpersonal relationships. After the initial interviews, aimed at focusing on and overcoming main conflicts in the patient's life, the psychotherapist helps the patient to gain insights into his/her body sensations. Generally, cardiac patients report a distorted and partial perception of their body, their body often perceived as foreign. The psychotherapist guides the patient to acquire full contact with his/her body, starting from the visceral zone, with the help of abdominal breathing and relaxation techniques. In the final phase of the individual meetings and whenever possible, the psychotherapist guides the patient into deeper insights through dream analysis. Generally, patients who have suffered a recent myocardial infarction report having experienced nightmares, often starting several months or even years before the acute event; or, alternatively, finding it impossible to remember dreams (often, patients only recall a few dreams from their childhood and/or adolescence). As the psychotherapist helps the patients to contact the central positive nucleus of their unconscious (the "In Se"), their nightmares cease and/or the patients resume remembering dreams related to their real-life problems. This reflects inner changes orchestrated by the patient.

The psychotherapeutic work done during the individual sessions is reiterated during group sessions, where the analysis and goals achieved in the individual sessions can be reinforced via *exchanges between group members. Group sessions, to which partners are invited, entail educational cardiological therapy (which includes a broader explanation of myocardial infarction and atherosclerotic processes, while accentuating the importance of cardiac risk factors prevention/reduction and lifestyle changes); music-guided breathing and muscular relaxation; comprehension of body signals; elements of oneiric language; and attention to specific partners/relationships.*

The aim of all these processes was to stabilize the pathology and promote global well-being within each patient."

As already said, the ontopsychological approach is based on a specific vision of the Human Being as a unification of bodily and psychic action. From this perspective, the unity of action is in great part unconscious to the subject, where the unconscious is defined as "*an active existential quantum which is not recognized by voluntary or responsible knowledge, both in the psychic and somatic aspect. It is entirely made up of the active and existing quantum of the subject, psychic and somatic, excluded from the consciousness and the responsibility of the Ego. The unconscious is the quantum of life and intelligence through which we exist, but which we do not know…*" [8]. The core of unconscious is seen here as a positive nucleus, which has been called "*In-Self*" (In Sé). It characterizes our specific identity, acting through the *vital boost* that drives human life. It might be considered the vitality, the criterion of nature, our specific identity which sustains us throughout life [3, 9]. It expresses itself in all the positive aspects of our life, from our biological needs (hunger, thirst, instincts) to more spiritual ones (intelligence, love, friendship, sociability, etc.). Therefore, to pursue happiness and health, one must follow her/his inner positive vital boost. In particular, one should in every moment listen to the signals that her/his In-Self expresses. It can be defined as "*our great wise*," which continuously communicates with our consciousness, to let one's Ego understand the best ways and solutions within the complex historical evolution of one's life. We could consider the In-Self as the psychic project throughout one's life, trying to bring a person to self-realization, in biological, affective, social, and spiritual dimensions.

13.4 Languages of the Unconscious

This positive nucleus expresses itself through both bodily and oneiric (dream-based) language. Related to body language, a body sensation may express itself as an emotional experience, and a dysfunctional somatic symptom may hide some inner conflict. In particular, the visceral zone seems to be an entry point for contacting emotions and instincts, which are expressions of the inner positive nucleus of the unconscious [10–14] (see also Chap. 4).

In my personal and clinical experience across many fields of psychotherapeutic application, I can verify that, in illnesses, patients have lost contact with their visceral zone. They feel their body as foreign, as something separate from their mind. Sometimes, this perception is concentrated within a specific part of the body, which is felt as heavy or painful. Cardiac patients often refer to the sensation of heaviness in their head, or in their chest corresponding to their heart, or the perception of only parts of their body. The body is never felt to be all together, as a unit.

The other In-Self signals are dreams. Dreams may be considered a symbolic language of the unconscious [15–17], reflecting its basic functional mechanisms, represented by projection. The inner and intimate world is projected in every aspect of life, and in every choice one makes. In the psychological context, dreams and drawings, utilized in projective tests (see Chap. 15), might be considered the product of unconscious projections registered by consciousness; for this reason, their analysis could help gain insights into the contents of the unconscious. We could consider dreams as "*…messages from our inner self…. They are not mere fantasies or hallucinations…they are the manifestation of the reality of the dreamer's life in all its dimensions—psychic and somatic, spiritual and material*" [18].

Many psychic components and dynamics contribute to the formation of oneiric symbols: complexes, the In-Self, the Super-Ego, affective and social relationships, signals from the environment, body illnesses, etc. [18, 19]. For this reason, dream analysis is the more complex task for a psychotherapist.

At this point, it is of utmost importance to underline how important it is for psychotherapists to have complete personal preparation, both for theoretical study and, above all, for personal analysis. Psychotherapists (more simply called "therapists"), who want to succeed at bringing another person to a better understanding of him/herself, and thereby achieve biological and psychological well-being, must have acquired a deep personal knowledge and coherence with the messages of In-Self. In particular, therapists must have acquired extensive knowledge of their own body sensations and reactions, a personal global perception as a healthy and holistic unity of body and mind. Therapists also must be engaged in a continuous analysis of personal life and dreams. Following the definition of ontopsychology, therapists must have achieved personal "*authenticity*," which means that they have acquired the capacity to develop following their intentionality of nature and intrinsic virtuality; in other words, they have to grow in a way that is in harmony with their own personal law of nature [3].

Therapists cannot undertake dreams analysis before they have completed continuous analysis to understand and verify the correspondence between symbols and psychic and real life, through their continuous personal experience [3]. In addition, they must conduct their own life in a way that is consistent with what they say and do to their patients. Only in this way can therapists take on the task of helping patients to understand themselves or guide them to experience the positive nucleus of their In-Self.

As explained earlier, in general, patients who have experienced an acute myocardial infarction "*report having experienced nightmares, often starting several months or even years before the acute event; or, alternatively, finding it impossible to remember dreams (often, patients only recall a few dreams from their childhood and/or adolescence)*" [2].

In my experience with cardiac patients, I can verify that dreams often manifest a psychosomatic dysfunction to the subject much in advance before the onset of the disease. Generally, by asking patients to recall dreams they have had in recent months or even years before their AMI, it is possible to verify that dreams initially indicate a psychological problem. It might be a problem that occurred in childhood or adolescence, or other problems in their personal life. It is a problem or conflict, related to patient's life choices, which hinders harmonic biopsychological evolution. The positive nucleus of the unconscious, the In-Self, highlights the problem continuously, possibly with recurring, repetitive dreams. Luckily, a complete dream indicates the possible solution too, often exposing the patient's historical potential and resources [18, 19]. If the dreamer understands these unconscious signals and changes, the dreams also change, reflecting a spontaneous change orchestrated by the person. But if the dreamer fails to understand and selects "wrong" choices or behaviors, the dreams will continue to give the same signal, the same symbols, and the same scenes. In this context, "wrong" choices/behaviors mean that the person follows values that are accepted or even encouraged by society, but contradictory to the indications of his/her In-Self (as revealed by dream analysis).

After a long period of time, if patients continue to not understand, they can lose contact with their inner world. At this point, patients start to feel unwell psychologically and/or at a somatic level, but they cannot resume the connection between their erroneous choices or behaviors and their personal suffering and/or physical dysfunction [13]. At this stage, patients usually cannot remember their dreams, or nightmares may begin, reflecting their internal discomfort and suffering. The psychological discomfort may then translate into various mood states: anxiety, depression, the sensation of stress, the fear of loneliness, the impossibility of having a happy personal affective and sexual relationship, difficulty efficiently carrying out social obligations or work, etc. It is of utmost importance that therapists help such patients to regain complete contact with their own natural identity, represented by their In-Self, so as to help them to overcome what internal difficulties exist.

13.5 Individual Psychotherapy

From a practical point of view, before starting their patients on psychotherapy, cardiologists and therapists should together explain to their patients their medical/heart condition, all the while emphasizing the importance of their full compliance with medical therapy, as well as how crucial it is for them to modify their lifestyle to reduce or eliminate problematic cardiac risk factors as part of secondary prevention. After this, they should also explain the importance of a survey of and therapy for their psychosocial risk factors, any one of which might contribute to a worsened cardiac prognosis [20, 21]. This can motivate patients to begin psychotherapy, a step they also might accept because of their own sense of discomfort. In patients who have suffered a recent myocardial infarction, it is often possible to trace back to some emotionally traumatic event (e.g., the loss of a job or death of a loved one). Sometimes, patients will recall this stressful event spontaneously and may, themselves, link the stressful event to their current AMI. Certainly, it might have played a precipitating role.

At the very beginning of psychotherapy, therapists can often sense their patients' interior suffering and discomfort; they may feel like their entire life has been blown apart and feel terrified to resume living a normal life and making personal decisions. Moreover, many patients feel objectified by medical care, and even how family members treat them, and this can contribute to their lost ability to make autonomous life decisions. They are often fearful about what has happened to them and petrified that further, even worse infarctions might occur. For this reason, many patients start to seek medical attention for every symptom they have, no matter how subtle or brief. They may feel like "a boat without a commander or direction." From a psychological point of view, therapists can acknowledge their patients' sense of having lost contact with their inner self, as well as their fear that they will never feel "normal" or happy again.

During the initial individual sessions, therapists should gently invite their patients to speak about their life, beginning either with their current medical problem or the distressing situation that they find themselves in: whichever seems more urgent to them. After patients have finished speaking about their main problem(s), and the therapists have attempted some initial analysis to help their patients identify some solutions, the therapists then should ask their patients to talk about their life, beginning with childhood. The personal story, as spontaneously related by patients, permits therapists to understand how the patients have survived emotionally, and to acquire a more comprehensive view of the patients' current situation and most important—whether happy or painful—memories, past events, and personal relationships.

Some patients exhibit no awareness of their own situation, cannot tell an adequate life story, and are unable to recognize past personal suffering or difficult situations. In such instances, therapists can be aided by other, already-collected information: in particular, psychometric and projective tests (see Chaps. 14, 15, and 20). The therapist may also be able to glean invaluable information through signals that stem from both verbal and nonverbal communication (see also Chaps. 16 and 17).

Of particular importance from an ontopsychological perspective is that the therapist is trained to be aware and take note of all components of the communication process, particularly specific aspects of unconscious communication, represented by the "*semantic field*" [3, 22]. The *semantic field*, a concept developed and justified by pioneers of the ontopsychological school, is a complex interplay of psychic and biological data that emanate unconsciously from every person during all interpersonal interactions.

Therapists can collect data within the semantic field by paying attention to their own bodily sensations (i.e., a so-called *organismic reaction*) as well as through the images that arise spontaneously in their own mind during the session. These images and sensations are therapists' symbolic and physical correlates of the verbal and nonverbal signals expressed by their patients, thereby revealing information about the patients' psychological and biological status, and constituting an essential component of the intuition process. Globally, the communication process is a fundamental and very complex part of the therapeutic setting, and therapists must be trained to be continuously aware of the disparate communication channels that develop during the therapeutic relationship, again both verbal and nonverbal. This training is particularly essential when verbal and nonverbal signals are incongruent, since accurately interpreting nonverbal signals is fundamental to grasping, with greater precision, the patient's inner dynamic during the psychotherapeutic encounter (see also Chap. 18). As with dream analysis, prolonged study and extensive experience is necessary for a therapist to precisely interpret the information released spontaneously into the semantic field, especially within the context of psychotherapy.

During individual psychotherapy, patients' lack of awareness of their personal situation and/or patients' resistance against psychotherapy may be so strong that they prevent any real potential for therapeutic progress. In such cases, therapists must respect the patients' will, and restrict their intervention to suggestions about lifestyle changes and offering ways to reduce or more effectively manage stressful situations, whenever possible.

In some cases, the main problem involves the patient–partner relationship. In such instances, it is wise and useful to also involve the partner during the course of psychotherapy, both in individual and couples sessions. I often offer the partner the option of starting their own personal psychotherapeutic sessions. In this way, I can help the partner and patient to begin making positive changes in their relationship. Over my many years working with cardiac patients, I have become convinced that it is optimal to involve the partner, whenever possible, because couples act as dyads [23, 24]. Without involving the partner, patients may start to see improvement while the psychological intervention is taking place; however, when the patients return home, the partners' anxiety and apprehension, or the reemergence of conflicts between them that predated the MI, may bring the patient back to square one.

This first phase of individual psychotherapy, during which the primary aims are to collect as much of the patients' personal story as possible and perform some initial analysis of their situation, may take three encounters or more, depending on the patients' situation. During these first few meetings, therapists should also explain to patients that, in a psychotherapeutic setting, they should no longer be passive, but an active participant who is there to regain control of and take responsibility for their own life, as well as to collaborate with the therapist to identify whatever solutions they can to restore them to a sense of personal equilibrium. The ability of the therapist to communicate is fundamental to overcoming any resistance and establishes a solid therapeutic alliance [25, 26]. Slowly the therapist must gain the patient's utter trust and confidence.

When any initial resistance that was present has been overcome, and when the initial history has been completely collected, explored, and analyzed, therapists must probe deeper in their analysis and motivate their patients to develop progressive awareness of their body sensations and emotions. At this point, therapists must start to educate their patients about essential psychological concepts to motivate and allow them to enter into deeper introspection. Therapists must particularly highlight how life events may have caused the patient to stray far from his or her inner self and natural identity and thereby can emphasize the importance of the patients resuming complete contact with their interior personal life to overcome their fear of disease and resume a personally fulfilling and happy life.

At this point therapists can start to invite their patients to explore their body sensations, starting with their visceral zone (i.e., abdomen) with the help of abdominal breathing. It is useful to invite patients to do a short relaxation exercise to better comprehend how they can sense their body, and whether certain body parts are not perceived consciously. The initial approach to perceiving bodily sensations, and in particular perception of the visceral zone, seems difficult for all patients who have suffered a recent myocardial infarction, particularly if the person is very old. Consequently, at this point therapists can explain about the existence of a *visceral brain*, which is continuously active throughout one's entire life (even if we have lost our conscious perception of it) and vitally important in its role as a mediator of inner emotions and feelings (see Chap. 4).

From a psychodynamic point of view, the inability to perceive the body as a unity of pleasure corresponds to the censorship of primary instincts, related to a conditioning suffered during one's first affective relationships (above all the mother, with reinforcement in familial and social contexts). Children learn all their lifestyle during their first years of life: how to be moved, how to love, how to relate to others, etc. [4]. We can say, in an extreme synthesis, that the origin of much psychopathological and psychosomatic dysfunctions may be related to a repression of a person's original instincts, where "instincts" refers to all the vital drives a person has, from biological to spiritual. On this dysfunctional psychological background, many other different life events may act as triggers to actual disease, including the specific case of an AMI. Admittedly, analyzing and modifying a dysfunctional psychological style may take a long time and can only be dealt with in a very precursory way during short-term psychotherapy.

Doing brief relaxation sessions, both within the psychotherapeutic setting and at home, helps a person to regain full perception of his/her visceral zone. This perception is generally, progressively, and spontaneously accompanied by the spread of perception to other body parts or the entire body. This brings a sensation of internal peace and well-being. Fear disappears and one's initial contact with the positive nucleus of the In-Self is reestablished.

Since, in the STEP-IN-AMI trial, we observed improvements in all of the psychological, cardiac, and other medical outcomes, we might hypothesize that the work done to restore patients' connections with their body via their visceral zone might have contributed to these results. In fact, the visceral brain is connected to the main systems that regulate the organism—the autonomic nervous, endocrine, and immune systems—and participates in their regulation (see Chap. 4). Our observation coincides with the results of other studies carried out in patients, post-AMI, utilizing relaxation therapy [27]. Further research should be conducted to confirm this interesting observation.

As previously stated, in accordance with current knowledge on psycho-neuro-endocrino-immunology, the visceral brain is connected to the functions of our most important bodily systems. From a psychological point of view, it is as if patients have restored a connection with the biological regulation of their body that nature automatically provided them. The patients overcome any internal rigidity, they have developed over time and no longer oppose the law of nature that normally regulates their body's harmonic functioning. This translates into a visible change in face physiognomy, their faces now appearing relaxed and radiant with sparkling eyes. Therapists must emphasize this result and encourage patients to continue in this positive experience. I was able to notice that, after this breakthrough, many psychological symptoms (e.g., anxiety, depression, anger) improved, and patients also became more motivated to take care of their health and change dysfunctional lifestyles.

At this point of the analysis, therapists may, whenever possible, guide the patients to deeper insights through dreams analysis. It is important to explain to patients the importance of remembering dreams, because they are an important message coming from their inner unconscious. During the initial phase, therapists should briefly survey their patients' dreams, while avoiding full analysis. It is usually important to avoid analyzing nightmares, because this could return patients to their anguish, without any improvement. In fact, therapists must always keep in mind the primary goal of psychotherapy, which is to restore the patient's sense of well-being, including full recovery and complete stabilization of their pathological situation. For this reason, therapists need to always reinforce their patients' positive resources, without excessively stressing negative issues. Patients will then be able to freely decide to change dysfunctional personal situations after completion of their psychotherapeutic course.

Therapists should wait patiently until their patients' nightmares cease and/or they start to refer dreams in relation to their daily life. Generally, as explained previously, this happens when the patients recover their perception of their visceral center, restoring contact with the central positive nucleus of their unconscious (the "In-Self"). This reflects inner changes orchestrated by the patients, a drop in their unconscious resistance, and complete openness to collaboration with the therapist. Only in this case the therapist highlights how dreams speak to them and how one's unconscious is able to adjudicate the dreamer's life situation. Most patients seem surprised by this interpretation, because they used to think that dreams were merely silly random thoughts lacking any real importance. If the therapists' analysis is performed correctly and coincides with the patients' real problems, this interpretation may push patients toward more meaningful changes and improvements in their personal life. Sometimes, if a patient is very old, he or she cannot change all the dysfunctional components and/or relationships in their personal life. However, awareness of the problem may help them to address their dysfunctional life situation in a more functional way.

When contact with the In-Self has been reestablished, the first phase, involving individual psychotherapy, is concluded, at least in the field of psychosomatics.

13.6 Group Psychotherapy

During the next phase, patients are invited to participate in group meetings, together with their partners if desired (in our study, a few patients did not favor this and refused to involve their partner from the very beginning). A few patients interrupted psychotherapy after the individual sessions, implicating personal commitments and a lack of time. A few partners refused to participate for the same reasons. However, the majority of patients in the STEP-IN-AMI trial participated in all of the scheduled sessions.

In group sessions, the psychotherapeutic work done during the individual sessions is reiterated and reinforced. From a practical point of view, from 6 to 20 people may be involved in each group and in each sequence of groups. With a limited number of participants, therapists can follow what everyone is saying and otherwise communicating more carefully. In our study, one or two nurses and one or two psychologists were involved in each group session. They participated in full and, when invited, could help the therapist to lead the group. Prior to beginning the group experience, patients are told that any details regarding their personal problems would not be shared in this setting, though they should feel free to speak of their own experiences if they desired. This explanation reassures patients and helps them to participate more serenely, without the fear of being subjected to others' judgments.

The group acts to reinforce the progress achieved in the individual sessions. However, to facilitate this, therapists must try to establish friendly relationships between participants and thereby dispel any initial shyness, fear, or other reluctance to promote enthusiastic group-wide participation. Patient partners who have been welcomed and agreed to participate may react differently. Generally in the STEP-IN-AMI groups, they were at ease if they had already engaged in individual psychotherapy. Conversely, partners for whom group sessions were their first participation often experienced difficulties; many of them expressed very important personal problems and conflicts. This observation supports the involvement of partners from the beginning of the psychotherapeutic process, whenever possible.

The sequence of five sessions, a standard number for such sessions, is conducted in the following way:

The first session is dedicated to introducing group participants and providing an initial description of the work that will be done over the following sessions. It is important to reiterate the importance of educational cardiology, including a broader explanation of myocardial infarction and the atherosclerotic process, while accentuating the importance of cardiac risk factors' prevention and lifestyle changes. An explanation about the role of psychosocial risk factors must be reiterated. Doing these things promotes more conscious participation by all. When the participants have been motivated and a friendly atmosphere has been established, the therapist should then lead them in a brief relaxation session, starting with abdominal breathing. After this brief relaxation session, everyone is invited to talk about their personal experiences. In this way, the therapist can observe initial reactions and the difficulties raised by the various participants.

The second session is completely dedicated to experiencing a relaxation technique. The relaxation phase lasts 25 minutes and is accompanied by melodic music, carefully selected by the therapist. It is very important that the therapist listens to and tries out the music beforehand, evaluating the personal organismic reaction it induces. Many different kinds of music can be selected for this; the important thing is that the music is not repetitive or monotonous and that it promotes sensitivity throughout one's entire body, in this way facilitating listeners' organismic perceptions and reducing their threshold for rationality. In the STEP-IN-AMI trial, Celtic pieces, classical music, and selections of Ontoart music (a modern, experimental form of music) were used [28–31]. The music acts by distracting one's consciousness, reducing one's super-ego, and enabling one to appreciate bodily sensations with total abandon. As explained previously, bodily perception, especially perception of one's visceral zone, is a very peaceful sensation that helps a person to regain full contact with the In-Self.

Also in this second session, after the relaxation exercise, every group member is invited to describe what they felt during the exercise. Patients who had already participated in the one-on-one sessions gained the most benefit from this session, even if they still had some residual resistance. Greater discomfort was generally reported by partners who had not partaken of the individual sessions. Many stated that they found it impossible to relax or that they experienced pain in certain parts of their body.

Some participants reported having spontaneous images during the relaxation exercise [19, 32]. These spontaneous images are similar to dream images and provide evidence that oneiric production is active throughout life, every moment of every day. After patients and partners verbalize what they have felt, therapists must start the important work of helping every group member to better understand their own bodily reaction and, when applicable, to also understand the meaning of the spontaneous images they had visualized.

The third meeting is dedicated to role play, during which issues that have already emerged can be reexplored. In this setting, participants are encouraged to talk about their own and their partners' difficulties, hopefully stimulating very useful exchanges in the group. If the work done over the first two meetings has been done well, group members may begin to feel like a very tight unit, wherein they can receive tremendous benefits from all the reciprocal exchanges.

During the fourth group meeting, oneiric (dream) material is analyzed, generally looking at dreams, which members have had over the last 2 weeks and briefly summarized in written form as per the therapist's suggestion.

The fifth and final meeting is again dedicated to a relaxation exercise, this time aided by different music than that utilized during the second group session. This last session always seems to be a wonderful surprise, both for group members and for myself. When residual resistance and body stiffness is overcome, members may experience a heightened sensation of well-being that spreads throughout their body. The body is then perceived as a unit of vitality. Often, whatever initial fearful or problematic images members may have had, have completely changed. Many spontaneously visualize peaceful, beautiful images depicting nature: a gently rolling sea, a lush forest, a flowery meadow, and a clear blue sky with a warm sun. These positive images testify to the tremendously positive changes that have transpired in their interior world, to their newfound contact with their organismic sensations, and to their arrival at a peaceful new level of bio-psychical equilibrium [32].

13.7 Conclusions

Ontopsychological psychotherapy encompasses many diversified techniques, ranging from individual to group psychotherapy and relaxation techniques.

The psychotherapeutic method utilized in the STEP-IN-AMI trial was a multidimensional psychotherapeutic intervention that represents a novel elaboration of the ontopsychological approach. Tested within the context of a randomized clinical trial, it was found to generally engender overall improvement in both medical and psychological outcomes. The implications of this are that knowledge of and experience with this approach could be very personally and culturally enriching for every health professional, who would like to broaden their practices. It also might lead them to find new, more effective ways to treat every patient they see.

References

1. Roncella A, Giornetti A, Cianfrocca C et al (2009) Rationale and trial design of a randomized, controlled study on short-term psychotherapy after acute myocardial infarction: the STEP-IN-AMI trial (Short term psychotherapy in acute myocardial infarction). J Cardiovasc Med 10: 947–952
2. Roncella A, Pristipino C, Cianfrocca C et al (2013) One-year results of randomized, controlled, short-term psychotherapy in acute myocardial infarction (STEP-IN-AMI) trial. Int J Cardiol 170(2):132–139. doi:10.1016/j.ijcard.2013.08.094
3. Meneghetti A (Eng ed 2004; It ed 1995–2008) Ontopsychology handbook. Ontopsicologia Editrice, Roma
4. Maslow AH (1962) Toward a psychology of being. Van Nostrand, New York
5. Black PH (2003) The inflammatory response is an integral part of the stress response. Brain Behav Immun 17:350–364
6. Besedovsky HO, Del Rey A (2001) Cytokines as mediators of central and peripheral immuno-neuro—endocrine interactions. In: Ader R, Felten D, Cohen N (eds) Psychoneuroimmunology, 3rd edn. Academic, Amsterdam
7. Bottaccioli F (2005) Psiconeuroendocrinoimmunologia. I fondamenti scientifici delle relazioni mente-corpo. Le basi razionali della medicina integrata. Red Edizioni, Como
8. Meneghetti A (Eng ed 1988–2004; It ed 1987–2001) Dictionary of ontopsychology. Ontopsicologia Editrice, Roma, p 260
9. Meneghetti A (1981–2002) L'In Sé dell'Uomo. Ontopsicologia Editrice, Roma
10. Gershon MD (1998) The second brain. Harper Collins, New York
11. Dander B (2001) Il primo cervello e l'Ontopsicologia. Nuova Ontopsicol 1:38–43, Psicologica Editrice (now Ontopsicologia Editrice)
12. Meneghetti A (English ed. 2004–2006; Italian ed. 1988–2000) Melholistics handbook. Ontopsicologia Editrice, Roma, p 97
13. Meneghetti A (1974–2008) La psicosomatica nell'ottica ontopsicologica. Ontopsicologia Editrice, Roma
14. Roncella A (2010) Dal criterio organismico il criterio di salute: il cervello viscerale. In: Di Carlo O (ed) Educazione alla Salute. Progetto per una nuova pedagogia sociale. Aracne Editrice, Roma, pp 41–59
15. Freud S (1900) The interpretation of dreams. Macmillan, New York (1913)
16. Jung CG (1974) Dreams (compilation from Collected Works, Vols. 4, 8, 12, 16). Princeton University Press, Princeton, NJ
17. Bonime W (1982) The clinical use of the dream. Da Capo Press, New York
18. Cangelosi A, Mencarelli C, Volpicelli C et al (2006) Dreams: in the depths of our reality. New Ontopsychol 2:30–61, Ontopsicologia Editrice
19. Meneghetti A (1994–2003) L'Immagine e l'Inconscio. Ontopsicologia Editrice, Roma
20. Rozanski A, Blumenthal JA, Kaplan J (1999) Impact of psychological factors on the pathogenesis of cardiovascular disease and implications for therapy. Circulation 27(16):2192–2217
21. Yusuf S, Rangarajan S, Teo K et al (2014) Cardiovascular risk and events in 17 low-, middle-, and high-income countries. N Engl J Med 28(9):818–827
22. Meneghetti A (1988, 2012) Campo semantico. Ontopsicologia Editrice, Roma

23. Moser DK, Dracup K (2004) Role of spousal anxiety and depression in patients' psychosocial recovery after a cardiac event. Psychosom Med 66:527–532
24. Joekes K, Maes S, Boersma SN, Van Elderen T (2005) Goal disturbance, coping, and psychological distress in partners of myocardial infarction patients: taking account of the dyad. Anxiety Stress Coping 18(3):255–267
25. Friedman L (1969) The therapeutic alliance. Int J Psychoanal 50(2):139–153
26. Meissner WW (1996) The therapeutic alliance. Yale University Press, New Haven
27. van Dixhoorn JJ, Duivenvoorden HJ (1999) Effect of relaxation therapy on cardiac events after myocardial infarction: a 5-year follow-up study. J Cardiopulmonary Rehabil 19:178–185
28. Cage J (1961) Silence: lectures and writings. Wesleyan University Press, Middletown, CT
29. Meneghetti A (Eng ed 2004; It ed 2000) Ontoarte. The In Sè of Art. Ontopsicologia Editrice, Roma
30. Grant Morag J (2003) Experimental music semiotics. Int Rev Aesthet Sociol Music 34(2): 173–191
31. Trappe HJ (2010) The effect of music on the cardiovascular system and cardiovascular health. Heart 96(23):1868–1871
32. Meneghetti A (1981–2012) Prontuario onirico. Ontopsicologia Editrice, Roma

Psychometric Tests: Epistemology, Rationale, Aims, and Applicability in Cardiology. Open Issues

14

Antonella Giornetti

... it is ... impossible ... to reach 1 by adding figures to the right of 0.99
Jean-Paul Sartre (Jean-Paul Sartre (1939) Sketch for a theory of the emotions)

14.1 Historical and Cultural Reference Points

The etymology of psychometrics leads us to a classic issue: the measurement (μέτρον) of the soul (ψυχή), whose immaterial nature has been distinguished from the material nature of the body. As pointed out by Solano, the distinction between the mind and body, and their reciprocal relationships, was made at a certain point in the history of Western culture. It is, therefore, a cultural construct, and not something that exists just as a matter of course [1]. Outlining the historical and cultural reference points within which psychometrics has established its scientific legitimacy allows us to identify the epistemological model and the social mandate that inspired the meeting of μέτρον and ψυχή.

A reference point is *positivist objectivization*. The foundations of psychology, in fact, date back to the second half of the 1800s, during the full flood of Positivism and spread of medicine, with rejection of all the therapeutic practices that had the slightest whiff of magic or lacked a sufficient, natural, scientific foundation [1].

The birth of scientific psychology was sanctioned by Wundt, a university professor with medical training. In 1879, he set up the first laboratory for psychological research in Leipzig, where ψυχή became an epiphenomenon and lost its meaning of soul in favor of a more deterministic meaning of mind. For the first

A. Giornetti, PsyD (✉)
Department of Cardiovascular Disease, San Filippo Neri Hospital, Via G. Martinotti 20, 00135 Rome, Italy
e-mail: antonella.giornetti@gmail.com

A. Roncella, C. Pristipino (eds.), *Psychotherapy for Ischemic Heart Disease*,
DOI 10.1007/978-3-319-33214-7_14

time, the mind was objectified through the breaking down of its processes and the categorizing of its basic functions via a method based upon systematized introspection. However, this methodology was later criticized for its subjectivity.

The acknowledged father of psychometrics was Sir Francis Galton, author of the unpopular *Hereditary Genius* (1869) [2], published after *On the Origin of the Species* (1859) [3] by his cousin Darwin, whose influence led him to establish the first anthropometric laboratory in London in 1884. The analysis and measurement of human powers was intended to "improve the race" by replacing natural selection with "rational" selection [4]. Galton brought into psychology the systematic use of questionnaires and new statistical research methods including, for instance, the definition of the still-used statistical term "correlation" [5].

This was therefore the epistemological context of individual psychology that saw the creation of a quick and easy way to administer a measurement tool, designed for the idiographic study of human differences [4]. The American James McKenn Cattell would call this new tool *test* and later, in 1890, *mental test*, after its modifications based upon elementary corporeal and sensory motor measurements [6].

The first psychometric laboratory was founded in 1886 at Cambridge by Cattell himself. His study was based on the quantification, classification, and comparative evaluation of mental processes. He was interested in the fundamental capacities and abilities that enable man to successfully adapt to his environment and in studying the suitability of these variables to predict the success of subjects in certain tasks [4].

The psychometric application assumed the role of certifying an individual's fitness for a given role, according to an expected model. It is no coincidence that it was developed primarily in schools and the army, two contexts where conforming to an expected model is essential to belonging to the context itself. Psychometrics spread in schools, after the first intelligence test by Binet and Simon in 1905 [7], and in the army, after the administration of the *Army Alpha* and *Army Beta* to thousands of American soldiers during the First World War [8, 9].

Following this line of reasoning, another reference point is *industrial efficientism*. In 1921, Cattell privately organized the company *Psychological Corporation Limited*, created to provide psychological consultations to industries and the public, specializing in standardizing and marketing psychometric tests [4]. In 1935, some of the most important psychometricians of the time banded together to form the *Psychometric Society* and establish the journal *Psychometrika* [10].

Psychology therefore developed as part of the cultural transformation triggered by the process of industrialization. At the beginning of the twentieth century, this process thoroughly permeated the whole economic and social system and also involved Western country latecomers. In other words, there was a regime of acceleration and efficiency in force, in which the new psychometric science responded to the social mandate by placing itself at the service of work and progress.

The concept of *fitness* had, on one hand, its most advanced application in the selection of personnel in production systems, which generated the famous Taylorist saying "the right man in the right place" [11]. In this field, strength is the use of the relationship between individual and context as a tool to identify the correspondence between personal skills and organizational needs: in other words, the matching of supply and demand. On the other hand, the concept of fitness underwent the process of "psychopathologizing" within health systems, where it was affected by the a-historical and a-contextual constraints of the nosological classification of the late nineteenth century.

The second half of the 1800s saw the modern definition of *illness*, based on alterations in the structure of organs and tissues. Each illness was defined in this way, not based on symptoms, as in the past. The nosographic insistence incorporated the mental sphere as well, so manifestations of psychological distress ended up being seen as symptoms of an illness [1]. This contributed to spread a new and still-used way to evaluate individuals that would identify the term *deficit* to describe any physical or mental manifestations that deviated from the expected average. Fitness thereby became a statistical and theoretical concept of normality—that is, the matching of individual and pathology—and gradually lost sight of its relationship with context. The last reference point therefore remained *psychopathology*.

An important turning point came in 1946 when Raymond B. Cattell, borrowing the idea of trait from Allport, constructed a personality questionnaire called the *Sixteen Personality Factor Questionnaire* (16PF), with which he measured 16 basic personality traits considered to be stable measurements of behavior [12]. This kind of psychometric test (PT), based on the theory of traits [12–16], would be used commonly in the medical field, where interest would be directed toward identifying the correlation between invariant aspects of individual's personality and physical illness.

An example is "*the pioneering work of Friedman and Rosenman, the two San Francisco cardiologists who in 1959 coined the term Type A behavior pattern (TABP)*" which was the first "*systematic investigation of the relationship between heart and mind. Since that time there has been a great deal of research on psychosocial factors and coronary heart disease*" [17]. However, TABP, in vogue for over 50 years as a negative prognostic factor, has for several years ceased to be associated with ischemic heart disease (IHD) [18].

As argued below, the application of psychometrics within the cardiology field today is still closely tied to the theoretical assumptions outlined so far.

14.2 Psychometric Tests Applied to Health Contexts: What Problems Do They Solve?

The year 1917 saw the publication of the first issue of the *Journal of Applied Psychology*, the sector's oldest journal, which highlighted the role of psychology applied to the world of work in terms of helping to solve real-life problems [4]. Almost a century later, in view of its great popularity, it can rightly be observed that PT became successful by pursuing the goal of solving practical problems, including those within health contexts.

The first problem solved was the *codification* of etiologies and symptoms into a conventional diagnostic code, which would facilitate communication between healthcare staff. In this sense, *the Diagnostic and Statistical Manual of Mental Disorders* (DSM) [19–21] has the undisputed merit of having organized a single coding system for psychological manifestations. Psychometric tests are based on theoretical constructs related to the DSM and, although it is constantly stressed that such tests do not replace clinical assessments [18], they are part of diagnostic practice, highlighting the presence/absence of intra-psychological dynamics and psychopathological aspects characterizing an individual's clinical case.

The second problem solved by PT concerns the *standardization* of the raw scores obtained on a test into comparable data, in and among different individuals and populations. A psychological test is a standardized situation in which a person's behavior is sampled, observed, and described [22], producing an objective, standardized measurement of a sample of behavior [23]. *Standardized situation* refers to a scenario where everything remains constant, except for changes in individual reactions; *measurement* refers to the product of the application of rules to classify or assign numbers to objects, so that the number represents the quality of the attributes or the degree to which a quality is present; *objective measurement* means that a measurement is replicable in the same experimental conditions if performed by the same or a different observer; and *standardized measurement* means that the single empirical datum is related to a more general system of reference [24].

The third problem that was solved was an economic-organizational one, concerning the *optimization* of structural and human resources in health contexts using efficientistic managerial logic. Psychometric tests are brief screening instruments, with precise instructions, easy for patients in acute conditions to read and complete; they can be managed by healthcare staff with both outpatients and inpatients, either after training or under close supervision by a psychologist [18], and therefore entail sustainable costs for the system in terms of time, materials, and staff. With regard to accessing psychological services, PTs can work as a stimulus [25], with the content of some items prompting an introspective attitude in patients, and as a filter, using the scores to establish treatment and referral priorities.

The problems of *codification*, *standardization*, and *optimization* are specific to research work in health contexts. The utility of a PT lies in its ability to standardize symptoms, data, and resources to create a diagnostic, statistical, and organizational code to facilitate scientific communication and the growth of knowledge regarding the psychological characteristics linked to diseases.

14.3 The Main Psychometric Tests Used in Cardiovascular Disease

The psychological macro-areas investigated in cardiology are the common emotive disorders, like depression and anxiety, and personality traits. In preventative and rehabilitative cardiology, such aspects may be revealed during screening with self-administered noncognitive PTs. A great number of PTs have been used in research on patients with cardiac disease. Some of the most widely used tests in international literature are cited below.

The *Beck Depression Inventory* (BDI) [26–28], of which the BDI-II (modified in 1996) is the latest version, consists of 21 items describing symptoms and behaviors observed during psychoanalytic psychotherapies with depressed patients [24] (feelings of guilt, sadness, discouragement, loss of interest, crying, etc). Other symptom-based measures of depression are the *Centers for Epidemiological Studies-Depression* (CES-D) *scale* [29] and the *Hospital Anxiety and Depression Scale* (HADS) [30] that has the feature of excluding somatic symptomatology and including hedonic tone.

The *Patient Health Questionnaire 9* (PHQ-9) [31] is a nine-item tool that is easy to both administer and score. The PHQ-2 [32] consists of the two first questions of the PHQ-9, which deal with mood and the lack of pleasure. According to a comparative study, these tools are as reliable as the BDI-II as a quick screen for depression [33].

To evaluate anxiety, the *Psychological General Well-Being Index-6* (PGWBI-6), designed specifically for the outpatient cardiology setting [34], is a brief six-item measure, highly correlated with other common scales and screens for anxiety, depressed mood, or self-control. However, the most often used instrument is the *State Trait Anxiety Index* (STAI) [35, 36] that is made up of two 20-item subtests: the first subtest is related to the patient's "state" of anxiety at the time of test administration; the second subtest measures anxiety as a "trait," that is, the subject's tendency to produce anxious reactions under specific conditions [24].

The *Distress Scale* (DS14) [37] is used to assess type D (distressed) personality, which has been identified as both a cause of psychological distress and an independent predictor of long-term mortality in patients with CAD, as well as of the greater stress observed in patients with acute coronary events (ACS) [18]. It consists of 14 items and is divided into two subscales: negative affectivity (NA) and social inhibition (SI). Individuals with increased levels of both NA and SI are referred to as having a type D personality.

Other very common PTs used to investigate personality traits are the *Multiphasic Minnesota Personality Inventory-2* (MMPI-2) [38], a very complex test exploring personality characteristics, whose 1st edition was elaborated upon by Hathaway and McKinley in 1940; the abovementioned 16PF [13]; and the *Eysenck Personality Questionnaire* (EPQ) [14]. These tests take a long time to administer and are, therefore, used further along in the clinical examination.

The assessment of quality of life and perceived state of health has an important role in cardiology and helps clinicians to analyze the construct of *chronic life stress*.

Various tools are available for this, of which the most frequently used are briefly mentioned here. The *36-Item Short Form Health Survey* (SF-36) investigates physical health (physical functioning, role-physical, bodily pain, general health) and mental health (vitality, social functioning, role-emotional, mental health) [39]. The *MacNew Heart Disease Health-Related Quality of Life Questionnaire* (MAC NEW) [40] is a 27-item tool that similarly evaluates emotional, physical, and social domains, but is easier to administer and score than the SF-36.

To delve into the construct of social support, one can use the *Multidimensional Scale of Perceived Social Support* (MSPSS). It is a 12-item instrument that assesses three sources of support: family, friends, and significant others. Validity has been established through the negative association between MSPSS scores and scores on measures of depression [41].

Cognitive or neuropsychological tests can be recommended for the assessment of intellectual functions and cognitive deterioration—for instance, after off-pump coronary artery bypass surgery—and therefore deserve to be dealt with separately.

14.4 Psychometric Outcomes in Psychological Interventions with Cardiac Patients

At this point, it is interesting to reflect on the relationship that the use of PTs creates between the psychologist, the patient, and the treatment pathway and to observe how the aim of a psychological intervention changes according to the epistemological paradigm adopted: the individualist approach designed to correct a deficit versus the relationship-based approach that aims to develop competence to guide a process.

As emphasized by Carli and Paniccia, when one adopts approaches that address individuals and their personal characteristics, intra-psychological dynamics, behavioral features, and cognitive structure, one ends up adopting a perspective of change, involving the individual relative to criteria of normalcy [11]. From the perspective of the individualist approach, the diagnostic usefulness of PTs supports the prescriptive relationship between the health context and the cardiac patient, which is established at the onset of the disease, and in which the psychologist also sets a treatment pathway. On one hand, there is an expert who prescribes a reduction in cardiovascular risk factors and a change in lifestyle (physical activity, diet, smoking, etc.) and, on the other hand, the patient, who can either comply with the recommendations or disregard them. Carli and Paniccia always clarify that the purpose of the individualist perspective is of a normative kind and leads to rehabilitation interventions that can modify the behavior of an individual or facilitate a deeper knowledge of that person's inner emotional dynamics. What marks this kind of psychological intervention, however, is the a-historical and a-contextual nature of the possible changes that are sought [11].

One alternative is the relationship-based approach, in which contextual and historical variables are used to guide the psychological intervention in the direction of development. In this case, the intervention's focus switches from the behavior of the individual to the relational process between the individual and context, in which *context* means anything about life (emotions, expectations, disease, therapeutic pathway, family, friends, work, background, etc). The psychotherapeutic goal is that the patient acquires competence to guide a process and to relate to their own inner world and, at the same time, to their own life context, of which he/she learns to explore the limits and resources.

From this perspective, the relationship between the psychologist and patient becomes the organizing principle of work [11] and implies a critical use of PTs and their outcomes.

As already mentioned, the utility of PTs facilitates the growth of knowledge among experts. However, such knowledge cannot be immediately made available and usable for the patient. Indeed, the diagnosis is powerful at categorizing illness, but can become an obstacle by conditioning the patient's experience. For instance, if a depressed patient is told he has depression, he is likely to immediately feel more depressed and justified in being so. Moreover, providing information to the patient about the correlation depression has with an increased risk of death from heart disease [42] and with poor therapeutic compliance [43] might worsen the emotional prostration of the patient. It is important to inform the patient about the risk of disease, but also important to reflect how to communicate it. Keeping in mind that healthcare staff members are always communicating with an individual within a context, which entails a personal system of expectations and representations of illness, then diagnostic coding must involve therapeutic decoding that makes the nosographic classification accessible in the patient's daily life.

With the relationship-based approach, the setting of the psychological intervention is a transformative relationship in which the psychological function can work like a *reducer*. In mechanics, a reducer, or gearbox, is a device situated between the drive shaft and the driven shaft to reduce the angular speed of the latter relative to the former. Similarly, the psychologist receives the speed of the diagnostic process (impersonal data in urgency) as input from the patient, whereas, as an output, he returns to the patient the calmness of the elaborating process, within which the polysemantic emotional meanings of illness are reconnected to the patient's values system and systems of coexistence (personal data in daily life).

Beyond the nosographic classification, a depressed patient is also a human in crisis with his/her own existence, in whom the heart disease may sometimes be the cause of the crisis, other times a symptom, and yet other times both simultaneously, in a vicious circle of implications both for the patient's health and for the psychological and medical treatments the patient is offered (see Chap. 1).

It is interesting to highlight how the etymology of crisis (κρίνω) concerns the decision-making that also concerns the psychotherapeutic process. In a study conducted at San Filippo Neri Hospital in Rome in 2004, forty patients with a recent myocardial infarction were enrolled to evaluate the efficacy of *writing therapy* [44]. The patients were randomly assigned into two groups: the experimental group (20 patients) and the control group (20 patients). Both groups were administered five PTs: the already-mentioned BDI to evaluate depression [26, 27], the *MACNEW Heart Disease Health-Related Quality of Life* questionnaire to evaluate quality of life [40], the *Symptom Checklist-90* (SCL-90) [45] to assess psychological distress, the 20-tem *Toronto Alexithymia Scale* (TAS-20) [46] to assess alexithymia (that is, the inability to recognize emotions and their subtleties and textures), and card C of the *Cognitive Behavioral Assessment Hospital Form* (CBA-H) [47] to assess for type A personality. The 20 patients in the experimental group were also invited to express their feelings about the most traumatic experience of their lives using Pennebaker's writing technique [48]. Twenty percent of them wrote about the acute cardiac event, while 80 % wrote about frustrating experiences in previous family or professional life. Nevertheless, the clinical-psychological criteria which unite all the analyzed writing is the failure of the patients' image of self and/or of own relational context. In fact, in both cases, the patients found themselves having to deal with change and the need to make new decisions. Sometimes this change was felt as a betrayal of the past and other times as diffidence regarding the future, but the feeling conveyed was of a disenchanted attempt to reorganize their system of expectations and representations of life. Furthermore, the writings disclosed their profound need to be able to strengthen their closest relationships and to feel renewed faith in themselves and in human relationships, also referring explicitly to their relationships with healthcare staff. In this study, the administered PTs failed to reveal any significance of the psychological variables. Consequently, the psychometric outcomes were unable to explain all of the poly-semantic emotional meanings that, instead, were revealed via clinical-psychological criteria in the patients' writings.

Emotional dimensions have a role in a patient's treatment pathway, and their analysis is therefore necessary to identify the personal, social, and cultural resources that patients can use to cope with their crisis. Indeed, starting just from these resources, the psychologist can guide the intervention and support a process in which potentialities prevail in a critical state, so that they will develop and not envelop [11], and in which the patient learns to understand failure as a chance to transform and choose, here and now, their ability to face up to the variability of existence. In short, the usefulness of PTs cannot disregard the theoretical and practical context of their use, either in research or in psychological interventions applied to cardiology. This means that there is a relationship between the theory of technique, the patient's treatment, and his/her resilience.

14.5 Open Issues

The way one construes one's situation of illness, especially if one is assailed by erroneous information and myths about the heart, can induce people to adopt behaviors that affect the outcomes of the illness itself [18]. Furthermore, the patients' expectations have been shown to be an important predictor of treatment outcome after a variety of surgical operations, which include coronary artery bypass graft surgery [49]. In other words, social representations [50] that shape reality into common thinking and expectations or, more precisely, affective symbolizations [11] that shape reality into an emotional-symbolic sense are respectively cultural and unconscious dimensions that belong to a community that shares the same context and has a role in the coronary artery disease treatment process.

Cultural influences are most understandable in the psychiatric field. For example, just as words appear and disappear from the vocabulary over generations, in the DSM since its first edition in 1952 [19], some disorders have been eliminated, as if they have fallen into disuse, while new ones have been introduced. Hysteria, so dear to Breuer and Freud, as well as the symptoms of sexual repression of that age, was ushered out in 1980, whereas internet addiction disorder (IAD) and selfism won a place in 2013 [20, 21], not surprisingly in the age of social networks, Photoshop, and evanescent appearances, such that our current time will be known as the "era of representation" [50].

Let us now take the example of two theoretical constructs whose assessment with self-administered PTs [39–41] is widespread in cardiology. The first is social support, which is measured to determine a patient's perception of being supported by a network of relationships versus being socially isolated. The second is chronic life stress, which is measured to determine a patient's stress level in daily life (illness, job, family, traffic, money, etc) or, in other words, to assess their threshold of tolerance to control and hold back emotions over time. It is interesting to highlight how emotions are our constant and primitive social dimension [51]. Following this line of reasoning, it could therefore be argued that chronic life stress concerns the deprivation of shared emotions in social relationships. This hypothesis seems supported by the demand for change expressed by the patients in the experimental group in the study cited earlier [44], specifically in terms of their profound need, after experiencing failure, to be able to feel renewed faith in oneself and human relationships.

Moreover, if one takes a broader view, extending the focus from the individual to the social incidence of social support and chronic life stress, then one is likely to see that *isolation* and *control* are manipulative mechanisms of the emotional "species-specific" variables both of the psychometric model and of the individuals belonging to the contemporary industrial context.

Could this then give rise to the hypothesis that individualism is an area of non-intentional symbolic-emotional intersection: in other words, a *collusion* [11] between the epistemological paradigm of psychometrics, as it is applied today in cardiology, and contemporary culture, of which coronary artery disease, besides being the most common cause of death in Western countries, would seem to be the symptom? This remains an area worth investigating for the potential implications of disease modeling in a systemic paradigm (see Chap. 1) and, therefore, to plan inherent therapeutic and preventative strategies.

14.6 Conclusions

Measurement in psychology and its application is therefore not a fact, but an unresolved issue. There is an unquestionable need to measure psychological dimensions, both to advance knowledge and to obtain indicators of the efficacy of psychological interventions. However, despite the invaluable corpus of theory from the past century in which psychometrics were born, mind–body and individual-context modeling have unresolved issues. Particularly in mind–body modeling, the unconscious and cultural dimensions are disregarded; meanwhile, in individual-context modeling, the modeling of replicable data interactions is impossible. Therefore, none of these perspectives, and hence also psychometrics, display a comprehensive picture. The uncertainty, after all, is a fundamental characteristic of the qualitative–quantitative complexity and not a side effect (see Chap. 1). Therefore, PTs can be useful in different clinical and research settings, but they cannot be reduced to the main instrument for the understanding of the multidimensional complexity of a person in his/her own life system, the definition of which remains an open issue in its qualitative/quantitative irreducible aspects that must be addressed from a systems science perspective (see Chap. 1).

As noted by Blanco, every man feels instinctively—and in this, primitive people from extremely varied cultures agree with those belonging to our scientifically evolved Western culture—that the visible physical manifestations of the psyche do not account for the whole psychic field, at least not very clearly [52]. If the uncertainty is therefore a fundamental characteristic of the knowledge, it is better to have a model to deal with it, than not to have it. Blanco consistently clarifies that unconscious fantasy is not intrinsically imponderable but, contrary to physical events, is susceptible to infinite measurements at the point at which the physical event is susceptible to only one measurement [52]. In this sense, it is important to support the futuristic work of the scientists and intellectuals of our time, who orient the study of how to measure ψυχή and update its meaning to the present day, so as to develop increasingly accurate instruments to account for such complexity. Its application would be desirable to provide orientation in the research and personalization of treatments, in the training of health staff, and in coronary artery disease education and prevention campaigns.

References

1. Solano L (2001) Tra mente e corpo. Come si costruisce la salute. Raffaello Cortina Editore, Milano
2. Galton F (1869) Hereditary genius, 1st edn. Macmillan, London
3. Darwin C (1859) On the origin of species by means of natural selection, or the preservation of favoured races in the struggle for life, 1st edn. John Murray, London, Retrieved 24 Oct 2008
4. Lombardo GP, Pompili A, Mammarella V (2002) Psicologia applicata e del lavoro in Italia. Studi storici, Franco Angeli Editore, Milano
5. Galton F (1888) Co-relations and their measurement, chiefly from anthropometric data. Proc R Soc Lond 45:135–145
6. Cattell JM (1890) Mental tests and measurements. Mind 15:373–380
7. Binet A, Simon T (1905) Méthodes nouvelles pour le diagnostic du niveau intellectual des anormaux. Année Psycho 2:191–244
8. Schrammel HE, Wood ER (1919) Army group examination alpha. Psychology Committee of the National Research Council, Bureau of Educational Measurements, Emporia, KS

9. Aa.Vv. (1920) Army group examination beta. Bureau of Educational Measurements Psychology, Committee of the National Research Council, Emporia, KS
10. The Psychometrics Centre, University of Cambridge (2015) http://www.thepsychometricscentre.com/page/36/the-society.htm
11. Carli R, Paniccia RM (2003) Analisi della domanda. Teoria e tecnica dell'intervento in psicologia clinica. Società editrice Il Mulino, Bologna
12. Cattell RB (1946) The description and measurement of personality. World Book, Yonkers
13. Cattell RB, Cattell AK, Cattell HEP (1993) 16PF fifth edition questionnaire. Institute for Personality and Ability Testing, Champaign, IL
14. Eysenck HJ, Eysenck SBG (1975) The eysenck personality questionnaire. Hodder & Stoughton, London
15. Guilford JP, Zimmerman WS (1949) The Guilford-Zimmerman temperament survey. Sheridan Supply, Beverly Hills
16. Costa PT, McCrae RR (1985) The NEO personality inventory manual. Psychological Assessment Resources, Odessa
17. Allan R, Scheidt S (1996) Empirical basis for cardiac psychology. In: Allan R, Scheidt S (eds) Heart and mind. The practice of cardiac psychology. American Psychological Association, Washington, DC, p 63
18. Giannuzzi P, Griffo R, Urbinati S et al (2006) Linee guida nazionali su cardiologia riabilitativa e prevenzione secondaria delle malattie cardiovascolari. Monaldi Arch Chest Dis 66:81–116
19. American Psychiatric Association (1952) Diagnostic and statistical manual: mental disorders—DSM, 1st edn. American Psychiatric Association, Washington, DC
20. American Psychiatric Association (1980) Diagnostic and statistical manual: mental disorders—DSM, 3rd edn. American Psychiatric Association, Arlington, VA
21. American Psychiatric Association (2013) Diagnostic and statistical manual: mental disorders—DSM, 5th edn. American Psychiatric Association, Arlington, VA
22. Korchin SJ (1976) Modern clinical psychology. Basic Books, New York
23. Anastasi A (1961) Psychological testing, 5th edn. Macmillan, New York (1982)
24. Boncori L (1993) Teoria e tecniche dei test. Manuali di Psicologia Psichiatria Psicoterapia. Bollati Boringhieri, Torino
25. Häuser W, Wambach S, Schiedermaier P et al (2001) Increased demand for psychosomatic consultation service (C-service) in a department of cardiology/pneumology due to psychometric screening. Psychother Psychosom Med Psychol 51(6):261–263
26. Beck AT, Ward CH, Meldelson M et al (1961) An inventory for measuring depression. Arch Gen Psychiatry 4:561–567
27. Beck AT, Kovacs M, Weissman A (1979) Assessment of suicidal intention: the scale for suicide ideation. J Consult Clin Psychol 47:343–352
28. Beck AT, Steer RA, Brown GK (1996) Manual for the beck depression inventory–II. Psychological Corporation, San Antonio, TX
29. Radloff LS (1977) The CES-D scale: a self-report depression scale for research in the general population. Appl Psychol Meas 1(3):385–401
30. Zigmond AS, Snaith RP (1983) The hospital anxiety and depression scale. Acta Psychiatr Scand 67:361–370
31. Kroenke K, Spitzer RL, Williams JB (2001) The PHQ-9: validity of a brief depression severity measure. J Gen Intern Med 16(9):606–613
32. Kroenke K, Spitzer RL, Williams JB (2003) The patient health questionnaire-2: validity of a two-item depression screener. Med Care 41:1284–1292
33. Ceccarini M, Manzoni GM, Castelnuovo G (2014) Assessing depression in cardiac patients: what measures should be considered? Depress Res Treat 2014:148256. doi:10.1155/2014/148256
34. Grossi E, Groth N, Mosconi P et al (2006) Development and validation of the short version of the psychological general well-being index (PGWB-S). Health Qual Life Outcomes 4:88

35. Spielberger CD, Gorsuch RL, Lushene RE (1968) State-trait anxiety inventory, Form X. Consulting Psychologists Press, Palo Alto, CA
36. Spielberger CD, Gorsuch RL, Lushene RE et al (1977–1983) State-trait anxiety inventory, Form Y. Consulting Psychologists Press, Palo Alto, CA
37. Denollet J (2005) DS14: standard assessment of negative affectivity, social inhibition, and type D personality. Psychosom Med 67:89–97
38. Butcher JN, Dahlstrom WG, Graham JR et al (1989) MMPI-2: manual for administration and scoring. University of Minnesota Press, Minneapolis
39. Ware JE Jr, Kosinski M (2001) SF-36® physical and mental health summary scales: a manual for users of version 1, 2nd edn. QualityMetric Incorporated, Lincoln, RI
40. Hofer S, Lim LL, Guyatt GH, Oldridge NB (2004) The MacNew heart disease health related quality of life instrument: a summary. Health Qual Life Outcomes 2:3
41. Zimet GD, Dahlem NW, Zimet SG, Farley GK (1988) The multidimensional scale of perceived social support. J Pers Assess 52:30–41
42. Frasure-Smith N, Lesperance F, Talajic M (1995) Depression and 18 month prognosis after myocardial infarction. Circulation 91:999–1005
43. Mayou RA, Gill D, Thompson DR et al (2000) Depression and anxiety as predictors of outcome after myocardial infarction. Psychosom Med 62:212–219
44. Giornetti A, Moroni F, Roncella R et al (2006) Effetti positivi di un intervento di scrittura dopo infarto miocardico acuto. In: Cicognani E, Palestini L (eds) Promuovere benessere con persone, gruppi, comunità, 28–30 settembre 2006, VII Congresso Nazionale di Psicologia della Salute. Università in Romagna, Società Editrice "Il Ponte Vecchio", Cesena, p 315
45. Magni G, Schifano F, De Leo D (1983) Assessment of depression in an elderly medical population. J Affect Disord 11(2):121–124
46. Bressi C, Taylor G, Parker J et al (1996) Cross validation of the factor structure of the 20-Item Toronto Alexithymia scale: an Italian multicenter study. J Psychosom Res 41(6):551–559
47. Zotti AM, Bertolotti G, Michielin P et al (2000) Linee guida per lo screening dei tratti di personalità, cognizioni e comportamenti avversi alla salute, manuale d'uso per il CBA Forma Hospital. Edizione Maugeri Foundation Books, Pavia
48. Pennebaker JW, Beall SK (1986) Confronting a traumatic event: towards an understanding of inhibition and disease. J Abnorm Psychol 95:274–281
49. Laferton JA, Shedden Mora M et al (2013) Enhancing the efficacy of heart surgery by optimizing patients' preoperative expectations: study protocol of a randomized controlled trial. Am Heart J. doi:10.1016/j.ahj.2012.10.007
50. Moscovici S, Farr RM (1989) Rappresentazioni sociali. Il Mulino, Bologna
51. Carli R, Paniccia RM (2002) L'analisi emozionale del testo. Uno strumento psicologico per leggere testi e discorsi. FrancoAngeli, Psicologia, Milano
52. Blanco IM (ed) (1975) The unconscious as infinite sets. An essay in bi-logic. Gerald Duckworth, London

Projective Tests: The Six-Drawings Test in Ischemic Heart Disease

15

Adriana Roncella and Silvia Scorza

Ways of determining the individual's private world of meanings, significance, patterns, and feelings. A culture-free field must be provided into which the individual can project his personal modes of reaction.

L. K. Frank (Frank L K (1939) Projective methods for the study of personality. The Journal of Psychology: Interdisciplinary and Applied 8:389–413)

15.1 Introduction

The *"words free association technique"* was first described by Carl Gustav Jung in the year 1910 [1]. Twenty-nine years later, in 1939, Frank published the first review on what he termed "*projective techniques*" and defined as various ways to access an individual's private world of meanings, significance, patterns, and feelings. He affirmed that a culture-free field had to be provided into which the individual could project his or her personal modes of reaction [2].

He believed that projective techniques were like X-rays, capable of generating pictures that revealed a person's inner self, a holistic image of his/her personality. Using projective techniques, patients can be analyzed as they "project," on the given "stimulus," their interior workings, sentiments, emotions, etc.

A. Roncella, MD (✉) • S. Scorza, PsyD
Department of Cardiovascular Disease, San Filippo Neri Hospital, Via G. Martinotti 20, 00135 Rome, Italy
e-mail: adrianaroncella@hotmail.it; silviascorza@libero.it

A. Roncella, C. Pristipino (eds.), *Psychotherapy for Ischemic Heart Disease*,
DOI 10.1007/978-3-319-33214-7_15

15.2 Development of Projective Tests

Since Frank's publication, projective techniques have been adopted by a number of different investigators, with different aims. For example, Kent and Rosanoff [3] utilized them to diagnose psychopathology, while Wertheimer [4] employed them in forensic medicine. Two early publications on this subject involved using the *Rorschach test* in 1921 [5] and Morgan and Murray's *Thematic Apperception Test* (TAT) in 1935 [6]. Over the next decade, there was more widespread use of projective tests, like the Wartegg's *Drawing Completion Test* [7], Düss's *Fairy Tales* [8], Rosenzweig's *Picture-Association Method* [9], Koch's *Tree Test* [10], Machover's *Human Figure Drawings* [11], and Corman's *Family Drawing* [12]. The success of these techniques in those early years was essentially determined by increasing interest in psychoanalysis and rising criticism of psychometric tests, which failed to provide a complete picture of an individual's personality.

However, just like enthusiasm over this approach flourished in the 1940s, over the next several decades, criticism started to spring up as a response to the indeterminate and disputable results of numerous empirical studies, which assessed the validity and effectiveness of these approaches. For this reason, in the 1980s, attempts were made to modify these techniques and standardize them, like psychometric tests. This led to continuous spirited debate regarding projective techniques' aims and modalities.

Now it is possible to categorize the various projective techniques in a variety of ways. One such way, proposed by Lindsay [13], bases their classification on the specific type of task that the subject is asked to complete:

1. To draw associations with ink blots or words: e.g., the *Rorschach test* [5], Holtzman's *Ink Blot test* [14], and Kent's *Verbal Association test* [3].
2. To compose a story: e.g., the TAT [6], Sharkey and Ritzler's *Picture Projection Test* [15], Blum's *Blacky Pictures Test* [16], and Wagner's *Hand Test* [17].
3. To complete sentences or stories: e.g., the *Rotter Incomplete Sentence Blank* [18].
4. To arrange or select pictures or words: e.g., *Sznodi's Test* [19].
5. To express themselves through drawings, games, or acting scenes out: e.g., Machover's *Human Figure Drawings* [11], Bucks' *House-Tree-Person Test* [20], *game techniques* [21], and Moreno's *Psychodrama* [22].

Childhood through adolescence has been the preferred patient age for application of projective techniques, e.g., asking child to express themselves through drawings [23, 24]. However, projective techniques have been also utilized in adult analysis, with the Rorschach test [4] one of the most commonly used tests in adult population. Less frequently, the TAT [5], Koch's *Tree Test* [9], and Machover's *Human Figure Drawings* [10] have been applied to adults. Published research includes psychosomatic studies using the Rorschach [25, 26] and Szondi's test [27]. Other studies have been conducted in patients with physical illnesses like psoriasis [28, 29], cancer [30, 31], and alexithymia [32–34]. The TAT and

Rosenzweig test have even been utilized to evaluate personality in patients with systemic arterial hypertension [35–37]. However, until now, projective techniques have not been formally assessed for use in patients with ischemic heart disease (IHD).

15.3 The Six-Drawings Test

One projective technique called the Six-Drawings Test (6DT) has now been utilized for the first time in patients with IHD, both within the context of a randomized clinical trial of adults with IHD (the *STEP-IN-AMI* trial) [38] and in our own outpatient Cardiac Psychology Clinic at San Filippo Neri Hospital in Rome, Italy (see Chap. 20). It is the first projective test to be formally evaluated in the setting of cardiac psychology, though this evaluation, both in the *STEP-IN-AMI* trial and our outpatient department, remains ongoing.

The Six-Drawings Test (6DT) is one of the psycho-diagnostic instruments used by the Ontopsychological clinical method [39, 40].

It is a nonstructured projective technique; only the subject of the six drawings—which the client can carry out freely, by following his fantasy—is given. The test material consists of six blank drawing sheets, on which no instructions are printed. Each of the six subjects must be drawn on a distinct sheet, in the following order: a tree, a person of the same sex of the client, a person of the other sex, the family of origin, the present situation, and the future purpose or future situation.

Though the picture topics are assigned, patients are encouraged to draw with total freedom, with no emphasis at all placed upon the quality, completeness, or any other characteristic of their drawings. As explained in Chap. 13, the underlying premise is that in each picture will be "projected" elements of the patient's deep, inner, unconscious self.

The word "*projection*" was used for the first time in 1896 by Sigmund Freud, who adopted it for use in Psychoanalysis, wherein he claimed that it entailed the mental process of looking outside of ourselves to identify our causes of grief or regret [41]. In 1915, his *projection theory* conjectured that individuals often need to express, in their external reality, unconscious psychic danger that their Ego is unable to manage [42]. In this way, Freud considered projection, above all, a pathological psychic mechanism.

Contrary to psychoanalysis, ontopsychology applies the concept of projection to the basic functioning of the unconscious, both in health and illness. We might say that we project our inner, intimate world in every aspect of our life, in every choice we make: "*The whole system of knowledge is based on the projection: the subject sees things according to the way he is. In a certain sense each of us chooses reality according to how we really are…*" [43].

The dreams and drawings utilized in projective tests might be considered the products of unconscious projections, which are registered by the conscious mind; for this reason, analyzing them could help therapists to trace back to the contents of the patient's unconscious (see Chap. 13). Our imagination is not free, but conditioned by personal conflicts and complexes. For this reason, someone asked to draw a picture will tend to reveal certain dynamics of their unconscious self. Therapists analyzing pictures drawn spontaneously by a patient must therefore do this as they analyze the images of dreams [39, 44].

It must be outlined that the first four "pictures" (the tree, the two drawings of human figures—male and female—and family) had already been utilized in other psychotherapeutic methods, as described in the introduction. Two major novelties of the 6DT are (1) that these four pictures were combined into a single test and (2) that the person's self-perceived present and future state/situation were added, rendering this test not only unique, but characteristic of the ontopsychological method. Another difference versus other tests is that different evaluation criteria are used, based upon the ontopsychological method's theoretical system of reference, as briefly described in Chap. 13. The union of six pictures allows the therapist to acquire a more comprehensive psychodynamic view of the patient's current state, a view that would be virtually impossible with a single picture. "*The 6DT shows a human being's general outline in the psychodynamic sense. It is a test that the subject himself creates; therefore it indicates his psychic graphology. At the basis we have the history of some figures, six fundamental ideas, which are very simple. From this essential simplicity, however, one can write an infinite series of characters*" ([39], p. 266).

Within the administrative process, the psychotherapist gives the client instructions on how to do the drawings. "*While carrying out the test, there are two conditions to observe: the drawing order... and the spontaneity, or immediacy in drawing them. The order is not determining; however it is better to follow this rule, because it arranges a kind of formalized introspection. It is as if the subject has to write an assay in order to present his own identity. The subject should not use an eraser and he should hand in the first drawings done; in any case the important drawings are the definitive copies that, at the end, he gives to the psychotherapist*" ([39], p. 267).

In the STEP-IN-AMI trial and the outpatient Cardiac Psychology Clinic at San Filippo Neri Hospital, we have thus far administered the test to adult cardiac patients between the ages of 31 and 82. We generally allow patients to use whatever sketching technique and colors they prefer (since the choice of technique and color may contribute to the images' interpretation). We also instruct them to draw the drawings spontaneously, without worrying about their artistic technique or aptitude. In the STEP-IN-AMI trial, the 6DT was administered by a psychologist at the time of subject enrollment, after the patient had provided signed informed consent, and after the medical/cardiac and personal history had been collected and psychometric tests completed. The 6DT was administered again after 1 year, together with the psychometric tests. In this way, the 6DT is a useful instrument for comparison, capable of being used again after a period of time (generally 6 or 12 months from the beginning of psychotherapy), which could allow clinicians to identify any client's changes that have occurred.

15.4 Six-Drawings Test Interpretation

After the test is completed, the psychotherapist provides only cursory explanations about the drawings, assuring the patient that more complete interpretations will be provided over the course of psychotherapy. To most accurately and comprehensively analyze the test, the psychotherapist must know the patient's full personal history. Therefore, it is wise to postpone any interpretation until after the beginning of the individual sessions, and to perform spontaneous, more in-depth analysis together with the patient only if and when required for psychotherapeutic purposes. In fact, the psychotherapist must always evaluate, for every single patient, what to explain and how, always remembering the aims of psychotherapy, which are to stabilize the patient's pathology and improve his or her quality of life. In reality, it is not always possible, within the context of psychosomatics, to perform complete personal introspection, as explained in Chap. 13.

In instances when the client exhibits resistance or fails to remember or describe his/her dreams, the 6DT might help the psychotherapist to gain initial insights into the patient's inner psychological state. During 6DT interpretation, it is important that the psychotherapist has been able to fully prepare him or herself to be on the lookout for and conscious of any possible personal projections he/she might make into the test analysis. This requires a prolonged period of preparation, both for theoretical study and personal analysis. Moreover, only therapists, who continuously engage in personal analysis to overcome their complexes and achieve a comprehensive knowledge of their own personal emotions and organismic reactions, can clearly recognize their clients' emotions, desires, drives, complexes, etc.

During the analysis phase, psychotherapists must initially adopt a panoramic perspective of the drawings, as well as acknowledge personal organismic reaction. That reaction might be a relaxing and expansive sensation in the visceral zone, or a sensation of organismic stiffness and closure. The drawings might seem well proportioned or disorganized and nonharmonic.

The therapist's first organismic impression of the drawings can provide initial, global insights into the artist's personality. After this initial evaluation, the therapist can begin a more analytical assessment.

Globally, the 6DT allows therapists to examine the following issues: the client's personality, past traumatic experiences, unresolved relationships based on conflict, the position of the person in his/her fundamental affective relationships, the current issue(s) and its (their) cause, the client's fundamental life goals, and drives by both ambition and growth.

The tree drawing generally represents the individual's psychobiological state [44]. The shape and the position of the tree may indicate the patient's global personality. Cut branches and holes in the trunk might represent traumatic life experiences. The presence of foliage and flowers may indicate the client's organismic state, with fruits potentially reflecting successes in life.

Drawing of a human figure the same gender as the artist reveals how the person sees him/herself, including self-awareness and organismic perception, that is to say, the patient's awareness of his/her own body. The human figure may be complete, corresponding to patients' complete subjective consciousness of their own body, or incomplete (without arms, legs, or even a torso, sometimes with missing or expressionless eyes, etc.). These very important details can help the therapist to understand the patient's subjective emotional life, as it relates to their own body, and thereby formulate a more effective therapeutic strategy.

In a specular way, the drawing of an opposite-gender figure reflects how the client sees members of the opposite sex, including possible inhibitions they have related to sex and/or intimacy. In both human figure drawings, it is useful to observe all the details: head and face, hair, facial expression, the complete or partial absence of limbs, clothing, etc. Every detail may provide further insights into the patient's underlying personality structure.

The family drawing may help in the therapist's evaluation of the patients' main affective relationships and position in their family.

The present situation drawing provides insights into the patient's current life, reflecting both the positives and negatives. It also may highlight the patient's current prevailing/emerging problem, one that can act as a precipitatory or causative element in their medical and/or psychological dysfunction. Generally, the problem highlighted by the patients in the drawing reflecting their present state/situation coincides with their fundamental life problem, which may reveal itself even further upon careful analysis during early psychotherapeutic encounters and dreams analysis. It is prudent for the therapist to avoid jumping to conclusions, however, as a more accurate interpretation of the patient's life issues is indeed likely with further detailed probing into their life.

The future goals or future state drawing allows the therapist to gain some perspective into the patient's fundamental life purpose, goals, ambitions, and intentions for personal growth.

In this way, each of the six drawings can contribute not only something, but something different to the therapist's understanding of the patient's hidden inner self and issues. Interpreting each and every image is therefore necessary to obtain as complete a picture as possible.

Note that a fuller description of the 6DT is beyond the scope of this chapter.

15.5 Observations in Patients with IHD

In patients with an acute myocardial infarction, it is possible to observe a wide range of 6DT drawings. Often they draw a distorted image of the same-sex figure, which corresponds to their own altered perception of their physical self, including perceived physical and psychological limitations and obstacles. Often, the other-sex figure is also distorted, potentially reflecting subconscious changes and inhibitions in the relationship they have with their partner. They might be unable to graphically depict their present and/or future state/situation, corresponding to uncertainties they have regarding their present and future life (for specific examples, see Chap. 18).

Work to validate and demonstrate the wide range of graphic and psychological information the 6DT can provide is currently under way. In the interim, albeit based purely upon our own anecdotal experience, we feel confident that the test can be very useful in the psychodynamic analysis of patients with ischemic cardiac disease.

It is now useful to highlight the main differences between psychometric tests and projective tests, and in particular the 6DT, in the psychological evaluation of patients with IHD. Psychometric tests measure a psychic symptom or a specific psychological characteristic. For this reason, they provide a more empirical rating of a condition or characteristic's frequency, severity, or impact, which can be used, for example, to measure the effectiveness of treatment, e.g., with cognitive-behavioral therapy. As such, psychometric tests quantify qualitative functions, which also can be very useful in scientific research and in the diagnosis of psychological illnesses. Moreover, they may be perceived by patients as an important commitment and, often, as their very first possibility to have a personal insight. In some patients, psychometric test completion may act as a form of beneficial catharsis (see also Chap. 14).

Nevertheless, this kind of test cannot help the therapist to grasp the patient's innermost self from a psychodynamic perspective, which hides under their clinically apparent psychological symptoms, like depression, anxiety, and anger. Moreover, psychometric tests are completed by the conscious part of a patient's Ego, whereas unconscious drives remain hidden to any conscious reporting. For this reason, psychometric test results can be distorted, if the patient exhibits strong defensive mechanisms and marked repression of his/her inner psychological self. In fact, in our experience, patients with very high levels of psychological dysfunction can score well on psychometric tests (which can clash with all the other data collected, in particular the 6DT). Similarly, patients who are relatively psychologically well may have psychometric test scores indicative of psychological dysfunction, which again will tend to clash with their good 6DT score. This phenomenon may reflect a higher level of consciousness and a more critical evaluation of their personal state. Otherwise, the 6DT provides direct psychodynamic insights and diagnoses, circumventing the mechanism of psychic repression.

It is possible to conclude that both kinds of test, psychometric and projective, can help therapists to acquire deeper insights into their patients' psychological state, but this requires that their results be integrated with the patient's personal history, as told by the patient in a psychotherapeutic setting, and analysis of their dreams.

References

1. Jung CG (1910) The association method. Am J Psychol 21:219–269
2. Frank LK (1939) Projective methods for the study of personality. J Psychol Interdiscip Appl 8: 389–413. doi:10.1080/00223980.1939.9917671
3. Kent GH, Rosanoff AJ (1910) A study of association in insanity. Am J Insanity 75:34–39
4. Wertheimer M (1957) Perception and the Rorschach. J Proj Tech 21:209–216

5. Rorschach H (1921) Psychodiagnostik Methodik und Ergebnisse eines wahrnehmungs-diagnostichen Experiments. Hüber, Bern
6. Morgan CD, Murray HA (1935) A method for investigating fantasies: the thematic apperception test. Arch Neurol Psychiatry 34:289–306
7. Wartegg E (1939) Gestaltung und Charakter. Ausdrucksdeutung zeichnerischer Gestaltung und Entwurf einer charakterologischer Typologie. Beih. 84 zur Zeitschrift für angewandte Psychologie. Barth, Leipzig
8. Düss L (1942) Die Methode der Fabeln in der Psychoanalyse. Z Kinderpsychiatr 9:12–24
9. Rosenzweig S (1945) The picture-association method and its application in a study of a reaction to frustration. J Pers 14:3–23
10. Koch K (1949) Der Baumtest. Hüber, Bern
11. Machover K (1949) Personality projection in the drawing of the human figure: a method. Charles C. Thomas, Springfield
12. Corman L (1964) Le test du dessin de famille dans la pratique medico-pedagogique. Presses Universitaires de France, Paris
13. Lindzney G (1959) On classification of projective techniques. Psychol Bull 56:158–168
14. Holtzman WH, Thorpe JS, Swarts JD, Herron EW (1961) Inkblot perception and personality: Holtzman inkblot technique. University of Texas Press, Austin
15. Sharkey KJ, Ritzler BA (1985) Comparing diagnostic validity of the TAT and a new picture projective test. J Pers Ass 49:406–412
16. Blum GS (1950) The Blacky pictures: a technique for the exploration of personality dynamics. Psychological Corporation, New York
17. Wagner E (1959) The hand test. Manual for administration, scoring, and interpretation. Mark James, Akron, OH
18. Rotter JB, Rafferty JE (1950) Manual: the Rotter incomplete sentence blank. Psychological Corporation, New York
19. Szondi L (1947) Experimentelle Triebdiagnostik Textband. Medizinischer Verlag Hans Huber, Bern
20. Buck JN (1948) The H-T-P technique a qualitative and quantitative scoring manual. J Clin Psychol 4:317–390
21. Staabs G (1964) The sceno test manual: a practical technique for understanding unconscious problems and personality structure. Hogrefe & Huber, Seattle
22. Moreno JL (1946) Psychodrama. Beacon House, New York
23. Widlöcher D (1965) L'interprétation des dessins d'enfants. Charles Dessart Editeur, Bruxelles
24. Rouma G (1912) Le language graphique de l'enfant. Misch-Throu, Bruxelles
25. Kanno S (1981) On the somatization of symptom in psychosomatic disease: consideration of Rorschach score. Shinrigaku Kenkyu 52:30–37
26. Pizarro JC (1956) The Rorschach test in relation to psychosomatic medicine. Dia Med 28: 1690–1699
27. Melon J, Dongier M, Bourdouxhe S (1971) Psychosomatic profile with Szondi's test. Considerations on the concepts of normality and of specificity. Ann Med Psychol 2:263–271
28. Noel J, Soule M, Bolgert M (1955) Use of projective tests in research on the psychosomatic origin of psoriasis. Sem Hop 31:1267–1271
29. Pfitzner R (1976) Psychodynamics of psoriasis vulgaris in the Rorschach test. Z Psychosoma Med Psychoanal 22:190–197
30. Sugiyama Y (1982) Psychosomatic aspects of cancer patients. Hokkaido Igaku Zasshi 57: 408–412
31. Mezei A, Nemeth G (1970) Studies on the psychosomatic factors in malignant tumors by means of the Rorschach test. Psychosom Med 18:265–270
32. Solano L, Toriello A, Barnaba L, Ara R, Taylor GJ (2000) Rorschach interaction patterns, alexithymia, and closeness to parents in psychotic and psychosomatic patients. J Am Acad Psychoanal 28(1):101–116

33. Clerici M, Albonetti S, Papa R et al (1992) Alexithymia and obesity. Psychother Psychosom 57:88–93
34. Acklin MW, Alexander G (1988) Alexithymia and somatization. A Rorschach study of four psychosomatic groups. J Nerv Ment Dis 176:343–350
35. Corani B, Livache R, Mallion JM et al (1985) Personality characteristics of hypertensive patients. Study of subjects with essential hypertension compared to a control population. Arch Mal Coeur Vaiss 78:1629–1632
36. Perini C, Rauchfleisch U, Bühler FR (1985) Personality characteristics and renin in essential hypertension. Psychother Psychosom 43:44–48
37. Perini C, Müller FB, Rauchfleisch U, Battegay R, Hobi V, Bühler FR (1984) Aggression inhibition and increased sympathetic nervous reactivity in the development of essential hypertension. Schweiz Med Wonchenschr 114:1851–1853
38. Roncella A, Pristipino C, Cianfrocca C et al (2013) One-year results of the randomized, controlled, short-term psychotherapy in acute myocardial infarction (STEP-IN-AMI) trial. Int J Cardiol. doi:10.1016/j.ijcard.2013.08.094
39. Meneghetti A (Eng. ed 2004; Ital. ed 1995–2008) Ontopsychology handbook. Psicologica Editrice, now Ontopsicologia Editrice, Roma
40. Meneghetti A (1994–2003) L'Immagine e l'Inconscio. Psicologica Editrice, now Ontopsychologia Editrice, Roma
41. Freud S (1896) Further remarks on the neuro-psychoses of defence. SE 3:162–185
42. Freud S (1915) The unconscious. SE 14:166–204
43. Meneghetti A (Ital. ed 1987, Eng. ed 2004) Dictionary of Ontopsychology. Psicologica Editrice, now Ontopsicologia Editrice, Roma
44. Meneghetti A (1981–2012) Prontuario onirico. Psicologica Editrice, now Ontopsicologia Editrice, Roma

Verbal Communication and Effective Communication: Communication in the Psychotherapeutic Setting

16

Oretta Di Carlo, Marinella Sommaruga, Maria Bonadies, and Adriana Roncella

Noli forsas ire, in teipsum redi, in interiore homine habitat veritas. Et si tuam naturam mutabilem inveneris, trascende et te ipsum. Illuc ergo tende, unde ipsum lumen rationis accenditur.

S. Agostino d'Ippona [S. Agostino d'Ippona, De Vera Religione, XXXIX, 72, 390 (Do not come out, return inside yourself; in the inner man dwells the truth. And if you find your nature mutable, transcend yourself as well. Reach towards a place where the same light of reason lights up.)]

16.1 Introduction

Oretta Di Carlo

The depth and complexity of communication is an ability that characterizes and is specific to humans, as opposed to all other living beings, and which is manifested in

O. Di Carlo, PsyD (✉)
Forma & Azione Cultural Association, Rome, Italy
e-mail: info@formaeazione.it

M. Sommaruga, PsyD
Clinical Psychology and Social Support Unit, Salvatore Maugeri Foundation, Care and Research Institute of Milan, Via Camaldoli 64, 20138 Milan, Italy
e-mail: marinella.sommaruga@fsm.it

M. Bonadies, PsyD
Associazione Italiana di Psicologia Analitica (AIPA), Via Fivizzano, 15, 00176 Rome, Italy
e-mail: mariabonadies@gmail.com

A. Roncella, MD
Department of Cardiovascular Disease, San Filippo Neri Hospital, Via G. Martinotti 20, 00135 Rome, Italy
e-mail: adrianaroncella@hotmail.it

A. Roncella, C. Pristipino (eds.), *Psychotherapy for Ischemic Heart Disease*,
DOI 10.1007/978-3-319-33214-7_16

the ability to know and reflect on what is known. Knowing is to "touch" new objects, inside and outside us.

It is communication that enables individuals to grasp and change the world around them: "*the process of development and realization of the each individual's potential is possible in an exchange, in the presence of a dialogue, characterized by the fact that an adult (parent or teacher), is interposed between the student and the outside world ... The progressive organization of the ego is the result of both neurobiological maturation and the interactions between the self-world of the others and the self-world of things.*" [1].

16.2 The Communication Process

Oretta Di Carlo

Only through communication with and mediation through adults does a child learn to recognize himself and the world around him. This explains why the first relationships in life are so important, as they affect the type of relationship one has with oneself and with the world.

Each word is a sheath through which the individual transfers quantums of information and action. The child learns words from physical contact; initially he uses the synchronous knowledge of mind and body and understands those words that he can connect with changes in his emotional and biological state. Then, progressively, the child loses this synchronicity, this psychophysical awareness, and proceeds to specialize in understanding and using words, one by one, split from their primary sense.

The overall approach to the study and interpretation of communication in relationships among individuals has greatly enriched the understanding of the cognitive and behavioral dynamics related to the exchange of information in different contexts.

A fundamental contribution to understanding a message's "intentionality" was that of the Mental Research Institute of Palo Alto [2] and of those psychotherapeutic trends that tend to describe personality disorders in terms of communication disorders: in other words that the former are the result of some deficiency or absence of authenticity in interpersonal communication. In this regard, it is relevant to mention the concept of *double bind* [3], a model of contradictory and pathological communication observed within families in whom schizophrenia is present; the characteristics of this kind of communication are applicable to many significant affective-relational relationships. For the purposes of our discussion, it is of particular interest to identify two levels of contradictory communication in the paradoxical communication model, a result of the hidden inconsistencies in language and thought: "*Every communication has a content aspect and a relationship aspect so that the latter classifies the first and thus becomes meta communication*" [4]. These semantic contradictions underline the impotence of the child, who is the recipient of the message, and lead to disconfirming the self; the double contradictory injunction places the individual in a situation with no way out. One way or another, for different reasons, it happens that the receiver of the message cannot escape this paradox, meta-communicating on it, and thus denouncing its paradoxical nature [5].

Such an innovative approach to the emblematic disease of the *"mal de vivre"* has profound implications, both for the etiology and the therapy of psychological distress and pathology in general, forcing science to undergo a *paradigm shift*: from the patient as the subject to the system that generates, and often feeds, the disease. The function of psychotherapeutic dialogue is precisely to make communication effective and reversible to known objects, that is, to restore the connection between the "labels" and the "content" transmitted by words [6].

16.3 Interference in the Verbal Communication Process

Oretta Di Carlo

As one delves deeper into the basic pattern of linguistic behavior, it becomes clear that there is a communication channel through which information is transmitted. Each message is generated and codified by a "source" and received and decoded by a receiver. Analyzing the structure of the communication process has revealed the presence of several elements that characterize the exchange of information between two or more parties. These include a source (sender), a message that is encoded and sent, and a recipient who will decode it and, consciously or unconsciously, react to it with either retro-information or feedback. During its passage from the sender to receiver, the message is exposed to a variety of effects that influence its transmission; the filtering of both parties and whatever "noise" there is in the area where the sender and the recipient are located can all interfere with the success of communication. The reciprocity between the communicating parties occurs through a preset linguistic code.

Different components affect the moment of message transmission and reception, contributed either by the sender or recipient. For this reason, human communication may be described within the following paradigm [7] (see also Table 16.1):

Table 16.1 The human communication paradigm

Emission		Destination
Private code ≫	M	≪ Private code
Semantic ambiguity ≫	E	≪ Semantic field
Syntactic ambiguity ≫	S	≪ Connotations of probability
Under code ≫	S	≪ Under code
Effects of feidelity ≫	A	≪ Effects of feidelity (or free interpretation)
Pre-supposed knowledge ≫	G	≪ Actual knowledge
Pre-orienting circumstances ≫	E	≪ Orienting (or deviating) circumstances

Private code: the way in which each individual makes use of the common code shared with the surrounding environment.
Semantic ambiguity: the way in which each word lends itself to having more than one meaning.
Semantic field: the areas of vocabulary whose elements are linked together by relationships of meaning. The area of meaning can be subjective and may change over time and in different contexts.
Syntactic ambiguity: the way in which the meaning of the discourse can change depending on the different connections and the causality of the different components.
Connotations of probability: the adjustment of a symbol to its most likely meaning.
Under code: the real intention of the speaker and of the listener. For example, propaganda or humor, which symbolize something of value or a thing intended to arrive at something else, or puns and metaphors that exploit a *double entendre* capable of emotionally engaging the speaker or listener.
Efforts of fidelity: a code according to the customary use imposed by the given language.
Free interpretations: when a word or speech is incomprehensible to its listener, the result is an arbitrary meaning which depends exclusively on subjective mechanisms. In extreme cases, it can happen that the speaker's linguistic code is reduced to mere noise in the listener.
Presupposed knowledge: knowledge that is presupposed or assumed to be existent in the listener by the speaker and upon which the entire speech is based.
Actual knowledge: only what is actually known has an effect on the listener.
Orienting circumstances: adaptation and development relating to all of the circumstances that might favor the speaker's discourse and that of the listener.

It is clear, then, that opportunities for misunderstanding abound. The greatest difficulty lies in the absence of an identity code. This code is, in fact, an unstable structure that is affected even by the slightest change in the social, cultural, environmental, emotional, etc., context. In fact, during each linguistic communication, a vast and imponderable degree of creativity occurs: at every level of meaning, there is a twofold process (1) of self-realization and (2) of the relationship with the other.

It is not our intention to delve more deeply in this chapter into the mechanisms amply highlighted by information theory [8], but rather to *explain the function of language as an instrument of anthropological authenticity*. The perceptibility of our senses is, in fact, a bridge between our mind and the entity upon which we are founded. As a result of research initially performed by the Mental Research Institute of Palo Alto, and successively further developed by several schools of psychotherapy, it has become clear that pathology may arise when this communication with the deep reasons of life is interrupted.

16.4 Dichotomy Between Language and the Intentionality of Nature

Oretta Di Carlo

Language is the instrument through which we understand and metabolize reality. It is part of our behavior, both as individuals and as members of a social group. Through speaking and listening, we build “bridges” between us and others and between ourselves and the world. Do the words of the psyche or the individual or collective unconscious communicate with our perception? And if they do communicate, how can they be recognized and processed for our rational history?

The analytical introspection on language that has been effected by psychology for over a century has shown a strong inconsistency between sign and fact, word and intention. The psychotherapeutic experience highlights the dichotomy between a verbal statement and the profound sense of the intentionality of nature, as outlined also in the Phenomenological Psychiatry of Binswanger [9], the Phenomenology of Husserl [10], and the Ontologic Existentialism of Heidegger [11].

Also for ontopsychology, often “*language does not coincide with the biological interactions of existence*” [12]. If we do not possess the criteria used by nature to communicate with our inner world and the external phenomena, we suffer from a lack of communication.

If the logical system of language retains its capabilities in legal, political, economic, and other spheres, it proves to be insufficient when applied to the science of psychology and especially to the psychotherapist–patient relationship. In this latter instance, the statement must *trace back to the intentioned object* of linguistic phenomenology and exist as an occasion of a functional rationality which operates via language.

Searching for a psychological science that does not objectify its protagonists, there have been studies with different orientations: the crisis of science and the need to reestablish psychology, as suggested by Husserl [13], Gestalt Therapy [14], the Theory of Systems [8], some exponents of psychiatry (Jaspers [15], Binswanger [16]) and those of anti-psychiatry (Laing [17], Cooper [18]), the “Client-Centered Therapy” of Rogers [19], and the Existential-Humanistic psychology of Maslow [20], May, Allport, and Feifel [21], up to ontopsychology [22]. In particular, the ontopsychological approach attempts to overcome the linguistic dichotomy that exists between nature and culture, the organismic intention, and the rational conscious image, providing a methodology equipped to retrace the order of sense, which formalizes the codes of existential interaction. In this context, “*organismic*” means a “*whole of material and psychic functions for a unity of action*” [23].

16.5 The Psychotherapeutic Dialogue

Adriana Roncella

Oretta Di Carlo

The premise behind a therapeutic relationship is a client's/patient's awareness of some need, degree of a suffering, or crisis in personal life that he/she is not able to overcome. Moreover, he/she cannot find a solution without the help of a professional. Patients usually neither precisely nor clearly understand the reason behind their suffering. It is for this reason that they seek assistance from a professional, often a psychotherapist, who might be able to guide them through a process of awareness.

All of the psychotherapeutic methodologies share common features, and the preliminary and necessary conditions to start a psychotherapeutic relationship may be synthetically described as follows:

1. Awareness of psychological suffering on the part of the client/patient, who asks for help and chooses a psychologist/psychotherapist whom he believes will be able to help him in that particular situation.
2. Confidence of the client/patient in the psychotherapist.
3. Acceptance of the client/patient by the therapist, including the therapist's ability to establish an empathetic relationship [19–20]; the therapist's unconditional acceptance for the patient he accepts to follow; it is not possible for the therapist to engage in an effective therapeutic relationship if he fails to feel unconditional love for and acceptance of the person/patient he has agreed to follow.

   The psychotherapist may have a broad base of psychological knowledge and experience, but when he is presented with the immediacy of a suffering person, the situation is often totally unique from anything experienced before, so that "*the priorities of science have no value but only the humility of contact and the therapist's participating attention to the extent of the absurd novelty*" [24].
4. Establishment of a solid therapeutic alliance between the therapist and the client/patient [25]. "*. . .the processes of developing and resolving problems in alliance are not simply prerequisite to change but rather the essence of the change process*" [25].

Every single step in the process just described is very complex, might require several encounters, and is thoroughly intertwined with the first phase of the psychotherapeutic process, during which the therapist must collect the patient's complete story and gain some initial insights into the patient's emotions, feelings, conflicts, dreams, etc. During this preliminary phase, aided by the material already collected (the personal story and the results of psychometric and/or projective tests), the psychotherapist might be able to grasp the core of the discomfort and suffering the patient is experiencing. The patient wants to feel well, to overcome his suffering, to solve his problems, and to be happy, but, paradoxically, he does not know how to overcome his uneasiness.

A deeper analysis of this preliminary phase of the psychotherapeutic process is beyond the scope of this chapter and has been analyzed in greater detail in Chaps. 13–15, 18, and 19.

The following sections briefly describe the therapeutic techniques used within the three main psychotherapeutic approaches that have been utilized most extensively in the field of Cardiac Psychology and, in particular, during the rehabilitation of patients with ischemic heart disease.

16.6 The Dialogue in Cognitive-Behavioral Psychotherapy

Marinella Sommaruga

Cognitive-Behavioral Psychotherapy (CBT) has been and remains the most commonly used methodology applied in the field of Cardiac Psychology, whether that be for research or practical application, especially among patients with ischemic heart disease, heart failure, arrhythmias, or an implantable cardioverter defibrillator (see also Chaps. 11, 19 and 22).

Over the last 30 years, research on clinical communication [26] has been predominantly conducted in medical settings, wherein the essential role that communication plays in high-quality health care has been repeatedly identified. The ability to effectively communicate with patients has been recognized as one of the core competencies of healthcare providers. In particular, the patient-centered approach [27] has contributed to changes in the traditional paternalistic approach. It requires that the physician simultaneously explores both the biomedical and psychosocial dimensions of illness. Patient-centered psychological and medical approaches are complementary and should be integrated into the interview process to elicit both personal and symptom data [27]. With such an approach, open-ended questions are largely used, as well as acknowledgement of the patient's feelings, emotions, beliefs, and opinions; moreover, patients are strongly encouraged to be active participants in their own health care [27].

Although there is no universal agreement on its definition [28], *patient-centered care* can be seen as a way of "*respecting and responding to patients' wants, needs and preferences, so that they can make choices in their care that best fit their individual circumstances*." [29].

Such communication skills can also be helpful to clinicians while they assess patients for psychotherapy. Psychotherapists, in particular, largely base their interventions on their verbal interactions with clients. Through words, it is possible for them to access, understand, legitimate, and enhance their patients' internal world. Communication is, therefore, one of the core instruments therapists have and can either compromise or enhance any intervention's effectiveness [30].

Studies systematically assessing clinician's use of communication skills are quite rare in psychotherapy settings. One review [31] revealed that techniques like exploration, reflection, noting past therapeutic success, accurate interpretation, facilitating the expression of affect, and attending to the patient's experiences can contribute positively to the therapist–patient alliance. Another study involving 23 psychologists administering cognitive-behavioral psychotherapy demonstrated that the effective use of passive and active listening skills, during the application of interventions, like summations, which structure the interview, were not used as frequently as they should be. A study conducted on a sample of 23 psychologists in cognitive-behavioral psychotherapy showed a good use of passive and active listening skills, while the application of interventions that structure the interview such as summarizing is not as frequent as they should be [32].

The main goals of a cognitive-behavioral assessment, from the very first encounter between the patient and therapist, are to diagnose disorders, discuss with the patient the goals of treatment, plan the treatment, and try to facilitate positive changes in the patient [33]. An essential part of the assessment is the process of data gathering. Without collecting adequate information, it is impossible for the therapist to understand the patient's problem(s); consequently, the patient's collaboration and trust may be compromised. Communication is, therefore, a key element in this stage of therapy and represents the bridge between the patient's perspective and the therapist's theoretical framework [33].

The goals of the CBT assessment interview are to collect all the relevant information necessary to allow for a better understanding of the patient's problem (s) and then, together with the patient, to come to some decisions about how to deal with the problem(s) (planning a therapeutic program). The therapist's ability to provide a clearly organized consultation and orient patients throughout the assessment phase becomes fundamental, whether for a single interview or an extended course of psychotherapy. These abilities become part of a process and are based upon several different skills, such as agenda setting, the use of orienting expressions, summarizing, transitions, and sign-posting.

The assessment phase can be divided into four different stages, each having specific goals. In the first stage, the therapist helps the patient to explore, define, and clarify problem(s) (exploring the patient's agenda). During the second stage, the therapist explores the patient's problem(s) from a cognitive-behavioral perspective while referring to theoretical models (exploring the therapist's agenda). Within the third stage, the therapist provides the patient with all the information that he or she deems relevant to the patient's problem(s) and tries to incorporate cognitive-behavioral theories and models into the patient's agenda (developing a new perspective reformulation). In the fourth and final stage, the therapist and patient set reasonable therapeutic goals and decide how to achieve these goals (decision-making) [33].

Goss et al. [33] suggest that, at the beginning of the interview, it is more useful for therapists to adopt an open-inquiry style, which allows the patient's narrative to be more freely expressed. The role of the therapist in this stage is to listen carefully and, if and when necessary, to guide patients through their storytelling. This being said, providing structure to the interview and explaining concepts may facilitate patients' overall comprehension, thereby affording them a greater opportunity to become more active in therapy. Structuring the interview therefore ensures efficient information gathering and enables the patient to feel involved in the therapeutic process.

Several communication skills are useful during the information-gathering process and for structuring the interview. They include listening, facilitations, reflections, clarifications, open- and closed-ended questions, checking, summarizing, reformulations, setting the agenda, time-framing and sequencing, and orienting expressions. Therapists may feel more natural and spontaneous using certain skills, whereas for others they may need more practice to feel comfortable with their use. When therapists expand their fund of knowledge and skills, it can significantly improve therapist–patient communication.

Rimondini [30] argued that the success of a communication exchange between patient and therapist depends on the co-presence of different elements, blended together and related to the psychotherapist's role: the robustness of his theoretical background, his previous clinical experiences in the field, and the degree to which the therapist is self-aware of his own emotional/cognitive functioning and appropriateness in the use of communicative micro-skills.

Even though considerably more evidence must still be collected in this field, psychotherapists' proper use of communication skills has already been demonstrated to positively impact clinical outcomes, as well as the patients' levels of satisfaction and collaboration.

16.7 The Dialogue in Psychodynamic Psychotherapy

Maria Bonadies

Psychodynamic psychotherapy is an empirical and speculative discipline that includes a wide range of theoretical models of mind and psychopathology and a wide range of psychotherapeutic techniques. Since it was first developed, derived from Freud's psychoanalytic theory, it has been contaminated by contributions from various theoretical approaches—such as ethology, the cognitive sciences, and the neurosciences. In the *Introduction to Psychoanalysis* (1915–1917), Freud outlined a theory of psyche characterized by a "*dynamic concept*" of the mind, where "*observable phenomena are conceived as signs of an interplay between forces that takes place in the psyche*" [34]. The psychoanalytic method proposed by Freud consisted of "*nothing more than an exchange of words between the analyzed and the doctor*." The words, "*if there is a special emotional bond between doctor and patient*," are the only working tool the analyst has. This core role of verbalization allowed psychoanalysis to be considered a *talking cure* that consists of the transformation of the dynamic and unconscious forces of the psyche into thoughts and words. Over the course of time, the psychoanalytic method became more complex, and, for Jung, "*psychotherapy, conceived as a simple and unidirectional method, turned into a kind of dialectic process, a dialogue, a confrontation between two persons*" [35]. Over the last few decades, in fact, contemporary psychodynamic theories have introduced a relational paradigm into psychoanalysis. However, certain distinctive features of the method last and specifically mark out the psychodynamic model of clinical intervention [36, 37].

The two pillars of the therapeutic session during psychodynamic therapy are (1) the free associations of the patient and (2) the analyst's free-floating attention. The analytical rule of free association consists of the psychotherapist's invitation, one that allows the patient to experience the most authentic and open self-expression, saying whatever comes into his/her mind without censure or judgment. While in the classical meaning, free associations were guided mostly by unconscious intra-psychic drives derived from conflicts that occurred during the patient's childhood, the current theoretical reformulation considers them a "narrative" that takes place in a "relational plot" [38].

As patients gain confidence in the therapeutic relationship and learn how to reflect on their emotions and affective reactions to guide their own behaviors, their stories' content will begin to exhibit an increasing ability to "associate," that is, to significantly connect emotions and memories, suffering and thoughts, and relationship experiences with others and the therapist. This activation allows the patient to make a "new self-experience," which Jung called an "individuation process" and Winnicott "development of the true Self" [39].

The therapist, on the other hand, must work with a "fluctuating attention," listening openly to the different forms of meaning within the patient's words and behaviors. Through this ability to "float" from the patient's verbalizations to her/his own inner resonance, thoughts, and emotions, the therapist hypothesizes new connections and constructs with the patient new bonds of meaning between somatic and psychic, subjective and objective, and conscious and unconscious content. In this sense, the interpretations of the therapist, connecting the present and future, and internal and external realities, erect bridges between different areas of the patient's affective and cognitive experiences, do represent an essential therapeutic component in psychodynamic therapy.

Hence, in the talking cure, language is the main instrument to spread feelings and emotions, to "give substance" to the patient's anxieties, expectations, desires, and emotions, both in a concrete and metaphorical sense. Language is the privileged therapeutic vehicle, especially in patients suffering from somatic diseases, like cardiovascular disease. Here the body is the mouthpiece of the patient's malaise. Then the therapeutic goal becomes "putting the discomfort into words." Despite these important premises, in recent decades the psychodynamic literature within cardiology reveals many gaps, as outlined in systematic review published by Jordan and Barde in 2007 [40]. The authors pointed out some of the methodological limits of prior studies (e.g., small subject samples and high dropout rates), as well as an obsolete psychodynamic perspective that considered cardiac events as trauma and focused on the defense mechanisms erected by the patient and his family. Furthermore, this perspective oriented the aims of the studies that were reviewed, focusing on the personality characteristics of patients with cardiovascular disease rather than on their treatment.

One good exception is a ten-year longitudinal study, the results of which were published by Lantz and Gregoire in 2003 [41], about the impact of a couple psychotherapy that combined the existential-phenomenological approach with the classical psychodynamic orientation. The existential treatment dynamics of holding, telling, mastering, and honoring couples after a heart attack were found to help to overcome the trauma of the disease. Twenty-four patients with post-myocardial infarction and their partners were treated. In this study, there was significant improvement in the patients' ability to elaborate on emotions related to their heart attack, their awareness of defense strategies adopted, and disease management. The partners' role in this study pertained to the patient's need to elaborate regarding the defense methods used by the couple or family to cope with the trauma of the heart attack. In fact, the trauma related to the acute cardiac event may often circumvent a couple's or family's ability to "transform" trauma pain into healthy manifestations of existence.

Finally, in this context, it is important to highlight how the psychodynamic perspective sets up a new vision about the importance of verbal communication while treating patients with somatic complaints, including those with cardiovascular disease. Multiple Code Theory and the phases of the referential cycle for effective therapy [42] outline a new relationship between somatization and verbalization. When a sub-symbolic activation, like a sensation, in fact does not turn into any kind of mental symbolic process, either by images or words, it can be expressed only through the body, by a symptom or some somatic pathology. And the greater the activation and disconnection, the more serious the symptoms will be [43]. Consequently, with psychodynamic therapy, symptoms represent a remarkable opportunity to create a new bridge between the body and mind, and verbal communication paves the way.

16.8 The Dialogue in Ontopsychological Psychotherapy

Oretta Di Carlo

Adriana Roncella

Ontopsychological psychotherapy [22] is a complex and novel method primarily derived from Psychoanalysis [34], Analytic Psychology [35], and Humanistic-Existential psychotherapy, as theorized by Maslow [20]. It has been utilized for the first time in Cardiac Psychology in the randomized controlled trial STEP-IN-AMI, in which 101 patients with an acute myocardial infarction treated with urgent percutaneous coronary angioplasty have been enrolled (see Chap. 13) [44, 45].

Ontopsychology borrows certain techniques from Psychoanalysis and Analytic Psychology, for instance, *dreams analysis*. Nevertheless, ontopsychology differs from other psychodynamic and humanistic-existential approaches on the basis of several highly unique characteristics, in particular, the epistemological criterion that is represented by the concept of *In Self* (more appropriately labeled, the *ontic In Self*) (also see the already-cited Chap. 13).

Through extensive experience in clinical psychotherapeutics, A. Meneghetti was able to verify that each person's psychic structure is sustained by a positive core, which he denominated the *"ontic In Self" ("In Sé ontico")*. The *ontic In Self* may be considered a person's *first reality*, the positive core of the unconscious, which coincides with the *project of nature* that is intrinsic to each person. It contains the drives for biological and psychical growth and self-realization throughout [22]. In this context, the *project of nature* refers to the In Self, similarly to biological DNA, containing all the psychological drives responsible for an individual's life-long development and self realization.

Other fundamental and distinctive concepts of ontopsychology include a different and more complex characterization of the *SuperEgo* than in Psychoanalysis and the tremendous importance given to the communication process, in particular nonverbal communication, represented both by Physiognomy–Kinesics–Proxemics and the *semantic field* (for a brief description of the semantic field, see Chap. 13). On the basis of its peculiar topographic and dynamic conception of unconscious, the meaning of symbolic dream images has also been largely recodified according to the *theory of interpretation* [6].

During the very initial phase of psychotherapy, the therapist concentrates entirely upon to listening to the patient's personal history, including his feelings, emotions, discomfort, suffering, and uneasiness. Subsequently, the therapist gradually focuses his or her analysis on the two main expressions of the unconscious drive: dreams and body language (for a detailed description, see Chap. 13). After a thorough analysis of the patient's situation, a very skilled therapist might be able to grasp the core of the profound suffering described by the patient and consequently help him/her to look for an initial solution whatever problematic situation underlies that suffering. The psychotherapist's effort is mainly concentrated to focus on the patient's *deeper reality*, represented by the ontic In Self. In this second phase of the therapeutic process, the use of dialogue by the psychotherapist is merely instrumental and exercised for the sole purpose of accessing the patient's most real and profound ego, which is inaccessible to the patient's consciousness. The clinical psychotherapist thereby acts as a "*mirror*" for the patient, neutrally reflecting a truer image that is closer to the patient's true identity, and language is an irreplaceable instrument to restore authenticity to the objects present in the consciousness of the Ego (for a more detailed explanation, see Chap. 13).

The entire psychotherapeutic process might be considered, above all, an instrument to help patients to regain full contact with their true identity, which fundamentally coincides with the intentionality of nature expressed by the ontic In Self. In this way, the psychotherapist is a tool guiding patients through this process of self-awareness. On the other hand, the "*true*" therapist and enactor of any change is actually the In Self. The psychotherapist helps the person to read and decodify messages expressed by the In Self and then aids in translating them into messages that are understandable at a conscious and rational level. Upon recontacting their own true identity, patients become the sole responsible subject, the only one who may decide *if* and *how* to change their personal life, lifestyle, relationships, job, economical choices, etc.

Being healthy means being oneself, that is, living in a way that corresponds to the specificity of identity required by one's nature. "*A healthy individual is one who works in self identity*" [46]; that is, he or she maintains his/her identity and grows as a person, with functional outcomes at both a biological and psychological level. Becoming "*sick*" means that one has strayed significantly from his/her project of nature, and symptoms are the language that indicates that the tolerance of nature's project has been exceeded. After the psychotherapeutic process, whether one remains sick or returns to health is ultimately the patient's choice.

16.9 Conclusions

Communication is a very complex and articulated process, which follows many parallel verbal and nonverbal paths that, in turn, may convey both coherent and incoherent messages. Health professionals (psychologists, physicians, nurses, etc.) are directly involved, at any given moment, in a complex communication process, which they must be able to understand if they want to help the patient to achieve the established goals of therapy. For this reason, all health professionals need to continuously enhance their general understanding of the communication process and particularly verbal communication.

Psychotherapeutic dialogue, entailing a more profound process of communication, has special features that distinguish it from all other types of communication and thereby ensure its effectiveness. For this reason, psychotherapists have the greatest responsibility of all to more fully comprehend the communication process. After all, the aim of psychotherapy is *to recover the awareness of the unity of action that is the patient and to implement it in his lifetime. The psychotherapist may be considered a "technician" who knows how to serve the human project.*

References

1. Vayer P, Destrooper J (1976) La dynamique de l'action éducative chez les enfant inadaptés. Doin, Paris, p 16
2. Watzlavick P, Beavin JH, Jackson DD (1967) Pragmatics of human communication: a study of interactional patterns, pathologies and paradoxes. Mental Research Inst./W.W. Norton, Paolo Alto, CA/New York
3. Bateson G et al (1956) Toward a Theory of Schizophrenia. Behav Sci 1:251–264
4. Watzlavick P, Beavin JH, Jackson DD (Italian edition 1971) Pragmatica della comunicazione umana. Astrolabio Ed, Roma, p 47
5. Mizzau M (1974) Prospettiva della comunicazione interpersonale. Il Mulino ed, Bologna
6. Meneghetti A (1994–2003) L'Immagine e l'Inconscio. Psicologica Editrice (now Ontopsicologia Editrice), Roma
7. Meneghetti A (1978) Ontopsicologia dell'uomo. Psicologica Editrice, Rome (Chap. "Language and Dialogue") (currently out of print)
8. von Bertalanffy L (1962) General system theory—a critical review. Gen Syst 7:1–20

9. Berrios GE (1989) What is phenomenology? A review. J R Soc Med 82(7):425–428
10. Husserl E (1970) The crisis of European sciences and transcendental phenomenology: an introduction to phenomenological philosophy. Northwestern University Press, Evanston, IL
11. Heidegger M (1927) Sein und Zeit [trans: Stambaugh J (1996) Being and time]. State University of New York Press, New York
12. Meneghetti A (Eng ed 2004; It ed 1987–2004) Dictionary of ontopsychology. Psicologica Editrice (now Ontopsicologia Editrice), Roma
13. Husserl E (1936) Die Krisis der europäischen Wissenschaften und die transzendentale Phänomenologie. Philosophia 1:77–176
14. Köler W (1929) Gestalt psychology. Liveright, New York
15. Jaspers K (1959) Allgemeine Psychopathologie. Springer, Berlin
16. Cargnello D (1977) Alterità e alienità. Feltrinelli Ed, Milano
17. Laing RD (1959) The divided self. Tavistock, London
18. Cooper D (1967) Psychiatry and anti-psychiatry. Tavistock, London
19. Rogers C (1961–1970) On becoming a person. A therapist's view of psychotherapy. Houghton Miflin, Boston
20. Maslow AH (1962) Toward a psychology of being. D Van Nostrand, New York
21. May R (1969) Existential psychology. Random House, New York
22. Meneghetti A (Eng ed 2004; It ed 1995–2008) Ontopsychology Handbook. Psicologica Editrice (now Ontopsicologia Editrice), Roma
23. Meneghetti A (It ed 1987–2004, Eng ed 2004) Dictionary of Ontopsychology. Psicologica Editrice, now Ontopsicologia Editrice, Roma, p 180
24. Meneghetti A (1973) Ontopsicologia dell'uomo. Pontificia University of St. Tommaso, Roma, p 47
25. Safran DJ, Muran JC (2009) The therapeutic alliance in brief. American Psychological Association, Washington, DC, p 7
26. King A, Hoppe RB (2013) Best practice for patient-centered communication: a narrative review. J Grad Med Educ 5(3):385–393
27. Smith RC (2002) Patient-centered interviewing. An evidence-based method. Lippincott Williams and Wilkins, Philadelphia
28. Illingworth R (2010) What does 'patient-centred' mean in relation to the consultation? Clin Teach 7:116–120
29. Institute of Medicine (IOM) (2001) Crossing the quality chasm: a new health system for the 21st century. National Academies, Washington, DC, pp 48–50
30. Rimondini M (2011) Background theories and main systems of analysis of communication in CBT. In: Rimondini M (ed) Communication in cognitive behavioral therapy. Springer, New York
31. Ackerman S, Hilsenroth M (2003) A review of therapist characteristics and techniques negatively impacting the therapeutic alliance. Psychotherapy 38:171–185
32. Rimondini M (2008) L'uso di tecniche comunicative in psicoterapia. Unpublished manuscript, Associazione Psicologia Cognitiva, Verona
33. Goss C, Rossi A, Moretti F (2011) Assessment stage: data gathering and structuring the interview. In: Rimondini M (ed) Communication in cognitive behavioral therapy. Springer, New York
34. Freud S (1915–1917) Introductory lectures on psycho-analysis. Hogart Press, London (1963)
35. Jung CG (1935) Practice of psychotherapy. Collected works of CG Jung, vol 16. Princeton University Press, Princeton, NJ (1966)
36. Gill MM (1994) Psychoanalysis in transition. The Analytic, Hillsdale, NJ
37. Shelder J (2010) The efficacy of psychodynamic psychotherapy. Am Psychol 65(2):98–109
38. Dazzi N, De Coro A (2001) Psicologia dinamica. Editori La Terza, Bari
39. Winnicott DW (1965) Maturational processes and the facilitating environment: studies in the theory of emotional development. Hogarth, London

40. Jordan J, Bardè B (2007) Psychodynamic hypotheses on the etiology, course, and psychotherapy of coronary heart disease: 100 years of psychoanalytic research. In: Jordan J, Bardé B, Zeiher AM (eds) Contributions toward evidence-based psychocardiology. A systematic review of the literature. American Psychological Association, Washington, DC
41. Lantz J, Gregoire T (2003) Couples, existential psychotherapy, and myocardial infarction: a ten year evaluation study. Contemp Fam Ther 25(4):367–379
42. Bucci W (1997) Psychoanalysis and cognitive science. A multiple code theory. Guilford, New York
43. Solano L (2013) Tra Mente e Corpo: Come si costruisce la salute. Raffaello Cortina, Milano
44. Roncella A, Giornetti A, Cianfrocca C (2009) Rationale and trial design of a randomized, controlled study on short-term psychotherapy after acute myocardial infarction: the STEP-IN-AMI trial (Short term psychotherapy in acute myocardial infarction). J Cardiovasc Med (Hagerstown) 10(12):947–952. doi:10.2459/JCM.0b013e32832fb477
45. Roncella A, Pristipino C, Cianfrocca C et al (2013) One-year results of the randomized, controlled, short-term psychotherapy in acute myocardial infarction (STEP-IN-AMI) trial. Int J Cardiol 170(2):132–139. doi:10.1016/j.ijcard.2013.08.094
46. Meneghetti A (1974–2008) La psicosomatica nell'ottica ontopsicologica. Ontopsicologia Editrice, Roma, p 207

Nonverbal Communication: The Forgotten Frame 17

Serena Dinelli and Sergio Boria

> *... expression in itself, or the language of emotions, as it has sometimes been called, is certainly of importance for the welfare of mankind ... we may conclude that the philosophy of our subject ... deserves still further attention, especially from any able physiologist.*
>
> Charles Darwin [Charles Darwin (1892) The Expressions of the Emotions of Man and Animals. John Murray, London, p. 387]

17.1 The Research on Nonverbal Communication: From the Beginnings to Recent Redefinitions

In the modern age, the scientific study of the nonverbal dimension that exists in behavior and communication started 150 years ago with Charles Darwin, who made important observations and theorizations from an evolutionist perspective [1].

Almost 100 years later, in the 1960s and 1970s, a revival took place, thanks to the development of *audiovisual technologies*. Whereas written text had always provided an effective means to analyze verbal productions, what lacked was something similar to analyze the rich but elusive dimension of nonverbal communication (NVC).

Dating back to this period, Paul Ekman's now classic studies focused on the analysis of facial expressions and their possible coding. These studies led to various

S. Dinelli, PsyD (✉)
Italian Association of Systemic Epistemology and Methodology (AIEMS), Via Guido Reni 35, 00196 Rome, Italy
e-mail: renadine@alice.it

S. Boria, MD
Italian Association of Systemic Epistemology and Methodology (AIEMS), Associazione Italiana di Medicina e Sanità Sistemica (ASSIMSS), Via Massimi 27, 00136 Rome, Italy
e-mail: sergio.boria@libero.it

A. Roncella, C. Pristipino (eds.), *Psychotherapy for Ischemic Heart Disease*,
DOI 10.1007/978-3-319-33214-7_17

findings. Notable among them is that there are a few emotions that have an innately common basis worldwide, both in terms of expression and interpretation. Happiness is unequivocally recognized. Moreover, most people can easily distinguish between a true expression of happiness and one which is affected and unnatural (curiously enough, the zygomaticus major muscle is only used during smiles that reflect *true* happiness). Other emotions that are generally recognized (even in cultures lacking specific words to label them) are sadness, anger, a combination of surprise and fear, and shame; disgust is sometimes mistaken for anger, for contempt, or a mixture of the two [2]. Important cultural determinants of facial expressions and their interpretation have also emerged from these studies.

Ekman and Friesen created the *Facial Action Coding System* (FACS) in 1978. The FACS allows for the classification and representation of any visible facial expression, in terms of a combination of action units of different parts of the face (the periocular region appears to be especially important and rich with differences). The FACS has also been used in research on medical relationships/contexts (an example is Vanessa Greco's work in pediatrics) [3].

Robert Rosenthal, a biologist at the University of Harvard, moved in a similar direction with his *Profile of Nonverbal Sensitivity* test and then with his research on gaze, tones of voice, kinesics, and so on [4–6].

Over the last 20 years, then, attempts to objectify the manifestations of NVC have led to prosperous developments in *computing*: one of these developments, *face tracking*, has been used to create algorithms to detect the faces of individual people, especially for security purposes; it has also been used to draw up sophisticated programs of artificial intelligence, notably in robotic devices [7–9].

The abovementioned research quickly revealed the close association between the NV dimension and emotions during communication between conspecific subjects. It is estimated today that almost 90 % of an emotional message is delivered through nonverbal channels.

17.2 The Origins of an Interactionist Perspective

Already in the 1970s, however, important developments were taking place, also spurred on by the ethological research of Hinde [10] and Eibl-Eibesfeldt [11]. Attention was drawn to a wider, interactionist perspective, to a whole body dimension, and to contextual components of this, like studies on kinesics and body motion communication by Birdwhistell [12] and studies on proxemics—which especially examines the value of physical proximity and/or distance between communicators—by Hall [13] and Morris [14].

Important studies on gaze also date back to this period. When two people converse, gaze has a regulative value for their coordination. The listener watches and observes much more than the speaker. The speaker looks at the listener only in key moments or at the end of his/her speech. The listener's gaze, however, together with nods and other gestures, is fundamental to the speaker, whose speech, lacking this kind of "mirrored" support by the listener, is likely to become incoherent. For this topic, one can consult studies published by Argyle and Cook [15] and Condon and Ogston [16]. These were also the years when Jean Cosnier and his collaborators started their important work at the *Laboratoire d'éthologie des communications* at Claude Bernard University in Lyon. Since the 1970s, the Laboratoire has conducted extensive research on NVC about doctor/patient relationships from an interactionist perspective [17].

17.3 A Wider Perspective on Nonverbal Communication: Relationship, Empathy, Coordination

17.3.1 Content and Relationship

Around the same time, a broader conception of NVC emerged, thanks to the studies by the Palo Alto group and to Gregory Bateson's work in particular. A well-known aspect of Bateson's thought is his distinction between verbal message—regarding content—and nonverbal message—regarding the relational aspects of communication. But Bateson actually posed the question in much broader and more significant terms [18]. He wrote:

> There is a general popular belief that, in the evolution of man, language replaced the cruder systems of other animals. I believe this to be totally wrong . . . it is very clear that the coding devices characteristic of verbal communication differ profoundly from those of kinesics and paralanguage (p. 411).
>
> . . .the kinesics of men have become richer and more complex, and paralanguage has blossomed side by side with the evolution of verbal language. Both kinesics and paralanguage have been elaborated in complex forms of art, music, ballet, poetry, and the like, and even in everyday life, the intricacies of human kinesics communication, facial expression, and vocal intonation far exceed anything that any other animal is known to produce. The logician's dream that men should communicate only by unambiguous digital signals has not come true and is not likely to.
>
> I suggest that this separate burgeoning evolution of kinesics and paralanguage alongside the evolution of verbal language indicates that our iconic communication serves functions totally different from those of language and, indeed, performs functions which verbal language is unsuitable to perform (p. 412).

In other words, Bateson strongly emphasized the specificity and extraordinary richness of the nonverbal dimension, both in itself and in the rich nonverbal dimensions that accompany any spoken utterance (paralanguage).

> . . . non verbal communication is precisely concerned with matters of relationship—love, hate, respect, fear, dependency, etc—between self and vis-à-vis or between self and environment and that the nature of human society is such that falsification of this discourse rapidly becomes pathogenic (ibid, p. 413).

In short, Bateson claimed that any communicative exchange occurs at two levels, which can be either *congruous or contradictory*.

17.3.2 NVC and Context

Another important contribution by the Palo Alto group and by Bateson especially is their reflections upon the concept of context. In Bateson's thought the word "context" encompasses a wide range of meanings: we can here define it as the overall situation where communication occurs—both "here and now," and as the "history" of the previous contact between the people concerned. If lacking context, words and actions do not have any meaning at all [19].

The doctor/patient communication is an excellent example of the importance of context: many of the gestures and exchanges occurring during a medical examination, for instance, would be typical of intimacy and familiarity in other social contexts. But in fact, the "medical examination context" affords them different values and meanings (and disrespecting the rules of such context can soon create ambiguities). It is also clear that the same way of communicating can have very different values and meanings depending on whether we are talking to a patient in fairly good health or to a patient in critical condition, whether we have known the patient for a long time or have never seen him/her before. Furthermore, communicating something painful has different values depending on whether the doctor/patient relationship has had a positive or negative and turbulent background.

Among the many contributions made by the Palo Alto group, we must also mention Virginia Satir's "in-family" therapy. She was the one who first pioneered the "sculpture" technique, in which family members express their emotions and relationships not in words, but through gestures and bodily attitudes.

17.4 Recent Studies and Redefinitions of Nonverbal Communication

Over the course of the 1990s, further research led to new discoveries and theories in child psychology, general psychology, the neurosciences, systemic psychotherapy, and the epistemological domain. These studies deeply redefined the scientific and philosophical paradigms of the *mind/body relationship*. Together with what we have already mentioned in this chapter, these new definitions can significantly change conceptions of what is commonly defined as "NVC." It is beyond the scope of this chapter to delve deeply into these vast fields of research and theorization, but we can point out four currents of clear interest.

17.4.1 At the Origin of Nonverbal Exchange

Throughout the 1980s, the mother/child relationship was explored in important observational studies. These revealed human inclinations toward NV exchanges from infancy, as well as their importance in the infant's well-being and growth: see studies by Threvarthen [20], Meltzoff [21] and Stern [22]. It is exactly thanks to nonverbal exchanges, rhythms, tones of voice, gazes, gestures, and so on that children and caregivers can become attuned to one another: perceiving both the other and themselves, at the level of emotions, intentions, shared attention, and moods, in a constant co-modulation of states of mind/attention/action.

17.4.2 Nonverbal Communication and Different Forms of Intelligence

Harvard psychologist Howard Gardner is famous for his theory of multiple intelligences. Among these we find intrapersonal intelligence and interpersonal intelligence. Gardner believes *intrapersonal intelligence* is the ability to understand one's own emotions and to channel them in socially acceptable ways. Conversely, *interpersonal intelligence* is one's ability to interpret other people's emotions, purposes, and states of mind, also thanks to the ability to "read" and understand NVC [23].

Daniel Goleman, another Harvard psychologist, based upon neuroscientific studies on the relationship between the brain and emotions (Joseph Le Doux's work in particular), has theorized that "emotional intelligence" is a meta-ability, determining how well we can use our other capabilities, including our intellectual ones. Furthermore, on the basis of perception studies, Goleman pointed out that, through our perceptions, we form intuitive judgments even before rational judgments [24]. Gardner's and Goleman's research drew attention to what occurs in the doctor/patient relationship and encouraged educational and preventative programs meant to improve emotional intelligence in children and adults alike. Education about reading NV messages is of crucial importance in these programs.

17.4.3 Nonverbal Communication and the Brain: The Mirror-Neuron System

One group of researchers at the University of Parma pioneered an important area of study on so-called *mirror-neurons*—a line of work that began by studying the brain of macaques, but ultimately was extended to work on humans. Mirror-neurons were discovered in specific localizations of the human brain, and this mechanism of mirroring between conspecifics was found to be so elaborate and complex that it was termed the "Mirror-Neuron System" (MNS) [25]. In short, when two people meet, the co-activation of neurons takes place in both the person who is enacting emotional expressions and the observer. In other words, the groups of neurons activated in the observer are the same ones activated in the one expressing emotions.

This is true for various dimensions of behavior, including those related to emotional facial expressions and to experiences like touch and pain [26–28]. The MNS is also deeply involved in immediate intuitive comprehension of the intentions underlying other people's actions [29].

In essence, the observer understands the other person's emotions and intentions thanks to a mechanism of *embodied simulation* and to a shared bodily state with the performer of the expression. As explained by Vittorio Gallese, these intersubjective dynamics of "empathetic" comprehension are automatic: they induce subjects to coordinate their actions and are also the basis for the development of more sophisticated social strategies [30, 31].

All of this emphasizes a crucial issue: the NVC actively involves both interlocutors, thereby allowing each to enter into the other's experience, often unconsciously.

17.4.4 Consciousness and Emotions

For decades, Antonio Damasio has conducted experimental studies in neuroscience, generating a vast amount of theoretical work over that time. He observes that, until recent times, both neuroscience and cognitive science afforded emotions a very cold shoulder. Emotions were too subjective, it was said; they were too elusive and vague, and reason was presumed to be entirely independent of them [32]. Contrary to this, Damasio's extensive experimental and theoretical work has been directed at reconstructing substantial relationships between the body, brain, emotions, and consciousness. Moreover, he does this from an evolutionist perspective, emphasizing the concepts of homeostasis and of organism. For these concepts, he took inspiration from Edelman and Bateson.

We cannot explore the whole body of Damasio's work. We can, however, point out that he believes emotion to be an integral part of reasoning and decision-making processes, for better or for worse. Having studied lesions in specific regions of the brain, he also claims that the selective reduction of emotions is at least as prejudicial against rationality as excessive emotions. Well-directed emotions can constitute a system of support without which reasoning cannot work effectively. He also emphasizes that spontaneous and genuine nonverbal signals are activated by complex cerebral structures outside our voluntary control. Moreover, the voluntary imitation of emotions is perceivable as false: there is always some inconsistency, either in the configuration of one's facial muscles or in one's vocal tone.

17.4.5 Body Language and Psychotherapy

The last 20 years have witnessed growing interest in NVC within the field of systemic/relational psychotherapy. Body language has proven to be particularly important in patients with psychosomatic disorders, that is, when emotional and relational conflicts turn into somatic symptoms. Among the various models of intervention, we recall the technique of "family sculptures": families give visual and spatial representations of themselves and of the relationships between the various members through gestures and gazes, games of distance and proximity, bodily use of space, etc. To examine this technique in further detail, one can review studies conducted by Virginia Satir [33], Philippe Caillè [34], and Luigi Onnis [35, 36]. Hidden aspects of emotional life are always deeply rooted in bodily perceptions; their reactivation is facilitated by emotional and body languages.

17.5 Some Aspects of Nonverbal Communication

The review we have conducted thus far reveals the complexity of the nonverbal dimension: perception and self-perception, emotions, relationships, and aspects of consciousness, all interplay within NVC. We now highlight some of the most important features of NVC:

a. First of all, it is *constantly at work*. We are immersed in NVC all the time. We cannot fail to communicate at this level, because we have a body; even keeping silent is, therefore, a form of communication. This is even more prominent in ambiguous situations like medical examinations. Patients go to see their doctors "because they do not know"; and the more they fear what they do not know, the more they try to interpret the doctor's signals, especially nonverbal ones.
b. *It is two-way*: I perceive the other, more or less consciously, but I also perceive myself, and the relationship between these two perceptions. I find myself smiling, for instance, if the other person is smiling at me; on the other hand, my facial and body muscles tighten if the other has a sharp, strained, and penetrating voice, thereby sending me messages of fear, rage, or hostility.
c. It has a *psychophysiological basis*: NVC concerns bodily dimensions linked to vital functions like breathing (affecting our tone of voice), heartbeat, skin temperature, secretions, the conditions of our face and body muscles, and so on.
d. It is largely *out of our conscious control* and often *translated into verbal terms with difficulty*. Apropos of this, Bateson wrote: *"If this general view of the matter be correct, it must follow that to translate kinesics or paralinguistic messages into words is likely to introduce gross falsification due not merely to the human propensity for trying to falsify statements about 'feelings' and relationship and to the distortions, which arise whenever the products of one system of coding are dissected on to the premises of another, but especially to the fact that all such translation must give to the more or less unconscious and involuntary iconic messages the appearance of conscious intent.... From an adaptive point of view,* ***it is therefore important that this discourse be carried on by techniques which are relatively unconscious and only imperfectly subject to voluntary control...*** " [37].
e. *It goes beyond the visual dimension.* In the world we presently live in, the visual dimension ("How do you see me?") is overestimated. With my eyes I can express emotions and, at the same time, grasp the other's state of tension or relaxation, his way of occupying space, the amplitude of his gestures, his reactions to touch, and so on. There are, however, other significant messages like a person's odor, depth and tone of voice, and rhythm of speech. Equally

significant are the messages I send and that I simultaneously perceive as a "feeling of myself."

f. *It is related to temporal dimensions, context markers, spatial relations, and more*. An example of the rhythmical and temporal dimension is alternating between active communication and silent listening—as is typical of a medical examination. Several studies have revealed, for instance, that doctors usually interrupt patients at the beginning of the visit, typically within 18–20 seconds; they do this to ask questions referring to protocols that might help them to characterize the patient's problem [38]. It can happen, however, that patients attribute other meanings to these interruptions. They might think, for example, that "the doctor isn't interested in what I am saying. . ." or that "the doctor is in a hurry, he has other matters to attend to." Consequently, patients might feel that the doctor is not really interested in them or their problem.

g. *As for context markers and spatial relations, medical consultations are very clearly* characterized. There is a clear gap between unfamiliarity and intimacy. Doctors and patients often hardly know each other or do not know each other at all. Nevertheless, their relationship classically involves dimensions that can be very private for the patient. Socially customary physical barriers break down, and personal emotional/psychological factors—whether manifested or hidden—come to be involved in both, the doctor and the patient. Distances, spatial movements, gestures, and tones of voice, therefore, take on contextual meanings.

h. *It has important cultural dimensions*. Nowadays, doctors typically see and treat patients from a broad array of distinct cultures, between which nonverbal signals can be conveyed and interpreted in very different ways. Based upon the results of a large study published in 1970, Watson classified cultures into either "contact" or "noncontact.'" In "contact cultures" (e.g., Arabs, South Europeans, Latin Americans), people are more likely to interact face-to-face, as well as to approach, touch, and look at each other much more often than in "noncontact cultures" (e.g., Asians, Indians, North Europeans). Gazes can cause misunderstandings. For example, a piercing glance can be considered insolent by Africans and Asians, while a poor gaze interaction can be considered a signal of inattentiveness or rudeness by Arabs and South Americans. The whole field of touch and physical approaches also varies according to different cultures [39].

i. *It has a complex relationship with verbal content*. As stated above, verbal and nonverbal messages do not necessarily coincide. Furthermore, they have different pragmatic implications. The nonverbal dimension can be a sort of comment confirming what is being said, but it can also either give special shades of meaning to the verbal content or it can clash with the very heart of the message. The expression "Relax!," for example, if directed at a patient about to undergo an unpleasant medical test, can totally clash with an authoritative or excited voice or with brusque gestures. Likewise, a request to an elderly patient to "cooperate responsibly" can be contradicted by a tone of voice that infantilizes him. A request for cooperation to a colleague can also be belied by subtle gestures of impatience, facial expressions exhibiting annoyance or contempt, or other forms of NVC.

On the other hand, however, NVC can be of help at difficult times. Bad news, for instance, can be made less painful if delivered with a grave but empathetic tone of voice. A simple gesture, a pause, or silence can also be of help, as occurs in the following dialogue between a patient and his doctor, who have had a long-lasting relationship (from Walter F. Baile et al. [40]):

> Doctor: *I am sorry to say the X-rays showed the chemotherapy does not seem to have worked (pause). Unfortunately, the tumor has advanced.*
>
> Patient: *I feared so (cries).*
>
> Doctor: *(moves his chair closer to the patient, offers him a napkin and waits) I know it is not what you would have wished to hear. I would have wished the news to be better.*

The nonverbal dimension, in other words, offers *a substantial contribution to doctor/patient coordination*, to information gathering, to sharing intentions, and to the general construction of the doctor/patient relationship. This is true both for the "here and now" and for the creation over time of a cooperative relationship of trust.

This is also true, of course, for the *relationships between healthcare workers* in various contexts. Those who work in operating theaters, for instance, know that most times a simple look, an excited or calm tone of voice, or the rhythm of the work being performed can all be specific signals either aiding with coordination or creating obstacles and tension.

Likewise, nonverbal and relational dimensions of communication, whether we recognize them or not, are constantly at work in the ordinary life of a hospital ward where, among other things, they affect the general work atmosphere, potential opportunities for (or obstacles to) cooperation, and the potential clarity or ambiguity of informative messages.

17.6 Obstacles to the Involvement of Nonverbal Communication in Medical Practice

In recent years, operational, scientific, and cultural environments in the healthcare world have evolved in terms that strongly hinder healthcare providers paying attention to NVC. Even if it is constantly present in the workplace, NVC remains a "blind spot" in healthcare workers' awareness and education. In a medical system based on the mechanization of its practices, awareness of NVC and its implications can be seen as an obstacle or a potential source of operational chaos.

After all, doctor/patient communications often take place in very unnatural situations: under strict time pressure, in the presence of a computer or medical equipment (from echocardiographs to respirators); and all of this may make the doctors look away from their patients. Considering what we said about the importance of gaze for coordination, this might make it more difficult for the patient to express him/herself and for doctors and patients alike to coordinate.

It often happens in hospitals that the emotional, nonverbal, and bodily dimensions are tacitly delegated entirely to medical attendants, who therefore contribute significantly to the flow of communication and to patients' well-being, often without having received adequate training in the awareness and good use of these dimensions.

On the other hand, the specific medical cultural context does not favor NVC. We have witnessed an eclipse of medical semeiotics, an overestimation of "data," and the conception of words as mere "content." Technology has tended to shift the whole of medical culture largely toward a visual dimension—and to diagnoses by images in particular—thereby neglecting other channels of information and communication. Furthermore, making diagnoses outside the boundaries of standard guidelines involves the risk of appearing "negligent," sometimes even with legal consequences.

Patients themselves are accustomed to a certain way of conceiving medicine: they share both the idea of the body as a machine and the illusion of its control, and they expect doctors to behave according to certain procedures. This is, however, in conflict with their need to be recognized as people; thus, they are often dissatisfied because they do not feel accepted. This is one of the reasons why "alternative therapies" are so successful: here a central role is played by relationships, empathetic communication, and patient empowerment (e.g., the co-construction and the sharing of decisions).

Last but not least, we can say that, notwithstanding the profound reasons why one chooses the medical profession, all the topics listed before might influence the vocational training of doctors. One interesting study compared the evolution of medical versus psychology students during their university education. At the beginning of their programs, their motivations were the same: feelings of empathy for those who were suffering and a desire to help them. However, by the completion of their curriculum, future doctors exhibited a considerable decrease in their level of empathy, whereas psychologist trainees did not [41].

17.7 Why Awareness of the Nonverbal Dimension Can Be Useful in Medical Professions

In conclusion, why should the issue of NVC be of interest to doctors? Let us now consider some possible benefits of such interest, particularly from the perspective of certain critical aspects of contemporary medical practice.

Crisis in authority: Today, before going to see a doctor, patients often gather information from various sources (e.g., online), thereby forming opinions about their problem, its possible treatment, and other issues. Doctors, then, cannot rely on the heritage of professional authority that they used to enjoy. Confidence and trust, therefore, must be created over the course of the doctor/patient relationship and regularly reaffirmed [42].

Reduced legal risks: If patients feel accepted and have a good relationship with their doctor, they generally will be less likely to develop a belligerent attitude and might therefore hesitate to file a complaint in cases of perceived or real medical error. They will probably be more understanding and more willing to accept human limits and share the distress of possible errors with their doctors.

Reduced burnout: In the long term, all helping professions cause chronic fatigue. This threatens the professional's health and increases their risk of making mistakes. If doctors are overburdened, or work in non-optimal conditions, their natural instinct could be to minimize relational engagement, merely following "objective" procedures, conforming more and more to routine guidelines—like relying on medical equipment and tests and sending patients to a number of specialists, etc. However, an increasingly mechanical practice is likely to worsen the problem. Conversely, willingness to develop relationships reintroduces vital dimensions into professional practice, in this way helping to reduce burnout. Doctors and patients can so bring richer dimensions into the context, dimensions that are nearer to their complexity as living organisms—and this is an important contributor to the health and well-being of both parties'.

Increased patient compliance: Several studies have shown that a good doctor/patient relationship has positive consequences for treatment. It also activates a positive dynamic, thereby increasing the patient's trust of their caregiver. A good relationship helps patients to be more willing to take their medicines as prescribed (co-construction of sense), reduce arbitrary interruptions, and deal with treatment side effects (*affecting compliance*). In cases of complex treatment, a good relational atmosphere helps patients to deal with possible feelings of rejection of treatment protocols, equipment, procedures, and so on. Some studies have shown that patients' knowledge or ignorance about treatments, together with their psychological state, affect both pharmaceutical action and therapeutic effects [43].

Placebo effects: Recent studies have also shown that the overall effectiveness of treatments is affected by cognitive and emotional processes, in which an important part is played by the "ritual," emotional and relational dimensions of the doctor/patient relationship. Particularly interesting in this scenario are studies on the placebo effect, which mostly works at a subconscious level [44]. Nonverbal components of the relationships can, therefore, play a significant role in how effective treatment is.

Diagnostic efficiency and the sustainability of medical services: In the past, doctors used to rely on their own personal sensorial skills to make diagnoses (through examination procedures like palpation and auscultation). They also relied upon their relationship with their patients to obtain therapeutic effects, keeping some sort of "shamanistic" tradition alive. These dimensions—which refer to the body, affectivity, and imagination and are constantly at work—have been clouded and replaced by technology. However, technology could and should support medical practices in an "and/and" framework instead. Conducting the typical semeiotic examination and letting patients go into the details of their symptoms and their onset means entering both the bodily/emotional and historic dimensions, allowing the clinician to access a broader range of information.

Related to this topic, we cite the importance of *Narrative Medicine*, as introduced and formalized by Rita Charon [45]. Narrative Medicine suggests that doctors build a better relationship with their patients, and helps them to do so, because the narrative dimension yields a more complete view of the patient's biopsychosocial context. In this way, pathology is not a casual accident in the patient's life, but can be understood in a wider dimension and with greater meaning. This, together with the evidence obtained by technology, can help both clinicians and patients grasp how the biopsychosocial and environmental dimensions are interwoven processes that give meaning to the disease. They might also contribute to avoiding unnecessary tests and examinations, in this way aiding the economic sustainability of medical services.

17.8 Conclusions

What we have considered in this chapter emphasizes the importance of NVC as a skill that is useful to all medical professionals. It is, of course, crucial to psychotherapists and psychologists, but also important to physicians, whether they are front-line general practitioners or specialists who see patients in either an outpatient or inpatient setting. Hospital attendants, social workers, and therapists who work in rehabilitation also can use NVC skills. What makes a difference is that they are aware of this dimension and of its relationships to the cognitive, emotional, and epistemological dimensions. In essence, clinicians need to learn how to spontaneously but respectfully communicate through nonverbal channels. This entails overcoming the operational and epistemological obstacles of the biomedical approach and deconstructing its scientific image. It also requires deep reflection at various levels (epistemological, anthropological, social, etc.). Otherwise NVC, even if constantly at work, will remain a blind spot in clinical perceptions and medical practice.

It is therefore important for medical students to receive such education that helps them to become aware of their own prejudices (both professional and personal) and emotional world. This does not entail producing "true" descriptions of emotions; it means instead attaining suitable language to talk about emotions and to create an agreed-upon dimension for them. It then means learning how to meta-communicate about one's own emotional responses, thereby reducing the risks of confusion, contradiction, conflicts, and misunderstandings.

In conclusion, health professionals should acquire narrative competences, so as to be able to talk and reflect upon themselves, integrating verbal and nonverbal codes in their relationships with patients and colleagues, allowing them to both communicate better with others and enhance their perceptions of self. The main training tool may be experiential workshops, which can offer activities like writing and autobiographical narratives, as well as experience observing how the body expresses itself.

With respect to psychotherapy, only formalized training (at least to the level of a *counsel*or) can afford the nonverbal dimension its proper frame. Indeed, being so deeply connected to emotional life, both on the side of the patient and therapist, NVC has an all-important role in the therapeutic process and should be attentively considered and experienced while therapists are in training. While the type of psychotherapy training one receives can vary depending on the methodology used, many schools pay special attention to the nonverbal dimension [46].

As stated above, NVC does not depend upon conscious control; there are, therefore, no easy "formulas" for mechanical use. What is important is "feeling," and not just "understanding," what goes on while communicating.

References

1. Darwin C (1982) The expression of the emotions of man and animals. John Murray, London, p 387
2. Ekman P. www.paulekman.com
3. Greco V (2008) La comunicazione tra pediatra e madre nella struttura ambulatoriale. Analisi svolta con il metodo F.A.C.S. di P. Ekman & W. V. Friesen. Riv Med Bambino 9:597–598
4. Rosenthal R, Hall J, Di Matteo MR, Rogers P, Archer D (1979) Sensitivity to nonverbal communication. The PONS Test. Johns Hopkins University Press, Baltimore
5. Hall J, Harrigan J, Rosenthal R (1995) Nonverbal behaviour in clinician patient interaction. Appl Prev Psychol 4:21–37
6. Harrigan J, Rosenthal R (2008) The new handbook of methods in nonverbal behavior research. Oxford University Press, Oxford
7. Damiano L, Lehman H, Dumouchel P (2013) Dicotomie instabili. Emozioni ed empatia sintetiche. Riflessioni Sistemiche 8:5–18
8. Damiano L, Dumouchel P (2009) Epigenetic embodiment. In: Canamero L, Oudeyer P-Y, Balkenius C (eds) Proceedings of the 9th international conference on epigenetic robotics. Modelling cognitive development in robotic systems. Lund University Cognitive Studies, Lund, pp 41–48
9. Pioggia G, Hanson D, Dinelli S, Di Francesco (2002) Importance of nonverbal expression to the emergence of emotive artificial intelligence systems. In: SPIE Proceedings, vol 4695
10. Hinde RA (1972) Non-verbal communication. Cambridge University Press, New York
11. Eibl-Eibesfeldt I (1989) Human ethology. Aldine de Gruyter, New York
12. Birdwhistell R (1970) Kinesics and context. Essay on body motion communications. University of Pennsylvania Press, Philadelphia
13. Hall ET (1979) Handbook for proxemic research. Society for the Anthropology of Visual Communication, Washington, DC
14. Morris D (1994) Bodytalk: the meaning of human gestures. Crown, New York
15. Argyle M, Cook M (1976) Gaze and mutual gaze. Cambridge University Press, London
16. Condom WS, Ogston WD (1967) A segmentation of behavior. J Psychiatr Res 5:221–236
17. Cosnier J, Grosjean M, Lacoste M (1993) Soins et communication: approche interactionniste des relations de soins. PUL éditeur, Lyon
18. Bateson G (1972) Steps to an ecology of mind. Ballantine Books, New York
19. Bateson G (2002) Mind and nature. Hampton press, Cresskill, NJ, p 14
20. Trevarthen C (1980) The foundations of intersubjectivity. In: Olson D (ed) The social foundation of language and thought. Norton, New York, pp 316–342
21. Meltzoff AN, Gopnik A (1989) The many faces of imitation in language learning. Springer, New York
22. Stern DN (1985) The interpersonal world of the infant. Basic Books, New York
23. Gardner H (1983) Frames of mind: the theory of multiple intelligences. Basic Books, New York

24. Goleman D (1996) Emotional intelligence: why it can matter more than IQ. Bantam Dell/Random House, New York, pp 60–61
25. Gallese V, Fatiga L, Fogassi L, Rizzolatti G (1996) Action recognition in the premotor cortex. Brain 119:593–609
26. Keyers C, Wickers B, Gazzola V et al (2004) A touching sight: SII/PV activation during the observation and experience of touch. Neuron 42:1–20
27. Hutchison WD, Davis KD, Lonzano AM et al (1999) Pain related neurons in the human cingulated cortex. Nat Neurosci 2:403–405
28. Singer T, Seymour B, O'Doherty J et al (2004) Empathy for pain involves the affective but not the sensory components of pain. Science 303:1157–1162
29. Iacoboni M, Molnar-Szachacks I, Gallese V et al (2005) Grasping the intentions of others with one's own mirror neuron system. PLoS Biol 3(3):e79. doi:10.1371/journal.pbio.0030079
30. Gallese V (2003) The roots of empathy: the shared manifold hypothesis and the neural basis of intersubjectivity. Psychopathology 36:171–180
31. Gallese V (2001) "Being like me": self-other identity, mirror neurons and empathy. In: Hurley S, Chater N (eds) Perspectives on imitation: from cognitive neuroscience to social science. MIT Press, Cambridge, MA, pp 101–118
32. Damasio A (1999) The feeling of what happens. Body and emotion in the making of consciousness. Harcourt Brace, New York (Chap. 1)
33. Satir V, Stachowiak J, Taschman HA (1994) Helping families to change. Jason Aronson, Northvale, NJ
34. Caillé P, Rey Y, Marche B, Taufour B (2004) Les objets flottants: méthodes d'entretiens systémiques: le pouvoir créatif des familles et des couples. Fabert, Paris
35. Onnis L (1996) Le langage du corps. Editions Scientifiques Françaises, Paris
36. Onnis L (1997) La palabra del cuerpo. Herder, Barcelona-Buenos Aires
37. Bateson G (1972) Steps to an ecology of mind. Ballantine Book, New York, pp 412–413
38. Bert G, Quadrino S (2002) Parole di medici, parole di pazienti. Counselling e narrativa in medicina. Il Pensiero scientifico Editore, Roma, p 32
39. Watson MA (1970) Proxemic behaviour: a cross cultural study. Mouton, The Hague
40. Baile WF, Buckman R, Lenzi R et al (2000) SPIKES—a six-step protocol for delivering bad news: application to the patient with cancer. Oncologist 5(4):302–311
41. Hoffman C, Formica I, Di Maria F (2007) Caregivers in formazione e alessitimia: un'indagine empirica su un campione di studenti dell'Università di Palermo. G Psicol 1(1)
42. Manghi S (2005) Il medico, il paziente e l'altro. Franco Angeli Editore, Roma
43. Benedetti F (2008) Placebo effects. understanding the mechanisms in health and disease. Oxford University Press, Oxford (Chapter 1)
44. Benedetti F (2008) Placebo effects. Understanding the mechanisms in health and disease. Oxford University Press, Oxford (Chapters 6 and 7)
45. Charon R (2006) Narrative medicine. Honoring the stories of illness. Oxford University Press, Oxford
46. Onnis L (2010) Lo specchio interno. La formazione personale del terapeuta sistemico in una prospettiva europea. Franco Angeli Editore, Roma

Psychotherapy for Cardiac Patients: Selection of Clinical Cases. Part I

18

Adriana Roncella

... the patient as a human being with worries, fears, hopes, and despairs, as an indivisible whole and not merely the bearer of organs—of a diseased liver or stomach—is becoming the legitimate object of medical interest.
Franz Alexander [F. Alexander (1950), Psychosomatic Medicine. Its Principles and Applications. W.W. NORTON and COMPANY INC. New York]

18.1 Introduction

Previous chapters have justified and demonstrated the role of psychometric testing and psychotherapeutic management in patients, who present with an acute cardiac event, like a myocardial infarction. In addition, various psychotherapeutic techniques and approaches have been described, including the six-drawings test (6DT), dreams analysis, psychoanalysis, and ontopsychotherapy, among others. In this chapter, one of the patients enrolled in the Short-TErm Psychotherapy IN Acute Myocardial Infarction (STEP-IN-AMI) trial [1, 2] is presented. This description incorporates both his medical/cardiac and psychological presentation, including formal psychometric testing, and his course throughout the entire psychotherapeutic cycle. As such, this can be considered a "complete case," which illustrates all the essential psychotherapeutic modalities we use in our Cardiac Psychology Clinic. Although we concur that every clinical case is unique, our hope is that observing how one patient is managed, from presentation to discharge, will help readers, whether psychologists or physicians, to better familiarize themselves with the underlying principles and practice of Cardiac Psychology.

A. Roncella, MD (✉)
Department of Cardiovascular Disease, San Filippo Neri Hospital, Via G. Martinotti 20, 00135 Rome, Italy
e-mail: adrianaroncella@hotmail.it

A. Roncella, C. Pristipino (eds.), *Psychotherapy for Ischemic Heart Disease*,
DOI 10.1007/978-3-319-33214-7_18

18.2 Clinical Case: Enrollment Phase

At the time of presentation to our unit, AR was a 51-year-old man. He was admitted to the emergency department for an acute anterior myocardial infarction with ST elevation (STEMI).

The time between the onset of his chest pain and arrival in the procedure room of the Interventional Cardiology Unit, where a coronary arteriography was performed, was approximately 180 min. The main arteriography findings were complete occlusion of the proximal segment of the anterior descending coronary artery and critical ostial stenosis of the first septal branch. The remaining coronary arteries exhibited noncritical atherosclerotic plaques. During the percutaneous coronary intervention (PCI), which was performed following coronarography, the patient's descending coronary artery was reopened via balloon inflations, followed by implantation of a drug-eluting stent. The first septal branch was a small and secondary branch; for this reason, it was not treated with a PCI.

After the interventional procedure, the patient was transferred to the Intensive Care Coronary Unit. Both before the PCI and throughout his stay in the hospital, the patient received comprehensive medical therapy, as per the most recent medical guidelines. The patient was highly compliant with all prescribed medical treatment throughout the duration of his hospital stay and 5 years of outpatient follow-up.

AR presented with the following biological risk factors for cardiovascular disease: (1) a family history of ischemic heart disease, (2) hypercholesterolemia, (3) prolonged cigarette smoking, and (4) excessive body weight. His only comorbid condition was second- to third-degree hemorrhoids. The echocardiogram performed a few days after the percutaneous trans-arterial coronary angioplasty (PTCA) revealed hypokinesis of the anterior and anterior septal walls, an ejection fraction of 40 % (a moderate reduction in overall ventricular function), and a wall motion score index (WMSI) of 1.88.

After transfer to the cardiology unit, the patient was invited to participate in the STEP-IN-AMI trial. He received a thorough explanation of the study's aims and of the importance of a complete evaluation of psychological risk factors for acute myocardial infarction. The patient accepted enrollment without hesitation. He spontaneously volunteered that, prior to his heart attack, he had felt like "*a completely full pot, which couldn't hold all its negative emotions… and that he would surely collapse…*" Luckily, the patient was randomized to the group treated with short-term psychotherapy.

The enrollment session in the STEP-IN-AMI trial was always very demanding for everyone—the doctor, psychologist, and patient—because of the huge quantity of data collected. First AR signed an informed consent form and all his cardiological and personal data were collected in a personalized folder.

This was his personal history, as collected during the enrollment interview:

AR was born in Egypt, of Italian parents. His father was now 76 years old; he had worked in company administration but had retired, though he remained in good health and still engaged in other jobs. His mother had been a housewife and died at the age of 67 from a ruptured aortic aneurism. AR was the second-born of three children; the eldest was a 53-year-old male and the youngest a 45-year-old female. AR had attended the first 4 years of secondary school, without completing the final (fifth) year. For the duration of his employment career, he worked in public administration. He was married to a 49-year-old woman who was working as a nurse at a public outpatient clinic. They had two female children; the older was 26 and was studying Psychology in university; the younger was 24 and had received a degree as a social assistant. For hobbies, AR was interested in hunting, fishing, and computer science.

The following psychometric tests were administered before the starting of the psychotherapeutic sessions, as scheduled as part of the trial research project [1, 2]: (1) Self-Evaluation Test, assessing the patient's global level of psychological distress over the preceding 2 weeks [3]; scores range from a minimum of 1 to a maximum of 10, which indicate not stressed and very stressed, respectively; (2) Modified Maastricht Questionnaire, specifically assessing levels of vital exhaustion [4]; (3) Social Support Questionnaire, evaluating each individual's perception of his/her social network [5]; (4) Recent Life Change Questionnaire, evaluating the presence and importance of occasional major life events and chronically recurring aggravations in daily life [6]; (5) Beck Depression Inventory (BDI), evaluating for symptoms of major or minor depression [7, 8], where a score between 10 and 15 is considered indicative of mild depression, and a score equal or superior to 16 is considered indicative of clinically relevant depression; and (6) The MacNew Heart Disease Health-Related Quality of Life Questionnaire, which assesses patients' quality of life across three specific domains—emotional, physical, and social—and generates a global QOL score [9]. For each domain, a score of "1" is indicative of a low quality of life, whereas a score of "7" indicates a high quality of life (for a broader description of psychometric tests, review Chap. 14).

The results of the psychometric tests, which were more helpful among others for the evaluation of the patient's psychological status at the time of enrollment, were as follows. His self-evaluation test score was 8, indicating a high level of personal distress. His BDI score was 8, indicating a tendency toward depression, being just below the threshold for mild depression. On the MacNew Heart Disease Health-Related Quality of Life Questionnaire, recalling that scores range from 1 to 7 and that higher scores indicate better quality of life, AR had an emotional dimension score of 5.0, a physical score of 5.2, a social score of 5.0, and a global score of 5.1. Overall then, this patient exhibited a high level of distress, with a slight tendency toward depression and reduced quality of life in all domains.

After psychometric testing, the 6DT was administered (see also Chap. 15). In brief, the 6DT is a nonstructured projective technique and one of the psychodiagnostic instruments settled upon for use in ontopsychological therapy [10, 11]. The test material consists of six blank drawing sheets, on which no instructions are printed. Each of six subjects must be drawn on a distinct sheet, according to the following order: a tree, a human figure/person who is the same sex as the patient, a person who is the opposite sex as the patient, the patient's family of origin, the patient's present situation, and the patient's future situation. Assessing all six of these pictures together allows the therapist to develop a reasonably well-rounded psychodynamic view of the patient's current psychological state. Analysis of these images is performed in the same way that dreams are analyzed. To see the six drawings submitted by AR at the beginning of psychotherapy (baseline), refer to Figs. 18.1, 18.2, 18.3, 18.4, 18.5, and 18.6. What follows are the therapist's initial interpretations of these six drawings.

AR's tree drawing (Fig. 18.1), which generally represents an individual's psychobiological state [12], clearly depicted a tree and was quite complete. Moreover, the tree appeared to be firmly rooted on the ground, was well centered on the sheet, had a thick trunk, and was richly foliated, indicating a full and strong personality, and good contact with reality (i.e., well-grounded).

The drawing of the same-sex figure generally reflects how the person sees him- or herself, including their self-awareness and organismic perceptions (see also Chaps. 13 and 15). Conversely, the drawing of the opposite-sex figure reveals how the person sees members of the opposite sex, and can uncover various inhibitions, which are present in the patient's intimate and sexual relationship (s) [10, 11]. In AR's test, the male (same-sex) representation was complete, depicting all major body parts, including the head, torso, and all four limbs (Fig. 18.2). However, it also was very small, relative to the sheet of paper, and

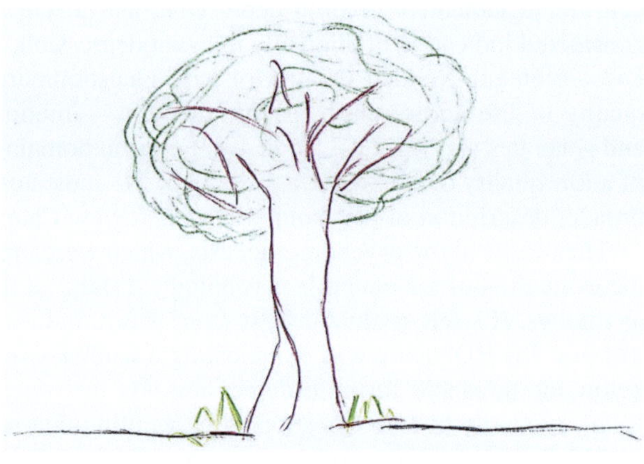

Fig. 18.1 Six-drawings test results for AR at baseline (before psychotherapy): Tree

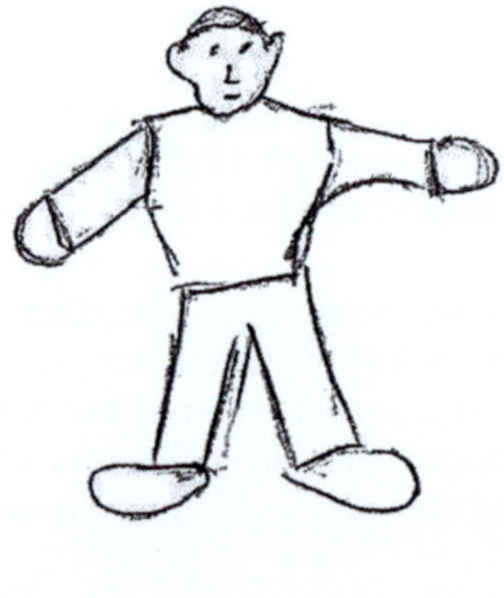

Fig. 18.2 Six-drawings test results for AR at baseline (before psychotherapy): Same-sex figure. In the original test the same-sex figure was much smaller and in the center of the sheet

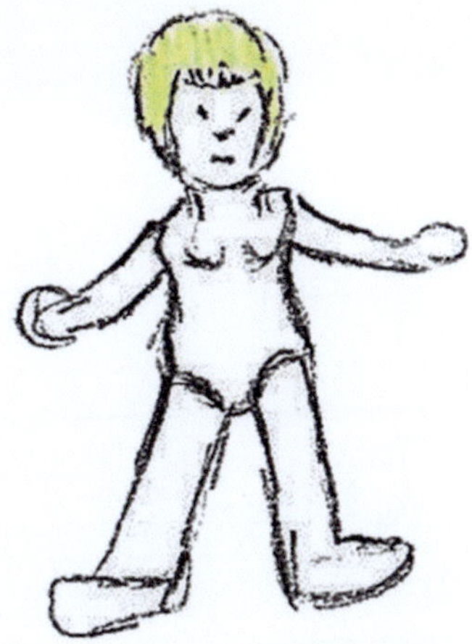

Fig. 18.3 Six-drawings test results for AR at baseline (before psychotherapy): Opposite-sex figure. In the original test the opposite-sex figure was much smaller and in the center of the sheet

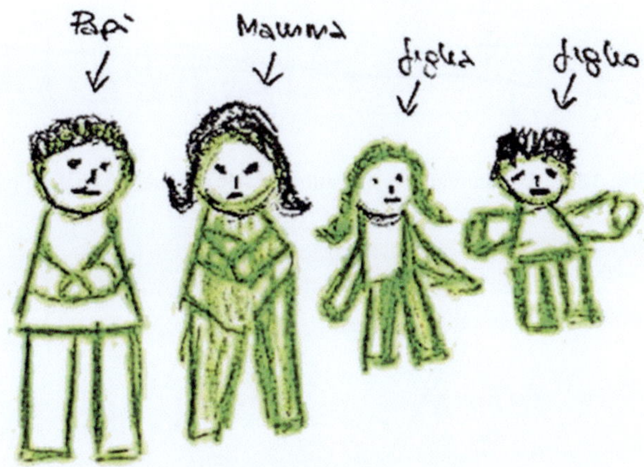

Fig. 18.4 Six-drawings test results for AR at baseline (before psychotherapy): Family. In the original test the family figure was much smaller and the shifted on the left side of the sheet

somewhat puppet-like, perhaps corresponding to a somewhat childlike personality. The drawing of the woman was similar (Fig. 18.3), potentially indicating that the patient had a somewhat immature relationship with his partner and/or remained fairly immature about sex/intimacy in general.

The patient's drawing of his/her family can help the therapist to evaluate the patient's main affective relationships and indicate his or her position and/or role in the family hierarchy [10, 11]. In AR's drawing, both the mother and father had folded arms, suggesting a lack of communication and/or closeness with each other and their children (Fig. 18.4). AR drew two children, a daughter and a son, which seemed odd, because in reality he had two daughters. The son might be indicative of an unfulfilled personal desire to have a son or might reflect an aborted son (see below).

The "present situation" drawing yields information about the patient's specific existential state, revealing both positives and negatives. It can also depict the main

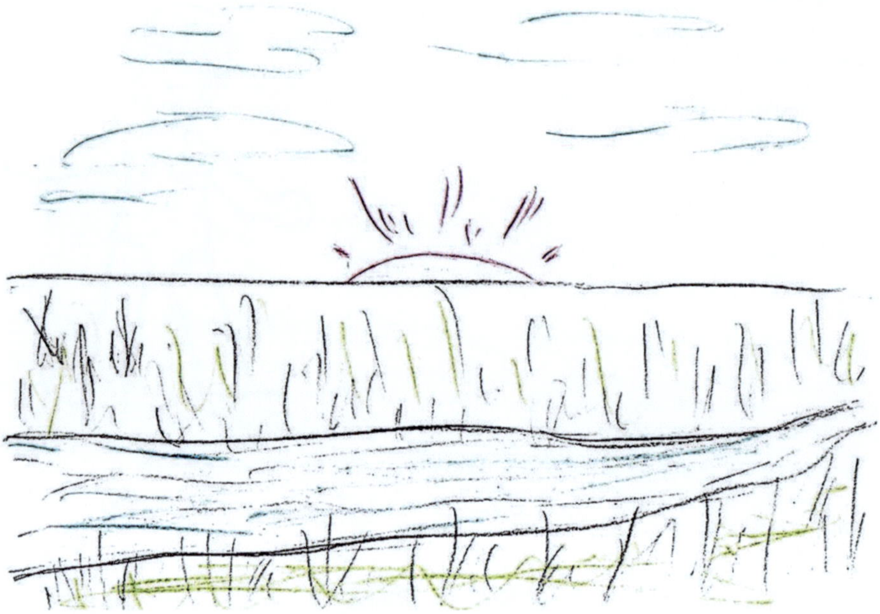

Fig. 18.5 Six-drawings test results for AR at baseline (before psychotherapy): Present situation

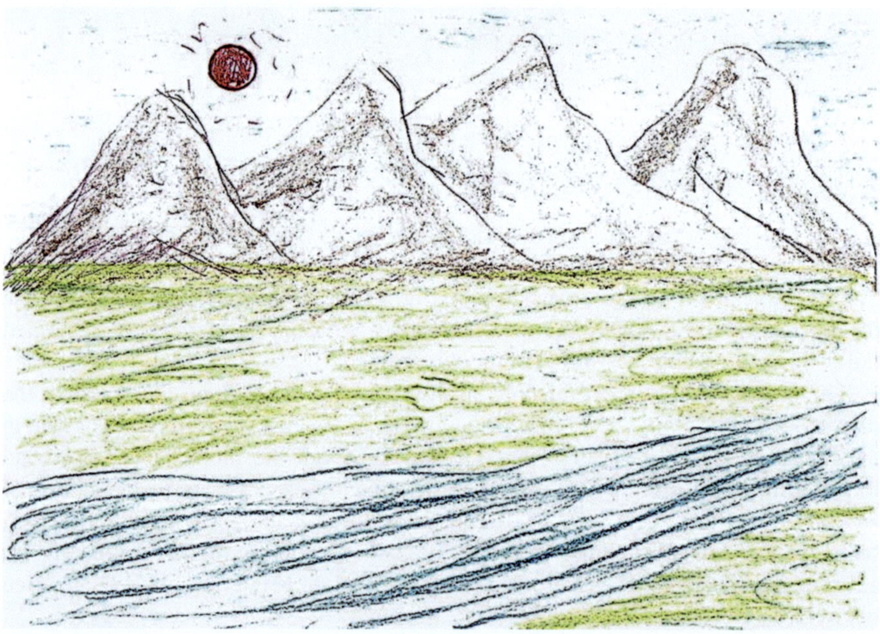

Fig. 18.6 Six-drawings test results for AR at baseline (before psychotherapy): Future life purpose or situation

problem or issue with which the patient is dealing, a problem or issue that could, over time, have led to or even precipitated his current as well as future medical and/or psychological dysfunction [10, 11]. For this drawing, AR painted a landscape with a black river (the color in the present reproduction might be slightly different than in the original) and a partial sun on the horizon (Fig. 18.5). A river usually represents someone's lifetime, and the river's characteristics indicate instinctual behavior [12]. The sun generally corresponds to a person's *In Self* and is typically a very positive symbol [12]. From an ontopsychological perspective, the *In Self* is the essence of one's unconscious, a person's innermost psychic project, and is the basis of every individual's psychological structure (see Chap. 13). In AR's drawing, the black river could be a projection of his health problem, which is now influencing the entire course (i.e., like a river's course) of his personal life. It might also be hypothesized that it represented the patient's unconscious projection of his diseased coronary artery. The sun, meanwhile is only partially depicted, suggesting that the patient's Ego, at that time, was quite distant from the interior positivity of his *In Self*.

The future purpose/future situation drawing can provide information on the person's fundamental life purpose, ambitions, and possible growth [10, 11]. AR drew a beautiful, sunny landscape, with a blue river, mountains, and a sun, which was complete in this scene (Fig. 18.6). This could reflect the patient's desire to overcome his psychological and physical problems and reintegrate himself into a full and rewarding personal life.

It is important to clarify that any hypothesis, which emerges from the preliminary analysis of such tests, must be always verified within the context of subsequent psychotherapeutic sessions.

18.3 Psychotherapy Sessions

After their first meeting, the psychotherapist and patient mutually agreed to begin psychotherapy sessions. The psychotherapy provided was based upon the ontopsychological method, specifically adapted to the context of Cardiac Psychology (for a detailed description of the psychotherapy administered, review Chap. 13).

During the first therapy session, AR seemed to be a good-hearted and helpful person. He said he appreciated being able to talk to someone, because this was the very first time he felt able to. His family was originally from Taranto, Italy. His grandfather initially emigrated to Egypt with the entire family, but then had to leave Egypt when AR was 3 years old. His older brother often recalled their life in Egypt, where they "*went to eat bananas*." His younger sister was born in Italy. AR had a good relationship with his parents, especially his mother, and both his brother and sister became quite jealous of this.

After AR's marriage, he and his wife lived near both his mother and his mother-in-law. This close proximity resulted in several sources of conflict, including conflicts between his wife and mother and between his wife's mother and sister.

AR's mother then died 4 years earlier from a stroke. AR claimed that he was not overly distraught at his mother's death, at any rate less than his brother and sister were. His mother-in-law also died a few years earlier. Antony and his wife had bought a plot of land from his mother-in-law without a bill of sale. After his mother-in-law's death, his wife's sister (AR's sister-in-law) refused to acknowledge the sale and "*dug in her heels*." Consequently, she sold the land to AR and his wife a second time. Later, AR and his wife built a house on the property, where he now was living with his family, as well as with his wife's aunt. One month before his acute myocardial infarction, AR started an unauthorized building modification to his house, which resulted in considerable difficulties with the surveyor and workers. This caused AR considerable stress.

At the end of the first session, the psychotherapist's impression was that whatever stress the patient had relating to his house modifications was only a small contributor to his overall distress. Basically, AR had been living in a highly matriarchal household (recall that both his children were female) and had become childishly dependent on it. This childish dependency resulted in a great personal loss of autonomy. The psychotherapist's analysis of nonverbal communication (i.e., physiognomy-kinetics and proxemics, and the patient's "semantic field"; for a definition of semantic field, see Chap. 13) confirmed the impression the therapist had gleaned from the patient's verbal story. In particular, AR seemed like a good-hearted and helpful person with no apparent aggressiveness or anger.

During the second session, AR spoke about the relationship he had with his wife. He had known her since he was 12 and she was 10, in primary school. They soon fell in love and started planning for their future as a couple. They were separated when AR left for military service, but resumed their relationship when he returned. AR claimed that his marriage was very good and that there were no problems. However, he also seemed very reluctant to delve deeper into his marriage, such that I, as the therapist, started to feel that, at some level, he was hiding something. At this point, I reviewed his family drawing with him and pointed out the lack of touching between the mother and father, as well as their folded arms. I explained that there seemed to be some sort of "disconnect" between the two. After I expressed my doubts, AR began to tell "*another story*."

His wife had had a very authoritative mother, so that she grew up fearful and had become quite closed-minded about many things. For example, she never used or allowed her husband to use any contraceptive method. For this reason, she ultimately had three procured abortions, one between the two daughters and two after the two daughters were born. She had undergone some psychotherapy, without any apparent benefit. Now the marital situation was somewhat improved, but AR and his wife virtually never had any intimate dialogue. On several occasions, AR tried to impose his directives on the family: "to *not have our children sleep in our bedroom and to make them play a sport, trying to help them avoid becoming as timorous as their mom, and to prevent their mom being like a broody hen*". He added: "*My wife really lives to suffer and my daughters are very spoiled children*."

At this point of psychotherapy, AR's story seemed complete enough to allow for a more accurate interpretation of his current psychological situation and state. It was possible for me to point out to him a third source of his distress: his marital relationship and difficulties dealing with his family. During subsequent sessions, we were able to begin working at a deeper level, thereby helping AR to start connecting with his unconscious dimension. In particular, it was possible to start his work analyzing and becoming more cognizant of his body's sensations and emotions. As explained in Chap. 13, "*a body sensation may express an emotional experience, and a dysfunctional somatic symptom may hide an inner conflict. In particular, the visceral zone seems to be an entry point for contacting emotions and instincts, which are expressions of the inner positive nucleus of unconscious, the In Self.*" During individual sessions, the psychotherapist gently invites the patient to pay attention to bodily sensations and emotions. Performing brief relaxation exercises, starting with abdominal breathing, helps patients to progressively attain fuller contact with their body, particularly their visceral zone. The body seems to be a conduit to the In-Self, and this passage immediately translates into a drop in psychic resistance. In fact, whereas AR failed to remember any dreams over his first four sessions, thereafter he started to do so. That he started to remember dreams indicated a real inner change. At this point, AR was deeply engaged in the psychotherapeutic process, as contact between his Ego and unconscious was reestablished. This is also proof that the psychotherapist had appropriately helped a patient to overcome his/her resistance and of the patient's acceptance of deeper introspection.

This was the dream AR described during his fifth session: "*I am going to a county fair with my wife. It is dark. Later my wife moves away from me onto a football pitch with a male doll*". This first dream is a clear projection of his marital relationship. "*I am going to a county fair with my wife. It is dark*"; that they are headed to a fair demonstrates their lack of any "authentic" relationship, and the darkness reveals their unhappiness. "*Later my wife moved away from me onto a football pitch with a male doll*"; this detail reveals his current situation with his wife, who is in fact playing with her femininity and motherhood (i.e., she is holding a doll like a little girl). The "*male doll*" also might have been reflected earlier in AR's 6DT family drawing, in which he did not draw the two daughters that he has, but a daughter and a son. As hypothesized earlier, the presence of a son in the drawing could reflect some inner desire AR has had to have a son or the loss of a son through abortion. In this setting, it was not possible to clarify what the drawn son actually represented, either with AR or his wife, who did not attend the one-on-one sessions.

During the seventh session, he spoke of the following dream: "*There is my brother, who is guiding me.*" (*Note that* AR described his brother as "*good and insecure*"). "*We enter a tunnel, which takes us into a castle. There are many meadows and green areas, but there's no way out. It leads always into a street, which ends in a ravine.*" In this dream, AR has delved into his early childhood, to the first relationships which structured his character, the basic structure of the "reflected matrix." The "reflected matrix" is defined by the ontopsychological school as "the codified base of specificity of complexes and stereotypes in the individual," which are the result of their very initial relationships in life, and will condition the individual's future psychological development [10, 13]. The brother in the dream may simultaneously represent AR's older brother and be a projection of his own personal characteristics (*good and insecure*). From an ontopsychological perspective, the castle represents the super-Ego related to the maternal relationship [12]. AR had developed, during his initial maternal and familial relationships, a dependent character; he was the "good baby" and "preferred child" of his mother (as he had already mentioned), but this form of relationship did not help him to grow into a responsible adult. This mode of relationships with other people and situations, which structured all his life, was going to be his ruination.

During the tenth session, he relayed this last dream: "*I am in a garage; there is a staircase, which leads down into the garage; the floor is covered with little stones and I have to shovel them all out. Directly outside the garage there is a street, which goes out from the garage. I have to tidy up the garage, so that water cannot enter it. In fact, the water flows out, without creating a marsh and without entering the garage*." This dream *again* confirms how AR had become deeply engaged in psychotherapeutic work and had started to really review his life. He is in the "*garage*" which is the deepest part of the house. The "*house*" may represent AR's existential space [12], and the deepest part of it is his projected representation of his unconscious. As such, AR is starting "*to tidy up the garage*"; that is to say that he is starting to put his personal life in order, beginning from his inner dimension "*so that water cannot go in*": in other words, so that familial relationships cannot invade his personal life again and overcome him. "*In fact, water flows out, without creating a marsh...*."

In all, AR attended ten individual and five group sessions. His wife took part in all the group sessions. Both were very enthusiastic about undertaking psychotherapy.

18.4 AR's Tests at the End of Psychotherapy

All psychometric tests were administered again 1 year after AR's enrollment visit, as established in the STEP-IN-AMI trial protocol.

AR's self-evaluation test score was four, a considerable reduction from his initial self-rated level of distress (baseline score = 8). His BDI score had similarly fallen, from a baseline score of eight to a follow-up score of two, demonstrating a marked reduction in any initial tendency he had toward depression. His MacNew Heart Disease Health-Related Quality of Life Questionnaire scores improved for all the domains. Specifically, his emotional score improved from its baseline 5.0 to 6.35, the physical score from 5.2 to 6.07, the social score from 5.0 to 6.15, and the global score from 5.1 to 6.19, indicating improved quality of life in all domains.

After the psychometric tests, the 6DT was administered (see Figs. 18.7, 18.8, 18.9, 18.10, 18.11, and 18.12 for AR's 1-year drawings). The tree drawing was larger and more robustly drawn than the first one, the tree occupying virtually the entire sheet of paper and being more artfully portrayed (Fig. 18.7). This could indicate an evolution and global, positive, harmonic reorganization of AR's

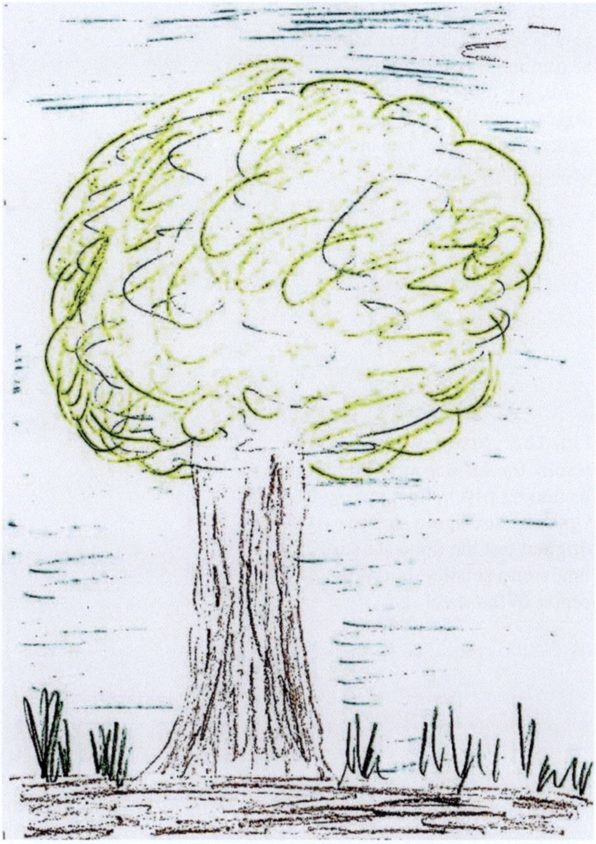

Fig. 18.7 Six drawings test results for AR one year after beginning psychotherapy: Tree

personality. This time, instead of a small, whole-body puppet-like drawing, the male figure drawing only included the head (Fig. 18.8) as did his drawing of a female (Fig. 18.9). At first glance, the absence of the body could be seen as a negative, but both faces are very expressive and they are no longer like little puppets. These two drawings could correspond to an expansion of his consciousness, and his increased capacity for personal introspection, and potentially to improved relations with his wife. The family drawing revealed a clear change in the family dynamics (Fig. 18.10), with the father and mother at the center, a child on each side, and all holding hands, providing evidence of renewed and much superior levels of communication.

For his present situation, AR drew a sunny landscape with a blue (instead of a black) river, a tree, and a full sun, all positive symbols of personal health and harmony (Fig. 18.11). Note especially how the sun is complete now, suggesting restored communication between the patient's Ego and In-Self.

For his future purpose/situation drawing, AR drew a beautiful seascape (Fig. 18.12). The sea is blue, but, strangely, the sky is cloudy and the sun broken by clouds. This image may indicate some doubt about AR's future evolution,

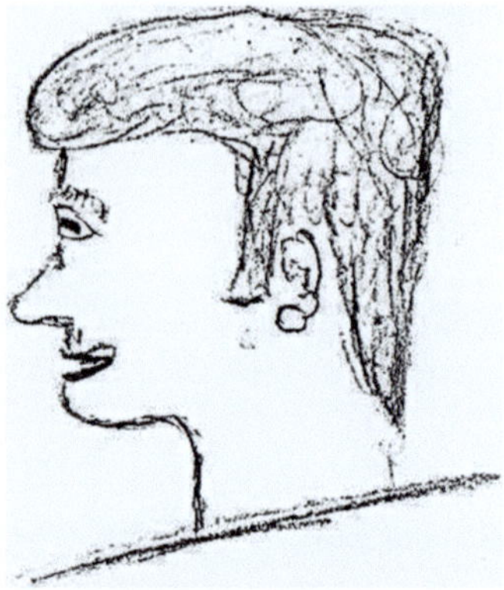

Fig. 18.8 Six-drawings test results for AR one year after beginning psychotherapy: Same-sex figure. In the original test the same-sex figure was smaller, but in the center of the sheet

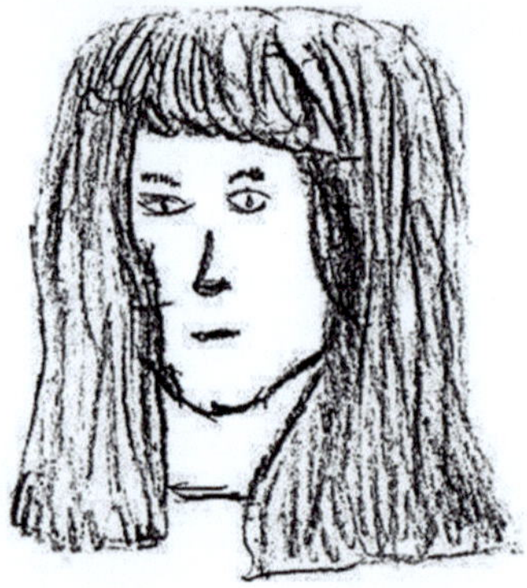

Fig. 18.9 Six-drawings test results for AR one year after beginning psychotherapy: Opposite-sex figure. In the original test the opposite-sex figure was smaller, but in the center of the sheet

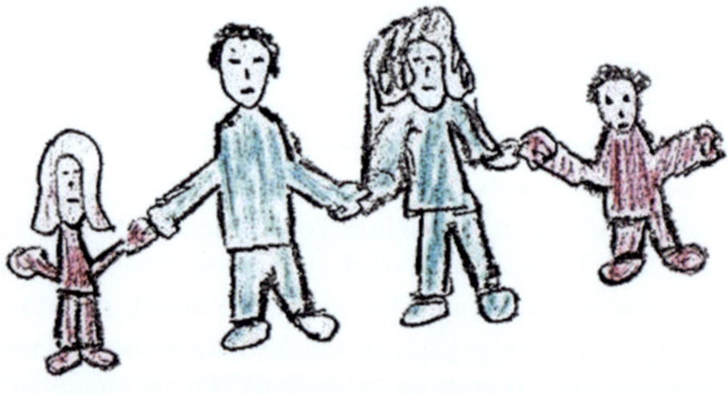

Fig. 18.10 Six-drawings test results for AR one year after beginning psychotherapy: Family. In the original test the family figure was smaller, but in the center of the sheet

appearing to depict future problems. Note, however, that AR had received only a short course of psychotherapy which, in my opinion, though efficacious, might only affect short-term improvements. To maintain personal physical and psychological equilibrium, it is advisable for each patient to thereafter partake of at least a brief course of psychological counseling on a yearly basis.

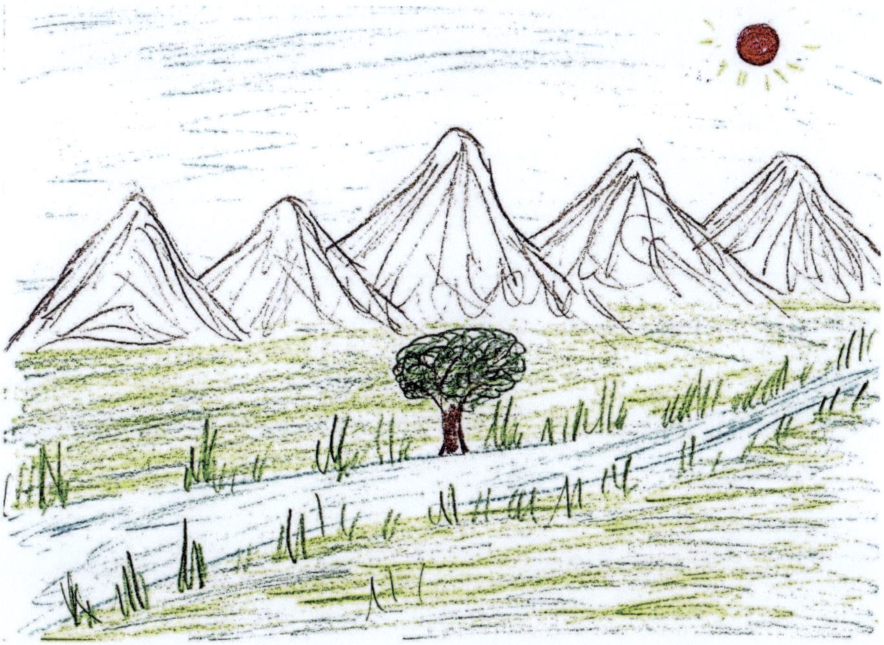

Fig. 18.11 Six-drawings test results for AR one year after beginning psychotherapy: Present situation

18.5 Medical and Cardiac Follow-up at 5 Years

Over the 5-year follow-up period, AR had no further cardiovascular events or new comorbidities. At the 1-year follow-up evaluation, he exhibited complete recovery of left ventricular function, the ejection fraction having increased from 40 % at baseline to 60 %.

18.6 The Future

Surely psychotherapy is neither divination nor magic. Nonetheless, looking at AR's last 6DT drawing, one might wonder what lies ahead for him. AR was not scheduled for further cardiac monitoring after completion of 5 years of follow-up, nor did he ask for monitoring within the hospital's Department of Cardiovascular Disease, where he had been treated and followed. The tenth year after the first acute myocardial infarction, he was admitted to our department for a second acute myocardial infarction, this time without ST elevation (NSTEMI). Coronary angiography, performed urgently, revealed patency of the stent that had been implanted in the left anterior coronary artery. However, there was critical stenosis in the

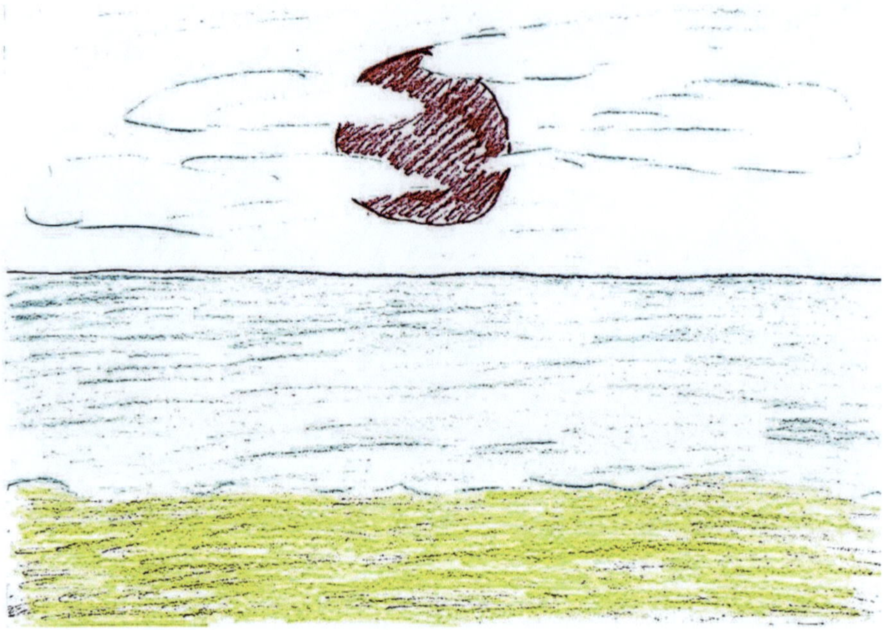

Fig. 18.12 Six-drawings test results for AR one year after beginning psychotherapy: Future life purpose or situation

second part of the right coronary artery. Consequently, a PCI was performed on the right coronary artery, during which a drug-eluting stent was implanted.

When I met with AR during his most recent hospitalization, I asked questions to determine his lifestyle over the last 5 years. He mentioned having completed a cardiovascular prevention program and having regular cardiac monitoring visits. His cholesterol and triglycerides were in the normal range and his arterial pressure was well controlled. He had not continued any psychological counseling after the study, because he believed that he had resolved all of his personal problems. It was not possible to further investigate this patient's personal situation at that time, so it is impossible to propose any hypotheses.

Outside of experienced psychotherapists, most would be surprised to discover as unconscious may speak about the whole situation of a human being, also if consciousness is not always able to grasp the psychobiological connections, which are preparing a new event in life, happy or sad, physical or psychological. Helping people to bring their unconscious drives to a conscious level can aid them to restore happiness and harmony in their life. The example presented in this chapter is clear evidence of this.

18.7 Conclusions

Our life is in continuous flux as we move from day to day and situation to situation. This requires our continuous ability to adapt in many complex ways, thereby influencing our physical health, psychological equilibrium, affectivity, social relationships, work commitments, physical environment, etc.

Ontopsychological psychotherapy might be considered a method that helps people to develop more complete awareness about their personal state, by learning how to interpret the continuous communication of their unconscious. This provides them with additional information in any situation and a greater capacity to cope with life's nonstop complexities. Our unconscious may guide us to seek out the best solution for each specific context. Continuously understanding and following the indications of our "unconscious intelligence" requires long-life learning and growth.

References

1. Roncella A, Giornetti A, Cianfrocca C et al (2009) Rationale and trial design of a randomized, controlled study on short-term psychotherapy after acute myocardial infarction: the STEP-IN-AMI trial (Short term psychotherapy in acute myocardial infarction). J Cardiovasc Med 10:947–952
2. Roncella A, Pristipino C, Cianfrocca C et al (2013) One-year results of the randomized, controlled, short-term psychotherapy in acute myocardial infarction (STEP-IN-AMI) trial. Int J Cardiol 170(2):132–139. doi:10.1016/j.ijcard.2013.08.094
3. Pignalberi C, Patti G, Chimenti C, Maseri A (1998) Role of different determinants of psychological distress in acute coronary syndromes. J Am Coll Cardiol 32:613–619
4. Apples A, Hoppener P, Mulder P (1987) A questionnaire to assess premonitory symptoms of myocardial infarction. Int J Cardiol 17(1):15–24
5. Choen S, Syme SL (1985) Social support and health. Academic Press/Orlando University, Orlando
6. Holmes TH, Rahe RH (1967) The social readjustment rating scale. J Psychosom Res 11:213–218
7. Beck AT, Ward CH, Meldelson M, Mock J, Erbaurgh J (1961) An inventory for measuring depression. Arch Gen Psychiatry 4:561–571
8. Beck AT, Kovacs M, Weissman A (1979) Assessment of suicidal intention: the scale for suicide ideation. J Consult Clin Psychol 47:343–352
9. Hofer S, Lim LL, Guyatt GH, Oldridge NB (2004) The MacNew heart disease health related quality of life instrument: a summary. Health Qual Life Outcomes. doi:10.1186/1477-7525-2-3
10. Meneghetti A (Eng ed 2004; It ed 1995–2008) Ontopsychology handbook. Ontopsicologia Editrice, Roma
11. Meneghetti A (1994–2003) L'Immagine e l'Inconscio. Ontopsicolologia Editrice, Roma
12. Meneghetti A (1981–2012) Prontuario onirico. Ontopsicologia Editrice, Roma
13. Meneghetti A (Eng ed 1988–2004; It ed 1987–2001) Dictionary of ontopsychology. Ontopsicologia Editrice, Roma

Psychotherapy for Cardiac Patients: Selection of Clinical Cases. Part II

19

Marinella Sommaruga and Antonia Pierobon

Symptoms of illness and distress, plus your feelings about them, can be viewed as messengers coming to tell you something important about your body or about your mind.
Jon Kabat-Zinn (Jon Kabat-Zinn (1990) Full Catastrophe Living: Using the Wisdom of Your Body and Mind to Face Stress, Pain, and Illness)

19.1 Introduction

Our model of psychotherapy covers a process of assessment, intervention, and follow-up, as mentioned in Chap. 11 and 22 and Fig. 22.1).

During the assessment process, after the first interview, the psychologist decides if any psychometric screening (Appendix 1) or further psycho-diagnostic evaluation is necessary. Then he/she chooses the specific tailored intervention for that particular patient.

The context of psychotherapy is cardiac rehabilitation, which entails individualized physical training, nutrition monitoring, psychological assessment, and psychotherapeutic interventions, as indicated (Appendix 2) [1–3].

Psychosocial screening reliably identifies the problematic macro-categories, especially if they are characterized by behavioral indicators, which facilitate detection. The psychological approach appears more suitable for better specifying

M. Sommaruga, PsyD (✉)
Clinical Psychology and Social Support Unit, Salvatore Maugeri Foundation, Care and Research Institute, Via Camaldoli 64, 20138 Milan, Italy
e-mail: marinella.sommaruga@fsm.it

A. Pierobon, PsyD
Psychology Unit, Salvatore Maugeri Foundation, Care and Research Institute, Via per Montescano, 27040 Pavia, Italy
e-mail: antonia.pierobon@fsm.it

A. Roncella, C. Pristipino (eds.), *Psychotherapy for Ischemic Heart Disease*,
DOI 10.1007/978-3-319-33214-7_19

macro-category characteristics, and for detecting less overt but still critical aspects of distress, thereby providing advice for and therapeutic management of any psychopathology. This may facilitate synergistic teamwork to address common priorities that respect both the point of view of the patient and clinical-rehabilitation purposes.

Each of the following two sections describes a typical clinical case involving a patient with ischemic heart disease treated in the cardiac rehabilitation ward.

19.2 Clinical Case 1: Mr. F. (Anxiety and Family Problems)

Mr. F. was a married sixty-one-year-old man with two adult married sons. He was working as a plumber with a demanding, high-paced time schedule and heavy workload. He had presented to the unit one year earlier for regular follow-up after a myocardial infarction. The patient was of normal weight (BMI = 23), but tended toward being hyperglycemic on a noncontrolled diet (fasting serum glucose = 120 mg/dl). Both his total and LDL cholesterol levels were elevated (total cholesterol = 230 mg/dl; LDL cholesterol = 150 mg/dl).

During *psychosocial screening,* performed during the first outpatient visit and involving the following tests—PCS, ASiHD, and HADS (described in Appendix 1)—the need for a full psychological interview became apparent. In fact, according to his Hospital Anxiety and Depression Scale (HADS) scores, Mr. F. suffered from high-level anxiety (HAD anxiety score: 14/21) and was near the threshold for borderline depression (7/21). Moreover, according to his ASiHD responses, a low level of perceived self-efficacy in behavioral adherence was evident, even though he appeared to have an appropriate level of illness perception and knowledge (see Fig. 19.1) [4–6].

During the *psychological interview*, the patient confirmed the low levels of adherence detected during screening. He admitted to not taking his medication punctually, not engaging in adequate physical exercise, not regularly following dietary prescriptions, and not being able to suitably manage stressful situations, despite his current heavy workloads. He expressed good knowledge of the cardiovascular risks that his severe lack of adherence to medication and lifestyle change recommendations subjected him to, and made no attempts to either minimize or deny his wrongful behavior. His high anxiety level appeared not to be a personality trait, but a conditioned reaction to family difficulties.

During the *psychological intervention*, Mr. F. claimed that he was "forced to work" as a result of debts contracted by his two sons and that, if it was not for his sense of duty, he would stop working and live on his annuities and other economic returns. However, he also strongly defended his moral responsibility to help his sons, even if both of them were adults and the resulting workload for him was beyond the safe limits of his clinical condition. His stress was worsened further by his deteriorating relationship with his sons, as well as their apparent ingratitude. It often happened that Mr. F. skipped meals to see clients, and this caused him to alter the timing of his drug doses. And even though Mr. F. appeared to be quite aware

QUESTIONS	ANSWERS
1. Do you accept your current state of health?	_ Not at all _A little ■Enough _Much _Very much
2. Do you accept the limitations related to your current state of health?	_ Not at all ■A little _Enough _Much _Very much
3. Does your family, friends and/or other people you know help you manage your current state of health?	_ Not at all _A little ■Enough _Much _Very much
4a. When you are at home, do you manage to take medicines punctually?	_ Not at all ■A little _Enough _Much _Very much
4b. When you are at home, do you manage to follow dietary prescriptions?	_ Not at all ■A little _Enough _Much _Very much
4c. When you are at home, do you manage to avoid smoking (if pertinent)?	_ Not at all _A little _Enough _Much ■Very much
4d. When you are at home, do you manage to control (moderate or eliminate) alcohol drinking (beer, wine, spirits)?	_ Not at all _A little _Enough _Much ■Very much
4e. When you are at home, do you manage to exercise following medical advice?	_ Not at all ■A little _Enough _Much _Very much
4f. When you are at home, do you manage to identify physical/psychological fatigue signs?	_ Not at all _A little _Enough ■Much _Very much
4g. When you are at home, do you manage to reduce stress sources?	■Not at all _A little _Enough _Much _Very much
4h. When you are at home, do you manage to control stressful situations?	_ Not at all ■A little _Enough _Much _Very much
4i. When you are at home, do you measure some clinical factors regularly (e.g., weight, blood pressure, heart rate, blood exams, amount of urine) as the doctors have asked you to do?	_ Not at all _A little _Enough ■Much _Very much

FONDAZIONE SALVATORE MAUGERI
CLINICA DEL LAVORO E DELLA RIABILITAZIONE
I.R.C.C.S.

ISTITUTO SCIENTIFICO DI MONTESCANO – 27040 Montescano (PV)

Fig. 19.1 ASiHD for clinical case 1 at time 0 (enrollment). Translated and adapted from Majani et al. (2007). ASiHD-R: Adherence Schedule in Heart Disease—Brief. These questions are about your state of health and treatment. There are no right or wrong answers. When responding, refer only to what you think about your state of health and what you think you are able to do to help yourself. Please put a cross by the answer you want to give. Clinical take-home message: From this schedule, we can illuminate difficulties pertaining to a patient's limitations and disease acceptance and low levels of behavioral adherence related to taking medicines, following dietary recommendations, exercising, and controlling stress at home

about the increased cardiac risk of his overextended lifestyle, he nonetheless felt as if he was stuck in a life that he could not change.

Starting with the therapist's suggestion that Mr. F. try to change at least one aspect of his life to start, the psychological work that was done reinforced his sense of self-value, efficacy, and work competence. He came to acknowledge that he could ask his clients to be more flexible when he scheduled appointments for them. Consequently, two adherence behaviors were modified in a positive way: the timing of his medications and his eating habits.

As to his family situation, he explained that the economic help that he was providing to his sons, completely supported by his wife, stemmed from the necessity to protect his preschool and school-age grandchildren from their fathers' bankruptcy. Therefore, during the therapeutic intervention, the patient's anxiety was explained and emotionally validated.

The intervention included five psychotherapy sessions. Each session focused on a different topic (Appendix 2) and was accompanied by relevant homework tasks. Mr. F. was invited to observe and record his stress behavior patterns over a whole week. At the beginning of each session, homework from the previous session was reviewed. In one of the exercises, the patient was asked to describe a situation that had provoked anxiety, and he did so. His stressful responses were then pinpointed and discussed. Cognitive-behavioral strategies were used in an attempt to alter his stress responses. In another exercise, behavioral strategies for problem solving were used in situations that were both perceived and described as threatening. The actual problem was observed, discussed, and reformulated by the patient.

One year later, the patient was clinically stable and his blood tests had improved (fasting serum glucose = 100 mg/dl; total cholesterol = 200 mg/dl; LDL cholesterol = 115 mg/dl). A *psychometric evaluation after one year* revealed a reduction in his perceived anxiety and depression symptoms (HADS scores = 10/21 for anxiety, 5/21 for depression) and an improvement in his behavioral adherence on the ASiHD scale (Fig. 19.2). In the end, Mr. F. was given the option of continuing on in the Psychology Unit for further sessions to further improve his illness management skills and maintain all the other progress he had made.

19.3 Clinical Case 2: Mr. B. (Depression and Work Stress)

Mr. B. was a fifty-six-year-old man who was married and had one adult daughter living with him and his wife. His job involved heavy manual labor. He also had been physically assaulted about four years earlier. He was a former smoker and had hypercholesterolemia. Five years previously, he suffered a heart attack and underwent coronary artery bypass. At the time of current presentation, he was hospitalized for a functional assessment and entry into a rehabilitation program following the onset of dyspnea over recent months. On admission, he appeared physically stable and remained so throughout the remainder of his hospital stay.

His initial inpatient *psychological and psychometric assessments* revealed several symptoms of anxiety and depression (HADS scores = 18/21 for anxiety, 18/21

QUESTIONS	ANSWERS
1. Do you accept your current state of health?	_ Not at all _A little ■Enough_ _Much _Very much
2. Do you accept the limitations related to your current state of health?	_ Not at all _A little ■Enough _Much _Very much
3. Does your family, friends and/or other people you know help you manage your current state of health?	_ Not at all _A little ■Enough _Much _Very much
4a. When you are at home, do you manage to take medicines punctually?	_ Not at all _A little _Enough ■Much _Very much
4b. When you are at home, do you manage to follow dietary prescriptions?	_ Not at all _A little ■Enough _Much _Very much
4c. When you are at home, do you manage to avoid smoking (if pertinent)?	_ Not at all _A little _Enough _Much ■Very much
4d. When you are at home, do you manage to control (moderate or eliminate) alcohol drinking (beer, wine, spirits)?	_ Not at all _A little _Enough _Much ■Very much
4e. When you are at home, do you manage to exercise following medical advice?	_ Not at all _A little ■Enough _Much _Very much
4f. When you are at home, do you manage to identify physical/psychological fatigue signs?	_ Not at all _A little _Enough ■Much _Very much
4g. When you are at home, do you manage to reduce stress sources?	_ Not at all ■A little _Enough _Much _Very much
4h. When you are at home, do you manage to control stressful situations?	_ Not at all ■A little _Enough _Much _Very much
4i. When you are at home do you measure some clinical factors regularly (e.g. weight, blood pressure, heart rate, blood exams, amount of urine) as the doctors have asked you to do?	_ Not at all _A little _Enough ■Much _Very much

FONDAZIONE SALVATORE MAUGERI
CLINICA DEL LAVORO E DELLA RIABILITAZIONE
I.R.C.C.S.

ISTITUTO SCIENTIFICO DI MONTESCANO – 27040 Montescano (PV)

Fig. 19.2 ASiHD of clinical case 1 at time 1 (1-year follow-up). Translated and adapted from Majani et al. (2007). ASiHD-R: Adherence Schedule in Heart Disease—Brief. These questions are about your state of health and treatment. There are no right or wrong answers. When responding, refer only to what you think about your state of health and what you think you are able to do to help yourself. Please put a cross by the answer you want to give. Clinical take-home message: From this schedule, we can illuminate difficulties pertaining to a patient's limitations and disease acceptance and low levels of behavioral adherence related to taking medicines, following dietary recommendations, exercising, and controlling stress at home

for depression), tendencies to experience negative emotions over time and to inhibit emotions and behaviors during social interactions, and characteristics consistent with a Type D personality (DS14 scores = 12/28 for affective negativity and 20/28 for social inhibition). Such symptoms were found to be associated with work-related stress, which is considered to be a risk factor for cardiovascular disease. The assessment also revealed that he possessed adequate knowledge and discrete awareness of his disease, especially in relation to physical effort. Discrete internal resources and family support, perceived as adequate for providing emotional and real support, were detected. Interviews with family members were also conducted, to better understand the patient's social support. Many depressive symptoms, including the onset of suicidal ideations as a result of a worsening employment situation, were detected. This dire psychological state warranted urgent pharmacological treatment, an urgent psychiatric assessment, and continued psychological support and monitoring [6–10].

A five-session individual psychological intervention was initiated. It included emotional counseling and cognitive-emotional-behavioral restructuring to especially reformulate his negative thinking and poor motivation for self-care.

During his hospital stay, Mr. B. also participated in six group sessions on health education, the main goals of which were to provide information, advice, and strategies to promote adequate management of risk factors and facilitate his reintegration into daily life.

At discharge, his *psychological and psychometric evaluation* demonstrated a slight reduction in both his anxiety and depressive symptoms (HADS scores = 14/21 for anxiety, 12/21 for depression). Moreover, he reported an increased sense of well-being. There also was an improvement in his functional status, documented as an increase in his walking test distance from 380 to 471 m, in the absence of any symptoms or major complications.

After discharge from the hospital, he participated in *ten cognitive-behavioral restructuring sessions* (once weekly for ten weeks) focusing primarily on stress management, modified eating habits, and improvements in his continued negative ideations and poor self-care motivation.

In the individual sessions, daily conflict situations were discussed. Mr. B. was introduced to various examples of situational conflict and asked to deal with them. True examples from the patient's own daily life were used, as well as fictional scenarios. He was informed that describing one's strengths at work and how this strength becomes visible within professional life is an important exercise. An exercise book with daily, concrete cognitive exercises, recognizing positive and negative emotions, was started and maintained throughout his period of rehabilitation.

Another goal was to have the patient characterize his own life situation. To do this, he was instructed to ask himself the following questions: "What is my life like now?" "How would I like it to be?" "How do I divide my time between work, leisure, friends, and family?" "What would I like this distribution of time to be?" "How much time do I save for myself?" "What is a good balance between these different life domains?"

Besides Mr. B. received ten sessions of progressive muscle relaxation training, with good results.

Educational materials on eating behaviors and stress management were also provided. The patient was handed a compact disc to allow him to continue to do his relaxation exercises at home. He also was instructed to try practicing relaxed behaviors at home, like walking slowly and purposely choosing the longest queue at the grocery store.

During this period, he was observed to develop enhanced disease awareness and improved internal resources to cope with problematic situations and objective difficulties at his workplace. During therapy sessions, an improved psychological state was observed, but it worsened again as he approached discharge, given persistent objective difficulties in the workplace.

His one-year *psychological and psychometric evaluation* revealed reduced perceived anxiety and depressive symptoms (HADS scores 9/21 for anxiety, 9/21 for depression).

Then, at three years of follow-up while participating in a further rehabilitation program, the patient exhibited further marked increases in well-being with HADS anxiety and depression scores of 0/21 and 3/21, respectively, following the resolution of his workplace difficulties. He also exhibited further improved functional status, documented as an increased walking test distance from 435 to 495 m, again in the absence of any symptoms or complications.

Appendix 1: Description of Psychometric Tools

- The *Psycho-Cardiological Schedule* (PCS) [5] was developed to detect critical behavioral cardiovascular risk factors or the presence of psychological, social, and cognitive problems. Administered by a nurse or cardiologist, in collaboration with a psychologist, the PCS identifies a patient's need for a more thorough psychological examination, whether that be clinical, via formalized psychometric testing, or both.
- The *Adherence Schedule in Ischemic Heart Disease* (ASiHD) [6] is one disease-specific tool among a group of Adherence Schedules for chronic diseases. The ASiHD was specifically designed to evaluate the cognitive, relational, and behavioral antecedents of adherence to treatment among patients suffering from coronary artery disease. It provides a useful synthetic schedule of psychological/behavioral variables that might influence perceived self-efficacy in disease management.
- The Hospital Anxiety Depression Scale (HADS) [6] is a 14-item questionnaire that identifies and rates the severity of a person's symptoms of anxiety (HADS-A) and depression (HADS-D). Response options range from 0 (no problems) to 3 (maximum distress), and each scale has set summation thresholds that indicate normalcy (summation score 0–7), borderline anxiety or depression (8–10), or likely pathology (summation score ≥ 11).

- The *DS 14 Distress Scale* [7–9] is a 14-item scale designed to identify Type D personality (DS14). It is comprised of two subscales: negative affectivity (NA) and social inhibition (SI), each containing seven items. Each item is answered on a five-point Likert scale that ranges from 0 (false) to 4 (true). A predetermined cutoff (9, in the Italian version) on both subscales is used to identify individuals with a Type D personality. The Type D (distressed) personality construct is characterized by a high score on two stable personality traits: NA and SI, the former denoting the patient's tendency to experience negative emotions across time and situations (individuals high for this trait tend to scan the world around them for signs of impending trouble) and the latter referring to the patient's tendency to inhibit the expression of these negative emotions during social interactions.

Appendix 2: Psychological Assessment and Psychotherapeutic Intervention

Areas of Psychological Assessment

- Baseline psychological characteristics of the individual: worry, depression, anxiety, low spiritedness, Type D behavior.
- Cognitive-behavioral styles (coping skills).
- Perception of the illness and consequent reactions: behavior relating to the prevention of coronary risk factors and psychological consequences related to the cardiac event.
- Levels of cognitive processing, emotional acceptance, and behavioral adaptation to the disease: psychosocial stress and physiological stress reactions, anger and hostility in response to daily stress exposure, problem-solving and cognitive strategies, coronary-prone stress behavior. Reviewing and testing patients' individual stress behaviors.
- Motivation for rehabilitation, treatment adherence, and lifestyle changes.
- Expectations regarding functional recovery.

Psychotherapeutic Intervention Strategies

Cognitive Level

- Reprocessing the perception of self (person-patient-person).
- Correcting erroneous processes of causal attribution and dysfunctional cognitive processing of the illness.
- Correcting inappropriate expectations regarding functional recovery.
- Identifying and strengthening cognitive resources and coping skills.
- Identifying positive interpretations of the illness.

Emotional Level

- Optimizing the recognition of psychophysiological signs.
- Facilitating the recognition of emotions and "giving them a name."
- Legitimizing emotional reactions to the disease.
- Helping to manifest emotions.
- Favoring and safeguarding gratifying interpersonal relationships and personal recreation.

Behavioral Level

- Correcting risk factors.
- Identifying and developing non-dysfunctional behavioral strategies.
- Being motivated to ask for help from supportive people, groups, or organizations; strengthening adaptive behaviors aimed at disease self-management.

References

1. Sommaruga M, Tramarin R, Angelino E, Task Force per le Attività di Psicologia in Cardiologia Riabilitativa e Preventiva, Gruppo Italiano di Cardiologia Riabilitativa e Preventiva et al (2003) Guidelines for psychology activities in cardiologic rehabilitation and prevention. Monaldi Arch Chest Dis 60(3):184–234
2. Griffo R, Urbinati S, Giannuzzi P et al (2008) Italian guidelines on cardiac rehabilitation and secondary prevention of cardiovascular disease: executive summary. G Ital Cardiol 9 (4):286–297
3. Pierobon A, Giardini A, Callegari S, Majani G (2011) Psychological adjustment to a chronic illness: the contribution from cognitive behavioural treatment in a rehabilitation setting. G Ital Med Lav Ergon 33(1 Suppl A):A11–A18
4. Majani G, Pierobon A, Giardini A, Callegari S (2007) Valutare e favorire l'aderenza alle prescrizioni in riabilitazione cardiologica e pneumologica. Pime Editrice, Pavia, pp 92–117
5. Pierobon A, Callegari S, Giardini A et al (2012) Presentation of the psycho-cardiological schedule and convergence levels analyses among the psycho-cardiological screening and the psychological assessment. Monaldi Arch Chest Dis 78(2):89–96
6. Costantini M, Musso M, Viterbori P et al (1999) Detecting psychological distress in cancer patients: validity of the Italian version of the hospital anxiety and depression scale. Support Care Cancer 7(3):121–127
7. Denollet J (2005) DS14: standard assessment of negative affectivity, social inhibition, and Type D personality. Psychosom Med 67:89–97
8. Gremigni P, Sommaruga M (2005) Personalità di Tipo D, un costrutto rilevante in cardiologia. Studio preliminare di validazione del questionario italiano. Psicoterapia Cogn Comp 11:7–18
9. Schiffer AA, Pavan A, Pedersen SS et al (2006) Type D personality and cardiovascular disease: evidence and clinical implications. Minerva Psichiatr 47:79–87
10. Sommaruga M, Della Porta P (2103) La patologia somatica: l'esempio delle malattie cardiovascolari. In: Ricci Bitti PE, Gremigni P (eds) Psicologia della salute, Modelli teorici e contesti applicativi. Carocci editore, Roma

A Model Integrating Psychotherapy into Medical Practices at San Filippo Neri Hospital in Rome, Italy

20

Adriana Roncella, Christian Pristipino, Vincenzo Pasceri, Silvia Scorza, Marinella Spaziani, and Giulio Speciale

> *. . .Molly was interested in the relationship between microbes and disease, in electricity as a treatment, in English doctors' practices. "It is good medicine," she said, "but it leaves dreams sick."*
>
> Wu Ming (Authors' translation from the Italian version: "Molly si interessava al legame tra microbi e malattia, all'elettricità come cura, alle pratiche dei dottori inglesi,'E' una buona medicina,- diceva,- ma lascia ammalati i sogni'". Wu Ming (2007, 2009). Manituana. Einaudi, Torino)

20.1 Introduction

Reading the novel "Manituana," one might be struck by a particular sentence that reads: "*It is good medicine. . .. but it leaves dreams sick*". One can borrow this sentence to describe the general formulation of modern medicine, which tries to take care of all the biological components of illness, often achieving good medical results, but often at most making the patient feel comfortable. This is because medical diagnostics and treatment often ignore the sick person's inner self, including his suffering, emotions, love and hate, and even his dreams, all of which can profoundly affect his biological and medical history and course (also see Chap. 1). An ill person's unconscious dimension expresses itself in many ways, and dreams are one of them. Ignoring the unconscious dimension means that the core of the suffering inner self remains untouched, continuing to adversely act out against the

A. Roncella, MD (✉) • C. Pristipino, MD • V. Pasceri, MD • S. Scorza, PsyD • M. Spaziani • G. Speciale, MD
Department of Cardiovascular Disease, San Filippo Neri Hospital, Via G. Martinotti 20, 00135 Rome, Italy
e-mail: adrianaroncella@hotmail.it; pristipino.c@gmail.com; vpasceri@gmail.com; silviascorza@libero.it; marinellaspaziani@hotmail.com; giuliospeciale@yahoo.it

A. Roncella, C. Pristipino (eds.), *Psychotherapy for Ischemic Heart Disease*,
DOI 10.1007/978-3-319-33214-7_20

person's linked psycho-emotional and biological dimensions, thereby perpetuating the vicious circle of disease.

Neglecting this aspect appears even more inappropriate when we consider that this qualitative and very vast inner world profoundly influences the biological dimension in a complex loop, where cause and effects form a unity of process and become tightly enmeshed and indistinguishable (see Chap. 1). Luckily, a huge quantity of research is currently being conducted in the fields of biology, medicine, psychology, epistemology, sociology, and ecology, all striving toward a contemporary, evidence-based integration of quantitative and qualitative practices [1–4] (also see Chap. 7).

At San Filippo Neri Hospital, on the basis of both the good results observed on 1-year follow-up in the STEP-IN-AMI trial [5, 6] involving medical, cardiac, and psychological endpoints, an outpatient Cardiac Psychology clinic has been created [7, 8], which is directly connected to the outpatient department of the Interventional Cardiology Unit. This unique and innovative concept was born out of the frequent, spontaneous requests of many patients admitted to the cardiovascular department for various clinical reasons. Indeed, the patients themselves often spontaneously mention stress and/or depression as either a cause or effect of their hospitalization and that they cannot envision ever returning to healthy personal, social, and working life without the help of a professional.

20.2 The Outpatient Cardiac Psychology Clinic

In actuality, the outpatient Cardiac Psychology clinic is dedicated both to clinical psychotherapy and to research on the role of psychosocial risk factors in cardiac diseases. Patients enrolled for clinical psychotherapy have generally been previously admitted to the cardiovascular department and referred for either depressive and/or anxiety symptoms. Patients can also be referred directly by any General Practitioner, who suspects some form of psychological disorder in a heart disease patient. Whereas enrollment in the STEP-IN-AMI trial has been limited to patients with acute myocardial infarction, patients admitted to the Cardiac Psychology outpatient clinic encompass all forms of ischemic heart disease (also see Chap. 1). This includes acute myocardial infarction with its disparate mechanisms, stable or unstable angina, treated or not treated with a percutaneous coronary intervention (PCI) or coronary artery bypass procedure, as well as patients with cardiac arrhythmias and/or chronic post-ischemic ventricular dysfunction.

Many of these patients present with highly complex clinical situations, including advanced and/or multiple comorbid conditions, which may share pathophysiological pathways with ischemic heart disease (e.g., diabetes mellitus, renal failure, chronic inflammatory disease, etc.).

Psychotherapy must be considered an adjunct to optimal medical and interventional therapy and can be applied only after appropriate and comprehensive secondary prevention measures have been put into place (e.g., lifestyle changes and the correction of modifiable biomedical risk factors). Only in this comprehensive way, embracing both the biological and mental dimensions, can psychological interventions be effective at improving cardiac and other medical outcomes, as well as the patient's psychological discomfort and quality of life, and promoting faster reintegration into family, social, and working life.

The Cardiac Psychology outpatient clinic is open 2 days per week. Its team is composed of three psychotherapists (two of them independent) and one nurse, all working in collaboration with cardiologists in the Department of Cardiovascular Disease.

Since the beginning of 2004, about 800 patients have been enrolled either for research or clinical purposes, and roughly 10,000 sessions scheduled, both individual and group.

Currently, three Italian congresses on "psychosocial risk factors in ischemic heart disease" have been organized, all in Rome, two in collaboration with the Italian Society of Psycho-neuro-endocrino-immunology (SIPNEI). These three congresses are as follows: (1) Psychosocial Risk Factors and Ischemic Heart Disease, January 2010, San Filippo Neri Hospital; (2) Psyche and Heart. Cardiology meets PNEI. November 2011, San Filippo Neri Hospital; and (3) Psyche and Heart. Cardiology meets PNEI, 2nd Session, January 2013, Hotel Marriott, Rome.

Whereas patients enrolled in research have generally been followed for between 1 and 5 years, depending on the study protocol, those referred to the outpatient clinic for treatment only are systematically evaluated until they complete their psychotherapy sessions, which generally last 6 months.

After the first visit, a patient who expresses a need for psychological support is accepted by the psychotherapist, who tries to explore the specific needs of the patient, as well as his or her desire and willingness to participate in either individual or group psychotherapy, or both, on a weekly basis. Very old or frail patients must be assessed to determine whether they can attend sessions on their own or accompanied by a relative.

After a mutual agreement has been reached as to the nature and length of therapy, all the patient's medical and cardiac data are collected into a folder by the cardiologist. In the same personalized folder, the psychotherapist collects all data related to the patient's personal history. In particular, the following data are requested: patient's place and date of birth; details about both parents (if they are living or dead; their actual age, or age of death; cause of death; previous and/or actual job); number of brothers and sisters, including birth order; patient's education; patient's previous and actual occupation; patient's marital status and age when married; current age of the partner and his/her name, education, and occupation; number of children and their ages, names, education levels, and occupations; favorite personal hobbies; and any other relationships or information about personal life that the patient feels is relevant.

After all relevant patient data are collected, psychometric tests and a projective test are administered to obtain a more comprehensive picture of the patient's current psychological state. The patient may be asked to complete these tests at home.

The psychometric tests currently used in our Cardiac Psychology clinic were selected from those that were statistically sensitive to change with treatment in the STEP-IN-AMI trial [5, 6]. These include as follows: (1) Self-evaluation test, assessing global level of psychological distress over the preceding 2 weeks [9]; (2) Social Support Questionnaire, evaluating each individual's perception of his/her social network [10, 11]; (3) Beck Depression Inventory (BDI), evaluating for symptoms of major or minor depression [12, 13], where a score between 10 and 15 is considered indicative of mild depression, and a score equal or superior to 16 is considered indicative of clinically relevant depression; and (4) The MacNew Heart Disease Health-Related Quality of Life Questionnaire, assessing the patient's quality of life across three specific domains—emotional, physical, and social—and providing a global QOL score [14]. In a subset of patients, the Type D Scale (DS14), assessing whether a patient has a type D personality, is added [15, 16].

Given frequent mention by some patients of anxiety and anger, recently two psychometric tests were added that explore these two characteristics: the State-Trait Anxiety Inventory (STAI) [17] and the State-Trait Anger Expression Inventory (STAXI 2) [18].

Also added is a projective test, the "Six-Drawings Test" (SDT), which is now being utilized for the first time, to our knowledge, in cardiac patients (see Chap. 15). It is one of the psycho-diagnostic instruments used in the ontopsychological clinical method [19, 20] and has been used in the STEP-IN-AMI trial (results not yet published).

Both the psychometric and projective testing are done at the beginning of psychotherapy, and again after completion of psychotherapy to identify any changes, which might have occurred.

20.3 Psychological Therapy

As in the STEP-IN-AMI trial, the main psychotherapeutic methodology used in this context is a novel form of short-term psychotherapy (STP) derived from the ontopsychological method and specifically adapted to the setting of Cardiac Psychology [19] (also see Chap. 13).

The initial evaluation requires at least one or two encounters, after which the psychotherapist arranges an appointment to begin individual sessions. Based upon our experience in the STEP-IN-AMI trial, a maximum of ten individual meetings are scheduled over a 3-month period. Generally, this number is enough to complete the first phase of psychotherapeutic work (see Chap. 13). As specified in Chap. 13, in some cases the main problem involves the patient's relationship with their partner. In this case, it is wise and useful to also involve the partner in psychotherapeutic sessions, if possible both in individual and couples meetings. Often the partner is offered the option of personal psychotherapy as well. In this way, we can help both the partner and patient to start to make positive changes in their relationship, if and as needed. Through our years of experience with cardiac patients, and given our reading of the published scientific literature, we feel strongly that it is best to have partners' participation, whenever possible, because couples tend to act as a dyad [21, 22]. Without this, patients may improve over the duration of the psychological intervention, but then relapse when they return home if nothing there has changed, including their partner's anxiety about their health. Anxiety and apprehension on the part of the partner, or conflicts between the patient and partner, that antedated the hospital admission, might negate gains and prevent any long-lasting, stable improvement.

The psychotherapeutic setting should consist of a comfortable office, with a desk or small table, one or more windows, a plant, and two armchairs opposite each other at a distance of about 2 m [19]. This being said, on many occasions, it has been necessary for us to use whatever space was available at a hospital, and then adapt it as much as feasible.

After the course of individual meetings has been completed, patients are invited to participate in group meetings, together with their partners if desired. In this way, the psychotherapeutic work accomplished during the individual sessions may be reiterated and reinforced. For the group to effectively reinforce the goals achieved in the individual sessions, the therapist must strive to establish a friendly atmosphere between participants, which can dispel any initial fears and promote enthusiastic participation. Patients' partners who elect to participate may exhibit a broad range of reactions. If they have already engaged in individual psychotherapy, they generally will be at ease in group sessions. Conversely, partners who are participating for the first time may have difficulty, many expressing important personal problems and conflicts. This observation has reinforced our conviction regarding how important it is to involve partners from the very beginning of psychotherapy, whenever possible.

20.4 Conclusions

After 15 years of experience in the field of Cardiac Psychology, we feel confident saying that illness can become a great opportunity for individuals to review and analyze their personal life, shrug off dysfunctional behaviors and poor lifestyle choices, and alter any personal and/or emotional rigidity that has encumbered them. For those patients who are able to use this critical period of their life to make positive changes, illness can be a real chance for inner rebirth and renewal.

References

1. Sommaruga M, Tramarin R, Angelino E, Gruppo Italiano di Cardiologia Riabilitativa e Preventiva et al (2003) Guidelines on psychological intervention in cardiac rehabilitation–methodological process. Monaldi Arch Chest Dis 60(1):40–44
2. Perk J, De Backer G, Gohlke H et al (2012) European association for cardiovascular prevention & rehabilitation (EACPR); ESC committee for practice guidelines (CPG). European guidelines on cardiovascular disease prevention in clinical practice (version 2012). The fifth joint task force of the European society of cardiology and other societies on cardiovascular

disease prevention in clinical practice (constituted by representatives of nine societies and by invited experts). Eur Heart J 33(13):1635–701
3. Rossini R, Oltrona Visconti L, Musumeci G, Italian Society of Invasive Cardiology (SICI-GISE), National Association of Hospital Cardiologists (ANMCO), Italian Association for Cardiovascular Prevention and Rehabilitation (GICR-IACPR), Italian Society of General Practitioner (SIMG) et al (2015) A multidisciplinary consensus document on follow-up strategies for patients treated with percutaneous coronary intervention. Catheter Cardiovasc Interv 85(5):E129–39. doi:10.1002/ccd.2572
4. Lazzari D (2007, 2012) Mente e salute. Evidenze, ricerche e modelli per l'integrazione. Franco Angeli, Milano
5. Roncella A, Giornetti A, Cianfrocca C et al (2009) Rationale and trial design of a randomized, controlled study on short-term psychotherapy after acute myocardial infarction: the STEP-IN-AMI trial (Short term psychotherapy in acute myocardial infarction). J Cardiovasc Med 10:947–452
6. Roncella A, Pristipino C, Cianfrocca C et al (2013) One-year results of the randomized, controlled, short-term psychotherapy in acute myocardial infarction (STEP-IN-AMI) trial. Int J Cardiol 170(2):132–139. doi:10.1016/j.ijcard.2013.08.094
7. Allan R, Scheidt S (1996) Heart and mind. The practice of cardiac psychology. American Psychological Association, Washington, DC
8. Allan R, Fisher J (2012) Heart and mind. The practice of cardiac psychology, 2nd edn. American Psychological Association, Washington, DC
9. Pignalberi C, Patti G, Chimenti C, Maseri A (1998) Role of different determinants of psychological distress in acute coronary syndromes. J Am Coll Cardiol 32:613–619
10. Choen S, Syme SL (1985) Social support and health. Academic/Orlando University, Orlando
11. Holmes TH, Rahe RH (1967) The social readjustment rating scale. J Psychosom Res 11:213–218
12. Beck AT, Ward CH, Meldelson M et al (1961) An inventory for measuring depression. Arch Gen Psychiatry 4:561–571
13. Beck AT, Kovacs M, Weissman A (1979) Assessment of suicidal intention: the scale for suicide ideation. J Consult Clin Psychol 47:343–352
14. Hofer S, Lim LL, Guyatt GH, Oldridge NB (2004) The MacNew heart disease health related quality of life instrument: a summary. Health Qual Life Outcomes. doi:10.1186/1477-7525-2-3
15. Denollet J (2005) DS14: standard assessment of negative affectivity, social inhibition, and type D personality. Psychosom Med 67:89–97
16. Emons WHM, Meijer RR, Denollet J (2007) Negative affectivity and social inhibition in cardiovascular disease: evaluating type-D personality and its assessment using item response theory. J Psychosom Res 63:27–39
17. Spielberger CD, Gorsuch RL, Lushene R, Vagg PR, Jacobs GA (1983) Manual for the state-trait anxiety inventory. Consulting Psychologist Press, Palo Alto, CA
18. Spielberger CD (1988) Manual for the state-trait anger expression inventory (STAXI). Psychological Assessment Resources, Odessa
19. Meneghetti A (Eng ed 2004; It ed 1995–2008) Ontopsychology handbook. Ontopsicologia Editrice, Roma
20. Meneghetti A (1994–2003) L'Immagine e l'Inconscio. Ontopsicologia Editrice, Roma
21. Joekes K, Maes S, Boersma SN, Van Elderen T (2005) Goal disturbance, coping, and psychological distress in partners of myocardial infarction patients: taking account of the dyad. Anxiety Stress Coping 18(3):255–26
22. Moser DK, Dracup K (2004) Role of spousal anxiety and depression in patients' psychosocial recovery after a cardiac event. Psychosom Med 66:527–532

Model to Integrate Psychology/ Psychotherapy with Medical Activities at the Hospital of Terni, Italy

21

David Lazzari and Ludovico Lazzari

Change does not take place with the passing of time but with the evolution of our thoughts
Leonard Orr, Konrad Halbig [Orr L, Halbig K (2011) Der verbundene Atem, Schirner Verlag, Berlin]

21.1 A Multidisciplinary Strategy

Interdisciplinary teams that incorporate psychologists help patients to reduce their risk of major chronic illness. This is accomplished both via the diagnosis and treatment of major psychological risk factors (PRF), like anxiety and depression, and by providing patients with stress management techniques that optimize the balance between the demand for services and healthcare resources. In other words, through such teams, patients receive more effective treatment associated with lower healthcare costs.

Providing mental and behavioral health services as part of a primary care model greatly increases access for underserved people, by acting as a basin for screening and start-up to therapy to reduce cardiovascular disease risk factors. To date, however, the role and effectiveness of such services has been undervalued. An integrated healthcare approach also helps to eliminate the negative stigma often attached to mental illness and increases awareness about the psychosocial aspects of health. Psychologists play a key role in integrated health care by helping people

D. Lazzari (✉)
Servizio di Psicologia Ospedaliera, Azienda Ospedaliera "S. Maria" Terni, Viale Tristano di Joannuccio 1, 05100 Terni, Italy
e-mail: lazzarid@aospterni.it

L. Lazzari
Università degli Studi di Perugia, Azienda Ospedaliera "S. Maria" Terni, UO Cardiologia, Terni, Italy
e-mail: ludovicolazzari@alice.it

A. Roncella, C. Pristipino (eds.), *Psychotherapy for Ischemic Heart Disease*,
DOI 10.1007/978-3-319-33214-7_21

to modify their behaviors and thereby either prevent or recover from health problems.

A multidisciplinary network able to adapt to patient needs, providing elements of diagnosis and start-up treatment paths over the duration of hospitalization (i.e., psychotherapy and/or behavioral interventions), can help patients to develop coping strategies and healthy behaviors that are effective at reducing certain factors associated with illness development. The aim is to replace the traditional medical model with a more integrated, comprehensive, biopsychosocial model of illness, in which the mind and body are no longer seen as separate.

Given the prevalence of anxiety and depression in the general population and, in particular, among patients with coronary artery disease (CAD), the potential public health impact of appreciating the nature of the relationship between anxiety, depression, and CAD to prevent the development and progression of the disease is enormous [1]. As already described in Chap. 7 of this book, there is a close causal relationship between PRFs, the development of CAD, and its prognosis. For example, cardiology patients, who have anxiety or depression during their hospital admission, are at increased risk of higher rates of in-hospital complications like recurrent ischemia, re-infarction, and malignant arrhythmias [2, 3]. They also have higher re-infarction and mortality rates after discharge [4, 5].

21.2 Our Experience at "Santa Maria" Hospital

As a general rule, a more integrated approach to health care requires that there is a certain degree of sharing of scientific and health knowledge. This can give rise not only to a common horizon of "values" and meanings (i.e., integration of knowledge), but also to the real potential for dialogue and operational collaboration between physicians, psychologists, nurses, and other healthcare professionals. This sharing of knowledge facilitates the proper recognition and use of specific scientific-professional expertise. The model, called "knowledge competences" [6], allows us to clearly decline the different operating modes of integration between medicine and psychology. It is evident, indeed, that the objectives are of three types, which are placed on different levels, but still interconnected and complementary:

1. To ensure that caregiving action is as "person-centered" as possible, medical, nursing, and other healthcare providers must be psychologically aware, and this requires adequate knowledge and training.
2. Optimizing the availability and proper use of therapeutic activities—like patient education and health counseling—that are based upon psychological theories and models requires the presence of psychologists and/or the specific training of other operators.
3. Finally, activities and interventions can (and must) be administered directly by psychologists or psychotherapists, whose competencies have been developed over years of extensive, specialized training.

Integrated approach to health care in collaboration with the cardiology team In the context of acute coronary syndromes, the cardiologist is involved in the management of an acute syndrome, the physician's primary aim being to quickly stabilize the patient with proper access to coronary revascularization. Often, a lack of time hinders the cardiologist's ability to delve into anything other than the patient's physical health history. Moreover, once stabilized, the patient is often quickly transferred to a sub-intensive therapy unit. However, the management of psychosocial risk factors and in-hospital stress is crucial. This is because the patient has been suddenly jarred from his/her stable, daily routine to a setting of sudden and intense medicalization and must somehow cope with a sudden loss of autonomy, intense stress, and an exaggerated increase in external stressors, often unbalanced by internal resources. As soon as the acute event has passed, the patient's concerns may be addressed via explanations about what has happened and is happening, accompanied by attempts to answer their questions about their prognosis and address their fears about the disease itself and their risk of relapse. The influence of external stressors is often astutely perceived by the patient, many of whom ask about how a state of chronic stress might have precipitated the acute cardiac event and what weight such stress might have in the future. This element of risk is often overlooked by physicians, however, in their need to medically manage the acute event, even though it should fall within the responsibilities of caregivers to provide or direct patients toward the external resources they need to manage their stress properly. Our experience helps us to overcome this imbalance between our patients' requests and our physicians' and organization's ability to provide the answers and support they need.

We have described the overall picture (see also Chap. 7) because, from these considerations, we started to promote the experience of "*laboratory of integration*" for cardiac patients and caregivers at Santa Maria University Hospital in Terni, Italy. There, collaboration exists between the hospital's Psychology Service and Cardiology Department, spearheaded by Professor Enrico Boschetti. This project, called "*with the Mind and the Heart*," entails the following stages:

(a) Knowledge sharing: This involves the sharing of initiatives regarding the overall rationale for the collaboration, including clinical experience and research evidence documenting the role of psychological factors in the onset and treatment of cardiovascular diseases. This sharing of knowledge particularly occurs through group meetings, training courses, and conferences.
(b) Observation: A period of observation was performed by two psychologists within the Cardiology Division, both in the inpatient unit and the CICU (Cardiac Intensive Care Unit). They also consulted and performed direct interventions on patients, as requested by other Cardiology team personnel.
(c) Training of Cardiology personnel. Completing the previous phases has resulted in a demand to train staff, in particular those who work in the CICU and postoperative intensive care unit (POCU). The main issues covered have been team working, managing emotions, relationships with patient and family

members who care for them, and critical care issues. These experiences have allowed us to improve these components of care and create an atmosphere of sharing with caregivers about the overall aims of the project.

(d) Work on patients. The operating protocol is presented in Fig. 7.2 of the already-cited Chap. 7 in this book. Our new protocol provides for the inclusion of patients (with acute coronary syndromes initially) along different gradients of intervention related to the patient's psychological screening, which is used for the assessment of levels of distress and adaptive balance linked to the disease and is used to address his or her personal needs. For the complete list of suggested intervention, see Fig. 7.1 of Chap. 7.

1. The first level of treatment its offered to patients who are high functioning and have low-level distress. It includes information on lifestyle, supplemented by psycho-behavioral guidance (e.g., practical behavioral information and techniques around issues like diet, smoking cessation, adherence to therapy, exercise, teaching of relaxation techniques, and stress management). Patients are motivated to maintain or develop social support and to correct their atherogenic lifestyle (by providing them with comprehensive information on how physical exercise and the management of risk factors are cornerstones for reducing their risk of recurrent ischemic events). The crucial message is: if you follow these tips, you are your first ally. This guidance is also behavioral, to the extent that does not contradict, but rather focuses upon issues like anxiety, depression, and stress reported by the patient, by identifying them as real risk factors. It also seeks to distinguish the patient's real physical limitations (in agreement with the clinical picture) from those imposed by the cited psychosocial factors to prevent patients from feeling "more ill than they really are" and self-limiting their own exercise, autonomy, and social relationships.
2. While the first level of intervention is easily managed by trained physicians and nurses, the following levels require the increasing presence of psychologists, to the point of the patient's exclusive involvement in psychotherapy. A psychologist integrates the other caregivers when the main concerns patients have relate to the significance and impact of their symptoms, their own disbelief or denial about having a cardiac problem, and catastrophic interpretations about the impact the disease will have on everyday life. Those elements guide the implementation of screening for anxiety and depression and pave the way for the next two steps.
3. Patients with moderate levels of function and distress are offered participation in empowerment groups that help to motivate them toward greater autonomy and self-efficacy. We proceed by identifying personalized (from both psychological and clinical perspectives) yet measurable objectives and then encouraging patients to achieve them (e.g., gaining autonomy or pursuing healthier behaviors). The use of groups is also inspirational and provides patients with a source of social support.
4. Those patients who are low functioning and have high-level distress are offered either individual or group psychotherapy. This, in addition to the intervention

described above, shepherds patients toward how to master and react to their illness and strengthen their social skills. This last step focuses on treating anxiety and depressive disorders through cognitive-behavioral therapy (CBT), which trains patients in the social skills necessary to enable them to better handle and resist stressful situations. This is achieved by showing them how to reduce negative moods and restructure anxiety-provoking thoughts, by helping them to learn relaxation techniques to counteract stress and anxiety, and by teaching them how to react to external stressors through the proper use of their internal resources. On the other hand, interpersonal psychotherapy intervenes by targeting symptom formation and social dysfunction, helping patients to alleviate their depressive symptoms and resolve any interpersonal crisis linked to their depression by focusing on and addressing one or more interpersonal problem areas that are identified as precursors to the depressive episodes.

The presence of a Psychology service in the hospital allows for the programming of activities and interventions for the different inpatient populations (oncology, cardiology, neurology, pediatric, etc.) as well as parallel activity with different professionals (training in listening, empowerment, relationship management, etc.) in collaboration with the departments involved. Particularly in the cardiology area, there are two dedicated psychologists, each one for 10 h per week. These two psychologists are on the Psychology Service but operate functionally within the Department of Cardiology. This includes attending and participating in departmental meetings, as appropriate.

Integrated approach to health care in collaboration with the cardiac surgery team

The Psychology Service at Santa Maria Hospital in Terni has developed, since 2011, an intervention for stress and pain management. As perceived stress has an impact on postsurgical outcome [7], we designed a study in order to verify the effectiveness and the subsequent transferability in daily practice of a psychological intervention designed to reduce stress by teaching the patient relaxation techniques together with methods of empowerment. We identified three strategic time points in the course of cardiac surgery patients at which to intervene with empowerment and stress management meetings. These time points are the time of admission and acceptance into the department (T1), hospital discharge (T2), and 3 months after surgery (T3). On each of these occasions, patients meet a psychologist specifically trained to administer psychometric tests and carry out psychological interventions. To reduce the risk of type 1 error secondary to a placebo effect, the mere result of dedicating attention to patients, a control group was added which was administered the same tests within short interviews with the psychologist, but received no intervention for psychological empowerment and stress management.

Both groups included patients undergoing elective surgery in the Cardiac Surgery Division of our hospital. Exclusion criteria were the presence of psychiatric conditions, taking medication for anxiety or depression, the presence of severe cognitive impairment, and the onset of complications that required any new surgical procedures or unforeseen treatments that might significantly impact on the patient's clinical course.

For the psychometric evaluation, we used the Hospital Anxiety and Depression Scale (HADS) and a shortened version of the Stress Balance Test [8], with the purpose of respectively measuring anxiety, depression, and the progressive evolution of the subjective "balance" between "demands" and "resources," both "internal" and "external." The psychological intervention consisted of a phase of empowerment and cognitive restructuring, and training in a psychophysiological technique called the "relaxation response (RR)," initially described by Herbert Benson, which we supplemented and amended [9]. The first component of the intervention was intended to provide patients with tools to analyze the dynamics of stress and its biopsychosocial dimension. It also promoted awareness regarding their potential to play an active role on their own managing stress and pain, through the balanced use of resources, both personal (internal) and informational, instrumental and relational (external). The second component included a sensitization phase, whereby patients learned to listen to and recognize their level of psychophysical tension and what triggers such tension, followed by training in psychophysiological relaxation and way to arrest any recurring unpleasant and intrusive thoughts they might have.

A diary was provided to patients so they could record the instructions for relaxation given by the psychologist during the session. Subjects were then asked to record the number of repetitions they spontaneously performed of each technique over the course of their hospitalization, under the premise that the beneficial effects of each psychophysiological technique are proportional to the skills that are acquired through the exercise. The full results of this intervention have been thoroughly detailed in Lazzari D, "Mente & Salute" [9], where we focus on insights into the perception of pain and days of hospitalization in patients receiving and not receiving the intervention (see Table 21.1).

Of 359 individuals enrolled ($n = 201$ in the experimental group and 158 in the control group), 54 % were men and 46 % women. The experimental group experienced a significant 83.3 % reduction in its perception of pain and days of hospitalization (mean = 7.8 days) relative to the control group, in which pain declined by 50.9 % and there were a mean of 11.5 days of hospitalization. Overall, comparing the experimental and control groups, the intervention was effective at (a) decreasing cardiac surgery patients' perception of the "burden" of their surgery; (b) increasing the patients' perception of internal resources, both during hospitalization and 3 months after the intervention; (c) significantly reducing their levels of anxiety; (d) preventing any increase in their depression; (e) decreasing their perception of pain; and (f) reducing the length of their hospitalization.

At follow-up, we observed a substantial difference between treated and untreated patients. Although we cannot present all the data here, it should be noted that the psychological intervention has resulted in a measurable reduction in the levels of anxiety and depression, which correlated with positive surgery outcomes such as pain reduction or reduction of hospital stay. Those results indicate

Table 21.1 Intervention in cardiac surgery patients

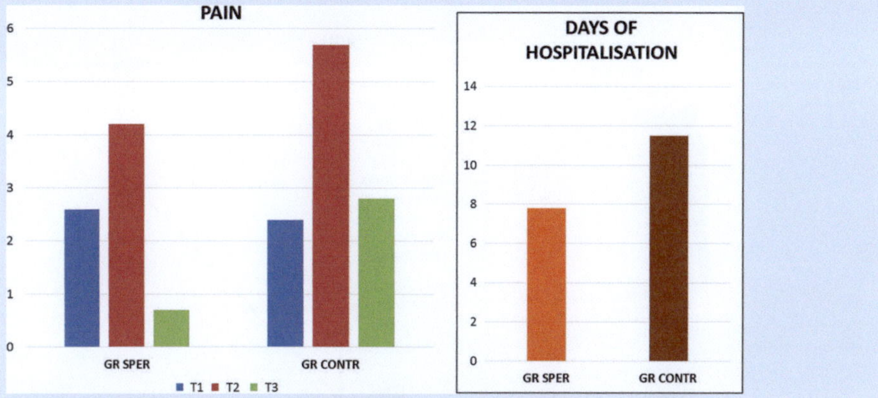

that our intervention reduced the imbalance between demands and resources. In particular, the intervention appeared to increase patients' internal resources [10]. The major statistically significant difference was the marked reduction in the length of hospital stay, which was almost four days (3.7) shorter in the intervention versus non-intervention group.

Based upon these findings, we came to the conclusion that the integrated intervention that we tested had significant, beneficial effects both on patient's outcome (e.g., perceived pain) and hospital resources management (e.g., reduced length of hospital stay).

21.3 The Balance Model

The Balance Model presently used at Santa Maria Hospital in Terni is an interpretive model used to frame the adaptive balance between patients and their distress [11]. In this model, adaptive balance is seen as the dynamic between "demands"—both external (e.g., illness) and internal to the patient (e.g., expectations and needs)—and "resources," which again can be categorized as either external (e.g., the support of caregivers) or internal (e.g., the patient's personal abilities and strengths). Imbalance between these four factors creates discomfort and distress and thereby is dysfunctional (see Fig. 21.1).

For greater clarity, visualize a balance scale with both external stressors, the demands of our environment, and internal stressors, the demands that we place upon ourselves in relation to our expectations and our perception of events on one side. On the other side are the resources at our disposal, which can come either from ourselves or from external support. Proper balance between the demands and resources allows us to manage stress appropriately, reasoning our way through difficulties while making optimal use of resources or reformulating the demands.

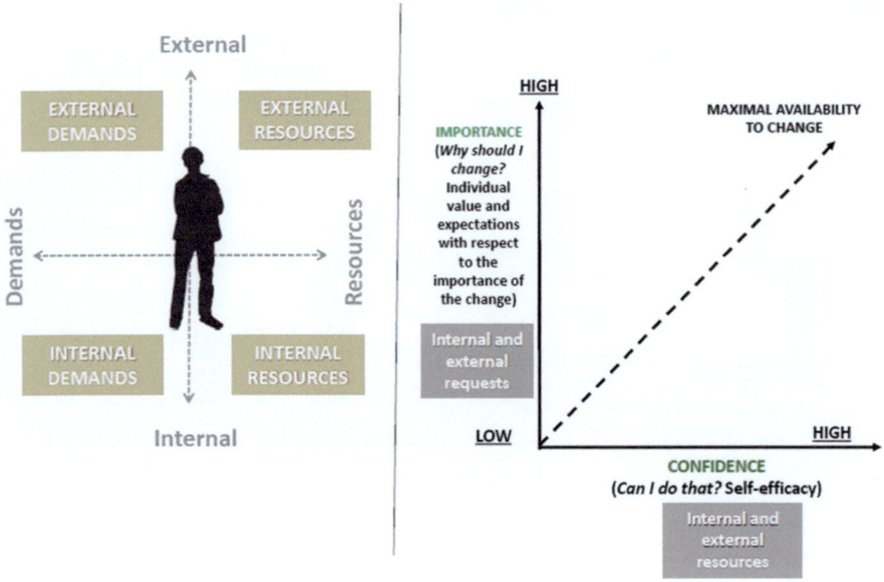

Fig. 21.1 Balance of adaptation/stress and motivation for change

When an imbalance between these factors and demands cannot be balanced by resources, there is a maladaptive response, a cognitive process that can result in a pathological thrust through neuroendocrine modulations that can disrupt the body's allostasis. The level of imbalance is measured with special instruments [12] that provide reliable scores related to four factors. The imbalance is correlated with the scores for anxiety, depression, and distress on other questionnaires.

The model is also used to target the interventions of psycho-education and empowerment, since resources are related to the "confidence" a person has to change their attitudes and behaviors, while demands appear to be related to the "importance" that is attributed to the change. Importance ("why change") and confidence ("I can do it") are predictors of adaptive changes in cardiovascular disease.

21.4 Conclusions

When a hospital has a Psychology Unit, it is possible to optimize activities and establish priorities for psychological interventions planning various activities through a "rationale" throughout the entire hospital. Such a program has been implemented at our hospital in Terni, launching a joint program of activities in cardiology that accommodates patients, caregivers, and healthcare workers. In this context, the functional presence of psychologists is modulated relative to the programs and needs that arise from time to time; it also provides a means to conduct research on cardiac surgery patients. Parallel activities are carried out aimed at supporting not only patients but also the cardiology staff in a logical and functional collaboration.

References

1. Moser DK, De Jong MJ (2006) Anxiety and heart disease. In: Molinari E, Compare A, Parati G (eds) Clinical psychology and heart disease. Springer, Italia
2. Zuidersma M, Thombs BD, de Jonge P (2011) Onset and recurrence of depression as predictors of cardiovascular prognosis in depressed acute coronary syndrome patients: a systematic review. Psychother Psychosom 80:227–237
3. Janszky I, Ahnve S, Lundberg I et al (2010) Early-onset depression, anxiety, and risk of subsequent coronary heart disease: 37-year follow-up of 49,321 young Swedish men. J Am Coll Cardiol 56:31–37
4. Whang W, Shimbo D, Kronish IM et al (2010) Depressive symptoms and all-cause mortality in unstable angina pectoris (from the Coronary Psychosocial Evaluation Studies [COPES]). Am J Cardiol 106:1104–1107
5. Nabi H, Shipley MJ, Vahtera J et al (2010) Effects of depressive symptoms and coronary heart disease and their interactive associations on mortality in middle-aged adults: the Whitehall II cohort study. Heart 96:1645–1650
6. Lazzari D, Marini C (2007) Il Modello conoscenze-competenze. AUPI Notizie 3
7. Tefikow S, Rosendahl J, Strauß B (2013) Psychological interventions in surgical care: a narrative review of current meta-analytic evidence. Psychother Psychosom Med Psychol 63 (6):208–216
8. Lazzari D (2011) Psicologia Sanitaria e Malattia Cronica. Pacini Editore, Pisa
9. Lazzari D (2007) Mente & Salute. Franco Angeli Editore, Milano, p 213
10. Bartoli S (2013) La gestione dello stress in Chirurgia. PNEI Rev 2:43–50
11. Lazzari D (2009) La Bilancia dello Stress. Liguori Editore, Napoli
12. Lazzari D (2014) I marker della psiche e quelli della vita. PNEI Rev 2:54–62

An Integrative Model of Psychotherapy in Medical Practice According to GICR-IACPR

22

Antonia Pierobon and Marinella Sommaruga

The doctor of the future will give no medication, but will interest his patients in the care of the human frame, diet and in the cause and prevention of disease

Thomas Alva Edison (inventor, scientist, and businessman, born on February 11, 1847, in Milan, Ohio—died on October 18, 1931, in West Orange, New Jersey)

22.1 Introduction

The Italian Association for Cardiovascular Prevention, Rehabilitation and Epidemiology (I.A.C.P.R.), previously named Gruppo Italiano di Cardiologia Riabilitativa (G.I.C.R.) has as its mission the promotion of excellence in research, education, and the organization of preventive and rehabilitative cardiovascular programs. The members of the GICR-IACPR are cardiologists, psychologists, physiotherapists, dietitians, and nurses, which attests to the society's innovative choice of a multidisciplinary approach [1].

Irrespective of whether a patient is being managed in an outpatient or inpatient setting, each individual's rehabilitative program is characterized by a multidisciplinary approach designed to address different patients' different needs. Continuity

GICR-IACPR stands for Il Gruppo Italiano di Cardiologia Riabilitativa e Preventiva—The Italian Association for Cardiovascular Prevention, Rehabilitation and Epidemiology.

A. Pierobon (✉)
Psychology Unit, Salvatore Maugeri Foundation, Care and Research Institute, Via per Montescano, 27040 Pavia, Italy
e-mail: antonia.pierobon@fsm.it

M. Sommaruga
Clinical Psychology and Social Support Unit, Salvatore Maugeri Foundation, Care and Research Institute, Milan, Italy
e-mail: marinella.sommaruga@fsm.it

A. Roncella, C. Pristipino (eds.), *Psychotherapy for Ischemic Heart Disease*,
DOI 10.1007/978-3-319-33214-7_22

of care is preserved via collaborations with general practitioners and local health services. The interdisciplinary approach to risk factors management demonstrates how the Cardiac Rehabilitation Unit (CRU), being responsible for secondary interventions, is also the most suitable environment in which to develop preventive interventions, especially in individuals at high risk for cardiovascular disease. With this double vocation, GICR-IACPR fully adheres to the policies of the European Association for Cardiovascular Prevention & Rehabilitation (EACPR).

In 2001, the GICR-IACPR Board, addressing a need to identify the essential characteristics of psychological interventions in cardiac rehabilitation and prevention (CRP) programs, based on scientific evidence, created a working group comprised of psychologists with specific experience in clinical research. The first task of this working group was to formulate specific Guidelines for Psychological Interventions in Italian Cardiac Rehabilitation. Until then, any descriptions of psychological interventions were either part of general cardiology guidelines or in papers based upon expert opinion [2–6].

The past and current operational proposal of the Psychology Working Group focuses on the identification and analysis of the following three issues:

- Efficacy and effectiveness of psychological activities in cardiac rehabilitation (in accordance with criteria published by the Task Force of the American Psychological Association, APA);
- Minimal and maximal standard criteria to which a psychological intervention must comply, with respect to human, professional, and structural resources;
- Educational professional training of multidisciplinary staff.

Then and now, the aim of the Psychology Working Group is to identify "which" (what psychological problems), "to whom" (which cardiac patients), and "how" (e.g., individual versus group treatment). The aim of this chapter represents a historical excursus of the PWG of GICR-IACPR from publication of the first guidelines on psychological activities in cardiac rehabilitation and their implementation to the current day [6].

22.2 Psychological Guidelines: Methodological Issues and Main Recommendations

The methodology adopted by the Psychology Working Group while drafting the first specific Guidelines for Psychological Practices in Cardiac Rehabilitation is consistent with National Guidelines Program Recommendations of the Italian Ministry of Health [7].

The guidelines for psychology practices in CRP are divided into three parts: an introduction, the main body of the text, and various appendices. In the introduction, the theme and context of the guidelines are described, preceded by a series of notes and user instructions. In addition, the intended audience is identified. The main body of the document is structured around the steps that characterize the interactions between the patient suffering from heart disease and the psychologist. The phases of this process are schematized as follows: selection, entry, evaluation, intervention, and follow-up (Fig. 22.1). For each of these phases, empirical evidence is given to support the evaluative and therapeutic tools that psychologists use in the context of CRP [8]. More specifically, Chap. 3 of the document describes the psychological characterization and specificity of psychological interventions in different cardiac patient populations. Considered are patients with ischemic heart

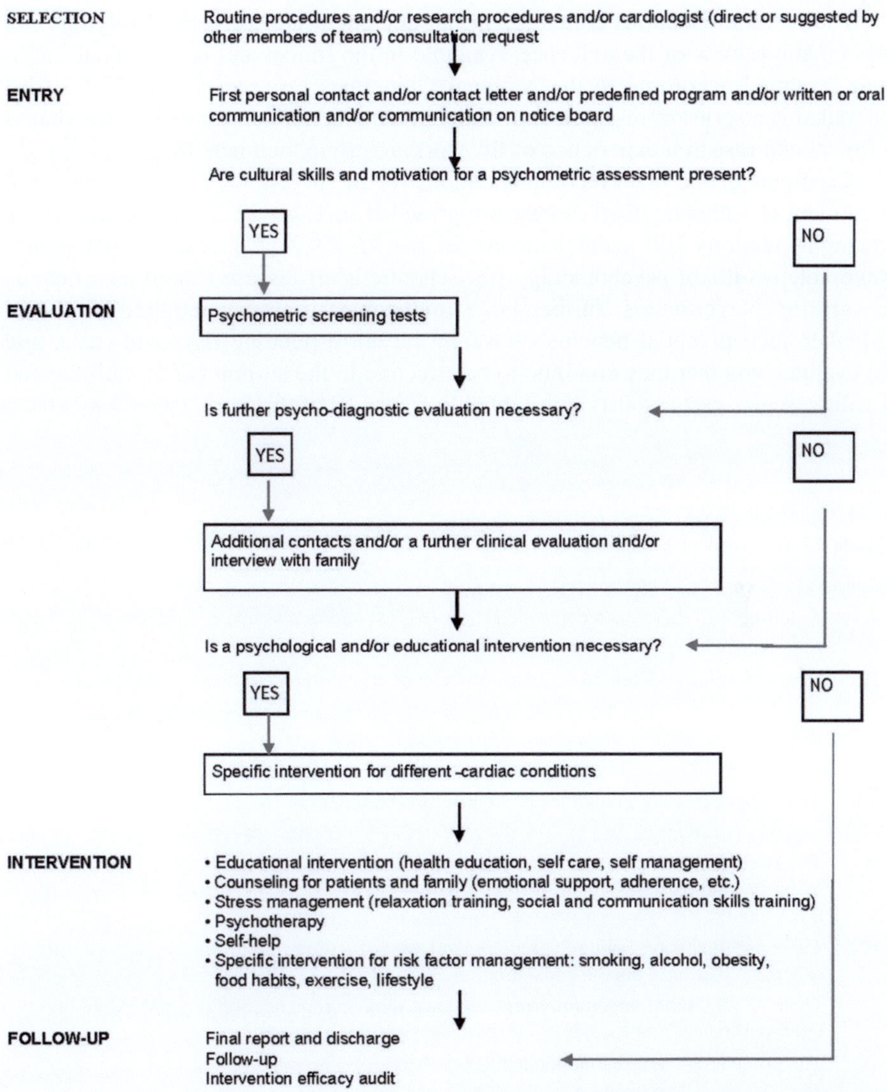

Fig. 22.1 Flowchart of the process of care (modified and translated from Task Force [8], p. 217)

disease, chronic heart failure, or chronic peripheral artery disease; postoperative patients after cardiac surgery, heart transplantation, or pacemaker or implantable cardioverter defibrillator placement; patients at high risk of cardiovascular disease; individuals over 75 years of age; and end-stage heart disease patients. The Psychology Working Group has been revising these guidelines as new evidence is identified [9].

The appendices to the document contain a synthesis of the scientific information, some tables, a glossary, and a section providing detailed information on specific topics.

The recommendations contained in the document are formulated relying on a systematic review of the evidence available in the Italian and international literature, codified according to the National Guidelines Program (Table 22.1). Also included is a series of research and clinical recommendations, based on the shared clinical and research experience of the working group members [8].

Examples of the main recommendations for the psychological assessment and treatment of ischemic heart disease are provided in Table 22.2. At this time, these recommendations still seem suitable for use in CRP [10], and the potentially favorable results of psychotherapy for ischemic heart disease should not come as a surprise. Nevertheless, further large multicenter trials are required to clarify whether such potential benefits outweigh the corresponding risks and costs, and to evaluate whether they continue to be effective in the current era of multifaceted cardiovascular care, as also highlighted in Chap. 10 of this book (see Chap. 10).

Table 22.1 Levels of evidence and grading

Levels of evidence	
I	A number of randomized controlled trials (RCTs) and/or a systematic review of RCTs
II	A single RCT
III	Nonrandomized cohort studies with concurrent or historical controls or their meta-analyses
IV	Retrospective studies (e.g., case control) or their meta-analysis
V	Case series without controls
VI	Expert opinion (like guidelines or a consensus conference)
Grades of recommendation	
A	The execution of a procedure or diagnostic test is strongly recommended. This recommendation is sustained by high-quality levels of evidence, though not necessarily level I or II
B	There are doubts regarding the recommendation of a procedure or intervention, but its execution warrants sincere consideration
C	There is substantial uncertainty for or against the recommendation of a procedure or intervention
D	The procedure is not recommended
E	The procedure is strongly discouraged

Modified and translated from Task Force [8], p. 189

Table 22.2 Principal recommendations regarding psychological assessments and interventions for ischemic heart disease patients

Recommendation A. The psychologist should assess the presence of behavioral risk factors, depression, low social support, psychosocial work characteristics, and anxiety in all ischemic heart disease patients
Recommendation A. All ischemic heart disease patients, in whom anxiety, depression, or low social support is diagnosed, should be treated appropriately
Recommendation D. Specific interventions to modify Type A behavior are not recommended as part of comprehensive cardiac rehabilitation programs
Recommendation A. Psychoeducational programs should be included in a multidisciplinary intervention
Clinical PWG recommendation. The psychologist should integrate his/her own intervention, tailored for the single patient, in the context of a comprehensive rehabilitation project, in close collaboration with the other members of the Cardiology team
Research PWG recommendation. Controlled studies evaluating the effectiveness of specific psychological interventions for psychological and cardiovascular endpoints are recommended

Modified and translated from Task Force [8]

22.3 Psychological Guidelines: Survey and Implementations

In 2005, in line with Italian National Guidelines Program indications, the Italian SurveY on carDiac rEhabilitation—Psychology (ISYDE-Psi) was conducted, its main objective being to evaluate the current state of knowledge and level of implementation of the Italian Guidelines for Psychological Practices in Cardiac Rehabilitation published in 2003 (PsyGL). The Psychology Working Group conducted this pilot survey on existing psychological practices in cardiac rehabilitation units (CRU) to improve PsyGL implementation through interactive training. A questionnaire was designed to gather information on organizational models and on the practices of those psychologists currently working in the surveyed Italian CRUs. The questionnaire collected detailed information on facilities, organization, staffing levels, professional backgrounds, and psychologist practices. The questionnaire was sent by conventional mail to the consulting psychologists in 107 CRUs (out of a total of 144 potential units), which in a previous survey, called ISYDE, had reported structured psychological programs. Data collection for ISYDE-Psi terminated at the end of March 2005, with replies from 70 of the 107 units assessed (participation rate 65.4 %) [11, 12].

Some of these results are summarized here (Figs. 22.2 and 22.3). Of the 70 CRUs, 55 (79.8 %) reported good knowledge of the published PsyGL, while 10.1 % of the psychologists claimed not to know the current PsyGL. The PsyGL was considered fully and partly applicable by 84.5 % and 15.5 %, respectively. Other data about psychological practices were collected. Psychological assessments were performed through clinical interviews in 94.3 % of the CRUs, with psychometric testing done in 81.4 %. Almost all of the units (92.8 %) used screening instruments to evaluate psychosocial risk factors, in particular anxiety and

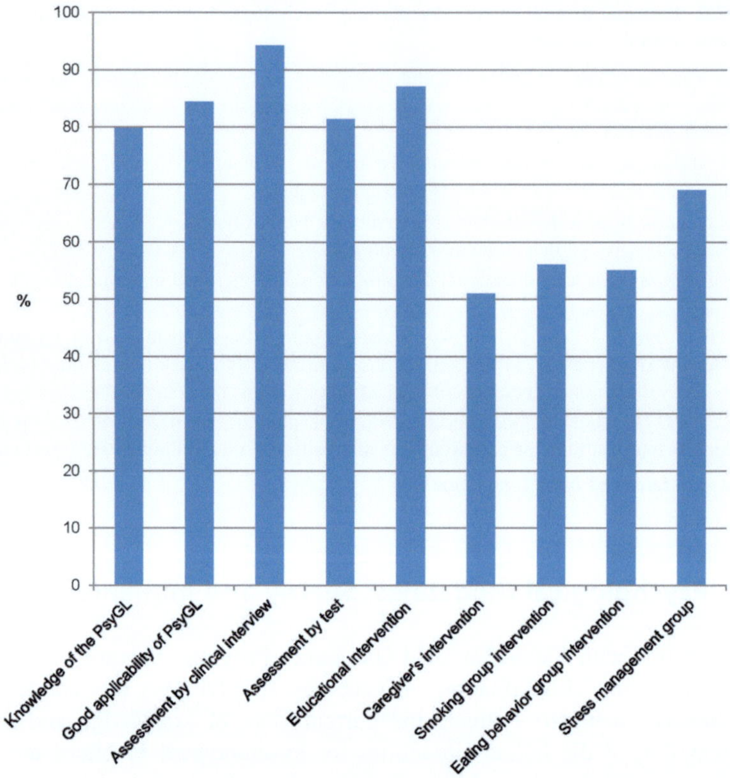

Fig. 22.2 Results of psychological activity in CRU from the Survey ISYDE-Psi—2008. Legend: *CRU* cardiac rehabilitation unit, *PsyGL* Italian Guidelines for psychological activities in Cardiac Rehabilitation, *ISYDE-Psi* Italian SurveY on carDiac rEhabilitation-Psychology

depression (64.3 %). However, only 22.8 % evaluated quality of life and 17.1 % cognitive impairment. Educational interventions were part of 87.1 % of the CRU programs. Education was extended to family members in 51 % of the units, while counseling was offered to family in 57 %. In terms of group interventions, specifically targeted behaviors were cigarette smoking (56 %), eating habits (55 %), and stress management (69 %). Psychological interventions tailored to individual patient needs were offered at 62.9 % of the CRUs. Final written reports were drafted by 88.6 %. After discharge, follow-up was carried out by 48.6 % of the CRUs, 15.7 % as part of a structured protocol. The survey also revealed wide discrepancies in the provision of psychological practices in Italian CRUs, especially between northern and southern Italy. Nevertheless, the psychological assessments and interventions offered to the patients seemed acceptably coherent with current national PsyGL for CRP [13].

Coherent with this data, the Psychology Working Group developed a training project for psychologists working in CRPs, sponsored by the Italian Council of

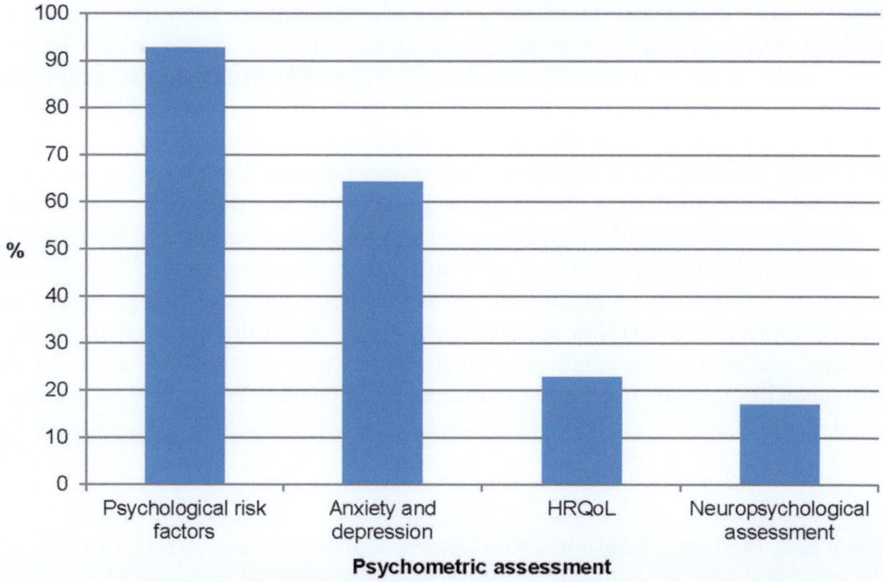

Fig. 22.3 Type of psychometric assessment in CRU from the ISYDE-Psi Survey—2008. Legend: *CRU* cardiac rehabilitation unit, *HRQoL* health-related quality of life

Psychologists, which was implemented in different regions of the country with the aim of PsyGL dissemination and the promotion of their correct application, despite existing regional organizational disparities [13, 14].

At the current time, there are no available measures of the level of adherence to PsyGL by the psychologists in CRPs. On the other hand, the PsyGL has become part of usual care and it is difficult to distinguish previous knowledge from that acquired through the PsyGL. Nonetheless, relative to the beginning of this process, over the last few years psychologists working in Italian CRPs have become more willing to utilize evidence-based practices and to update their clinical and scientific knowledge to remain current.

22.4 National and International Updates on Psychological Interventions

The Italian Guidelines for Psychological Practices in CRP were updated in 2005, inside the National Cardiac Rehabilitation Guidelines issued by the Italian Program for Guidelines. The full text of this document is available online [15]. The document was an update of the Guidelines of the SIGN (Scottish Intercollegiate Guidelines Network) with a specific focus on ischemic disease. The psychological contribution focused, above all, on anxiety, depression, and other psychosocial and behavioral risk factors. It also demonstrated growing interest in issues like illness beliefs, self-efficacy, and type D personality (distressed personality, resulting from interpersonal interactions characterized by social inhibitions and negative affectivity). Furthermore, it stressed the need to tailor treatment to address individual patient needs and problems. It was becoming increasingly clear that psycho-educational programs for coronary artery disease (CAD) patients do not increase event-free survival, but that the intervention can improve depression, social isolation, adherence to therapy, health-related quality of life (HRQoL), and overall prognosis. A number of appendices and educational materials for both health operators and cardiac patients are available. As an example, Table 22.3 contains an updated appendix 2 regarding the most frequently used psychological tests in Italian CRUs [1, 15–17]. For a more recent review about the impact that psychotherapy and ancillary psychological interventions may have on the prognosis of patients with ischemic heart disease, readers are encouraged to review the already-cited Chap. 10.

Table 22.3 Psychological and neuropsychological tests. References and descriptions of the tools are available at www.gicr.it in the psychological area-tools section [1]

• *Screening and outcome*
– Cognitive Behavioral Assessment-Hospital Form (CBA-H)
– Anxiety and Depression-Revised (AD-R)
– Hospital Anxiety and Depression Scale (HADS)
– Beck Depression Inventory-2 (BDI-2)
– Mini Mental State Examination (MMSE)
– The Montreal Cognitive Assessment (MoCA)
– CORE-OM
– Psychological General Well-Being Index (PGWB-S)
• *Personality*
– Cognitive Behavioural Assessment 2.0 Scale Primarie (CBA-2.1)
– Multiphasic Minnesota Personality Inventory-2 (MMPI-2)
– SCID I-II (DSM-IV-R)
– Distress Scale (DS14, Type D personality)
• *Knowledge and adherence*
– MaugerI CaRdiac preventiOn-Questionnaire (MICRO-Q)
– Adherence Schedule in Heart Disease—Brief (ASHiD-R)
• *Care-giver*
– Family Strain Questionnaire (FSQ)
– Disease Impact On Caregiver (DIOC)
• *Neuropsychology*
– Esame Neuropsicologico Breve-2 (ENB-2)
• *Coping, self-efficacy and positive variables*
– Coping Orientations to the Problems Experienced (COPE)
– General Perceived Self-Efficacy Scale, Italian version (GPSES)
– Revised Life Orientation (LOT-R)

The Fifth Joint Task Force of the European Society of Cardiology (ESC) Guidelines confirmed well-known psychological risk factors and highlighted other psychosocial factors that contribute to the risk of developing cardiovascular disease (CVD) and having a worsened clinical course. Low socioeconomic status, lack of social support, stress at work and in family life, depression, anxiety, hostility, and a type D personality act as barriers to treatment adherence and worsen the prognosis of CVD. Mutual mechanisms link psychosocial factors to increased CVD risk: factors that include an unhealthy lifestyle (frequent smoking, poor diet, and less physical exercise), increased healthcare utilization, financial barriers to health care, and low adherence to behavior-change recommendations or cardiac medications. In addition, persons and patients with depression and/or chronic stress show alterations in autonomic function (including reduced heart rate variability), in the hypothalamic–pituitary axis, and in other endocrine markers, which affect hemostatic and inflammatory processes, endothelial function, and myocardial perfusion. Enhanced risk in patients with depression may also be due in part to the adverse effects of tricyclic antidepressants [18, 19] (see also in this book: Chaps. 1–3, 9).

The recommendations regarding psychosocial factors emphasize the importance of both assessing them via clinical interviews and/or standardized questionnaires (Table 22.3) and managing them with tailored individual or group interventions. It is further recommended that interventions are mediated by cognitive behavioral strategies, such as motivational interviewing, stress management, psychological counseling, and effective communication to facilitate behavioral change and the therapeutic alliance. More precisely, it is declared that combining the knowledge and skills of clinicians (e.g., physicians, nurses, psychologists, and experts in nutrition, cardiac rehabilitation, and sports medicine) into multimodal, behavioral-cognitive interventions can help to optimize preventive and rehabilitative efforts [18].

According to ESC Guidelines, the aim of the last position paper promoted by GICR-IACPR is to provide specific recommendations to assist CR staff in the design, evaluation, and development of their healthcare delivery organization. The position paper should also assist healthcare providers, insurers, policy makers, and consumers in the recognition of quality of care requirements, standards and outcome measures, quality and performance indicators, and the professional competence of personnel involved in preventive and rehabilitative programs [20].

Furthermore, a multicenter, prospective, longitudinal survey carried out by the GICR-IACPR in patients on completion of a CR program after coronary artery bypass grafting (CABG) and percutaneous coronary interventions (PCI) confirms that participation in CR after revascularization can yield excellent results, as does a healthy lifestyle and good medication adherence at 1-year follow-up. The rates of various behaviors have been compared between the beginning of hospitalization and at 1-year follow-up. They include rates for smoking of 19 % versus 10 %, respectively; healthy eating habits—42 % versus 72 %; and physical activity more than three times per week—6 % versus 46 %.The Italian survey on CardiAc RehabilitatiOn and Secondary prevention after cardiac revascularization (ICAROS) results offered a portrait of the "real world" of clinical practice concerning patients after CABG and PCI. Many patients after revascularization leave the acute wards without optimal prescriptions for preventive medication, whereas the prescription of cardio-preventive drugs and risk factor control tends to be excellent after completion of a CR program. Last but not least, ICAROS demonstrated that certain characteristics (percutaneous coronary intervention, PCI, as the index event; living alone; poor eating habits; smoking at a young age; old age; and, most notably, associated comorbidities) can identify patients at risk for poor behavioral modification at medium-term follow-up. For these patients, further support may be warranted [21].

A recent consensus conference on clinical management after acute coronary syndrome (ACS) by GICR-IACPR and the Italian Association of Hospital Cardiologists (Associazione Nazionale Medici Cardiologi Ospedalieri—ANMCO) generated a joint proposal for the management and follow-up of patients discharged alive after an ACS. The document highlights the important role that psychologists have within the interdisciplinary cardiac team, in terms of optimizing patient adherence and their adaptation to chronic disease [22]. In fact, patients suffering from a chronic cardiovascular illness continuously revise their lifestyle, adapting themselves to the behavioral limitations imposed by their clinical status. This incessant adjustment work causes profound psychological changes and a reformulation of self, in a more or less conscious way [23]. During this process of self-redefinition, the psychologist has various tasks:

- To evaluate and legitimatize the patient's emotional state (depression and anxiety)
- To recognize the patient's stage of adaptation and reformulation of self (from patient to person)
- To facilitate the patient's acceptance of their clinical condition
- To stimulate the patient's redefinition of life goals
- To motivate the patient to correct cardiovascular risk factors that remain present (e.g., smoking, poor dietary habits, a sedentary lifestyle, high stress, etc.)
- To support the patient's coping skills, internal-external resources, and positive outlook
- To reinforce the patient's adaptive behaviors directed toward self-care and clinical adherence
- To help the patient to reappraise their social and intrafamilial relationships and roles, so as to be congruent with their current level of illness

These issues are typical components of cognitive behavioral treatment in the setting of cardiac rehabilitation, with a constant focus not only on limitations but also on resources, as per the biopsychosocial model of illness and the International Classification of Functionality [23–28]. Accordingly, evidence-based cognitive-behavioral psychological interventions, which target patients with depressive symptoms, are likely to be more efficacious at improving CAD outcomes than those that offer generic stress management and general support for all patients, regardless of their life history and psychological status. Future trials are needed on psychological interventions in CAD patients with moderate to severe depression, who are the most likely to benefit from them. To determine whether this leads to improved cardiac and survival outcomes, the studied intervention should be sufficiently intensive to modify psychological outcomes [29, 30].

Even more avant-garde is treatment based upon "positive psychology" and "mindfulness." Positive psychology and psychotherapy may provide interesting insights into the mechanisms underlying psychological well-being that significantly reduce cardiovascular mortality in healthy populations and death rates in those with chronic disease [31–33]. On the other hand, mind–body practices have yielded encouraging results in patients with various cardiac and cardiovascular diseases [34]. In a recent review, practices based on mindfulness-based stress reduction, transcendental meditation, progressive muscle relaxation, and stress management were found to potentially improve certain specific outcomes in cardiac patients; among these enhanced outcomes were physical and mental quality of life, depression, anxiety, and both systolic and diastolic blood pressure [35] (also see Chap. 12).

Addressing these issues, the present Psychology Working Group performs ongoing updates of the Italian Guidelines for Psychological Practices in CRP that were published in 2003 [8]. In 2014, preliminary data were published at the Annual Congress of the GICR-IACPR [9]. This updated PsyGL, like the previous version, is different from the majority of psychological guidelines published in the literature, especially because it takes into account not just ischemic heart disease but several other cardiac diseases, in accordance with a recent position paper published by Ladwig et al. [19, 36].

22.5 Minimal Psychological Care Going Toward a Consensus Conference

Minimal care (MC) refers to the implementation of an evidence-based process of care in rehabilitation settings, with the participation of nurses, physiotherapists, dietitians, and psychologists in close cooperation with cardiologists. This preliminary position paper is a first attempt to delineate certain minimum, robust, and essential standards for any evidence-based CR program. The document details the practices that should be carried out in each CR program phase, including pathways for nurses, physiotherapists, dietitians, and psychologists. MC pathways were identified and divided—according to the types of patient who access the CRP program—into high, medium, and low complexity. Phases of care include an initial assessment, intervention, evaluation, and final report, as defined in the PsyGL [37, 38].

Further educational work on minimal care is being performed by the Psychology Working Group within a collaborative network that incorporates nurses, physiotherapists, dietitians, and cardiologists. Listed on the GICR-IACPR website are several educational events that were organized across Italy, from north to south, in 2014 and 2015. The educational interdisciplinary course seems to be an efficient strategy for other clinicians to implement an increasing number of patient-tailored interventions and, thereby, join the efforts of different professionals in CRP [18]. The next step will entail discussing and establishing a criteria-based definition of minimal care for CRP programs at a consensus conference that will lead to a final position paper.

22.6 Conclusions

In accordance with an operational proposal drafted in 2001, the Psychology Working Group has now achieved several of its predetermined goals. Over the past 15 years, psychologists in CRP programs have started to work more and more in collaboration with cardiology teams, developing tailored interventions to address the needs of both patients and their caregivers. They also have orchestrated educational sessions on stress burnout and compassion fatigue, two scenarios that are not at all uncommon among healthcare professionals. Our desire is to spread and aid in the implementation of evidence-based psychological "know-how" in these CRPs, by involving psychologists who are already working with cardiac patients, as well as those interested in attaining specialized skills in the field of cardiac psychology.

References

1. GICR-IACPR Italian Association for Cardiovascular Prevention, Rehabilitation and Epidemiology. http://www.iacpr.it/. Accessed 7 Apr 2015
2. Task Force on Promotion and Dissemination of Psychological Procedures (1995) Training in and dissemination of empirically-validated psychological treatments: report and recommendations. Clin Psychol 48(1):3–23
3. Linden W (2000) Psychological treatments in cardiac rehabilitation: review of rationales and outcomes. J Psychosom Res 48(4–5):443–454
4. Zotti AM (1999) Strategie e modelli di intervento psicosociale in riabilitazione. In: Giannuzzi P, Ignone G (eds) Riabilitazione nelle malattie cardiovascolari. UTET, Torino
5. Linee Guida per la riabilitazione cardiologica (2000) Giornale di riabilitazione, XVI
6. Sommaruga M, Tramarin R (2001) Proposta operativa per l'accreditamento dell'intervento psicologico in area cardiologica. Giornale di Riabilitazione 17:9–80
7. Sommaruga M, Tramarin R, Angelino E, Gruppo Italiano di Cardiologia Riabilitativa e Preventiva et al (2003) Guidelines on psychological intervention in cardiac rehabilitation—methodological process. Monaldi Arch Chest Dis 60(1):40–44
8. Task Force per le Attività di Psicologia in Cardiologia Riabilitativa e Preventiva, Gruppo Italiano di Cardiologia Riabilitativa e Preventiva (2003) Guidelines for psychology activities in cardiologic rehabilitation and prevention. Monaldi Arch Chest Dis 60(3):184–234
9. Pierobon A, Abatello M, Balestroni G et al (2014) L'attività psicologica in cardiologia riabilitativa e preventiva: Linee Guida 10 anni dopo. 12° Congresso Nazionale GICR-IACPR "Cardiologia Preventiva 2014", Genoa
10. Sommaruga M (2009) Psychological guidelines in cardiac rehabilitation and prevention. In: Dwivedi A (ed) Handbook of research on information technology management and clinical data administration in healthcare. Medical Information Science Reference, IGI GLOBAL Hershey, New York

11. Urbinati S, Fattirolli F, Tramarin R, Gruppo Italiano di Cardiologia Riabilitativa e Preventiva et al (2003) The ISYDE project. A survey on cardiac rehabilitation in Italy. Monaldi Arch Chest Dis 60(1):16–24
12. Sommaruga M, Tramarin R, Balestroni G et al (2005) Task Force on Psychological Interventions in Cardiac Rehabilitation. ISYDE-Psi first step of the implementation of guidelines for psychology activities in cardiac rehabilitation and prevention. Italian SurveY on CarDiac REhabilitation-Psychology. Arch Chest Dis 64(1):53–58
13. Sommaruga M, Tramarin R, Balestroni G et al (2008) Organization of psychological activities in Italian cardiac rehabilitation and prevention. Survey on the implementation of guidelines for psychological activities in cardiac rehabilitation and prevention. Monaldi Arch Chest Dis 70(1):6–14
14. Ordine Nazionale Psicologi. http://www.psy.it/. Accessed 7 Apr 2015
15. Linee guida nazionali su cardiologia riabilitativa e prevenzione secondaria delle malattie cardiovascolari, PNLG/ISS (2005). http://www.snlg-iss.it. Accessed 7 Apr 2015
16. Rees K, Bennett P, West R et al (2004) Psychological interventions for coronary heart disease. Cochrane Database Syst Rev (2):CD002902
17. Writing Committee for the ENRICHD Investigators (2003) Effects of treating depression and low perceived social support on clinical events after myocardial infarction: the enhancing recovery in coronary heart disease patients (ENRICHD) randomized trial. JAMA 289: 3106–3116
18. Perk J, De Backer G, Gohlke H et al (2012) European Association for Cardiovascular Prevention & Rehabilitation (EACPR); ESC Committee for Practice Guidelines (CPG). European guidelines on cardiovascular disease prevention in clinical practice (version 2012). The Fifth Joint Task Force of the European Society of Cardiology and Other Societies on Cardiovascular Disease Prevention in Clinical Practice (consisting of representatives from nine societies and invited experts). Eur Heart J 33(13):1635–1701
19. Pogosova N, Saner H, Pedersen SS et al (2015) On behalf of the Cardiac Rehabilitation Section of the European Association of Cardiovascular Prevention and Rehabilitation of the European Society of Cardiology. Psychosocial aspects in cardiac rehabilitation: from theory to practice. A position paper from the Cardiac Rehabilitation Section of the European Association of Cardiovascular Prevention and Rehabilitation and the European Society of Cardiology. Eur J Prev Cardiol 22(10):1290–1306
20. Griffo R, Ambrosetti M, Furgi G, Gruppo Italiano di Cardiologia Riabilitativa e Preventiva et al (2012) Standards and outcome measures in cardiovascular rehabilitation. Position paper GICR/IACPR. Monaldi Arch Chest Dis 78(4):166–192
21. Griffo R, Temporelli PL, Fattirolli F et al (2012) ICAROS (Italian survey on CardiAc RehabilitatiOn and Secondary prevention after cardiac revascularization): temporary report of the first prospective, longitudinal registry of the cardiac rehabilitation network GICR/IACPR. Monaldi Arch Chest Dis 78(2):73–78
22. Abrignani M, Bedogni F, Berti S et al (2014) Documento ANMCO/GICR-IACPR/GISE L'organizzazione dell'assistenza nella fase post-acuta delle sindromi coronariche. G Ital Cardiol 15(2 Suppl 1):3S–27S
23. Pierobon A, Giardini A, Callegari S, Majani G (2011) Psychological adjustment to a chronic illness: the contribution from cognitive behavioural treatment in a rehabilitation setting. Giornale Italiano di Medicina del Lavoro ed Ergonomia 33(1 Suppl A):A11–A18
24. WHO (2001) International classification of functioning, disability and health. WHO, Geneva
25. Donoghue PJ, Siegel ME (2000) Sick and tired of feeling sick and tired: living with invisible chronic illness. Norton, New York
26. Stanton A, Revenson T, Tennen H (2007) Health psychology: psychological adjustment to chronic disease. Annu Rev Psychol 58(1):565–592
27. Dobbie M, Mellor D (2008) Chronic illness and its impact: considerations for psychologists. Psychol Health Med 13(5):583–590

28. Bettinardi O (2015) Costi e benefici dell'intervento psicologico in cardiologia riabilitativa. In: De Isabella G, Majani G (eds) Psicologia in medicina: perché conviene. Franco Angeli, Milano
29. Goldston K, Baillie AJ (2008) Depression and coronary heart disease: a review of the epidemiological evidence, explanatory mechanisms and management approaches. Clin Psychol Rev 28(2):288–306
30. Dickens C, Cherrington A, Adeyemi I et al (2013) Characteristics of psychological interventions that improve depression in people with coronary heart disease: a systematic review and meta-regression. Psychosom Med 75(2):211–221
31. Seligman M (2009) Positive health. Appl Psychol 16:444–449
32. Chida Y, Steptoe A (2008) Positive psychological well-being and mortality: a quantitative review of prospective observational studies. Psychosom Med 70(7):741–756
33. Sommaruga M (2010) Affettività positiva e salute cardiovascolare. Monaldi Arch Chest Dis 74:1–8
34. Abbott RA, Whear R, Rodgers LR et al (2014) Effectiveness of mindfulness-based stress reduction and mindfulness based cognitive therapy in vascular disease: a systematic review and meta-analysis of randomized controlled trials. J Psychosom Res 76(5):341–351
35. Younge JO, Gotink RA, Baena CP et al (2015) Mind-body practices for patients with cardiac disease: a systematic review and meta-analysis. Eur J Prev Cardiol 22(11):1385–1398
36. Ladwig KH, Lederbogen F, Albus C et al (2014) Position paper on the importance of psychosocial factors in cardiology: update 2013. Ger Med Sci 7(12):1–24
37. Gruppo di lavoro sulla Riabilitazione, Ministero della Salute, approvato in Conferenza Stato Regioni (2011) Piano di indirizzo per la Riabilitazione. http://www.statoregioni.it/. Accessed 7 Apr 2015
38. Bettinardi O, da Vico L, Pierobon A et al (2014) First definition of minimal care model: the role of nurses, physiotherapists, dietitians and psychologists in preventive and rehabilitative cardiology. Monaldi Arch Chest Dis 82:122–152

MIX
Papier aus verantwortungsvollen Quellen
Paper from responsible sources
FSC® C105338
FSC
www.fsc.org

If you have any concerns about our products, you can contact us on
ProductSafety@springernature.com

In case Publisher is established outside the EU, the EU authorized representative is:
Springer Nature Customer Service Center GmbH
Europaplatz 3, 69115 Heidelberg, Germany

Printed by Libri Plureos GmbH
in Hamburg, Germany